Cosmopolitan and *Playboy*. She is ... York and Key West.

Her other books include *Jealousy* (also published by HarperCollins*Publishers*), *Men in Love*, *Women on Top* and *My Secret Garden*.

Also by Nancy Friday

JEALOUSY
MEN IN LOVE
WOMEN ON TOP
MY SECRET GARDEN

NANCY FRIDAY

My Mother/My Self

The Daughter's Search for Identity

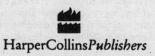

HarperCollins*Publishers*

HarperCollins*Publishers*
77–85 Fulham Palace Road,
Hammersmith, London W6 8JB

This paperback edition 1994
5 7 9 8 6

Previously published in paperback by Fontana 1979
Reprinted sixteen times

First published by Delacorte Press, USA 1977

Copyright © Nancy Friday 1977

The Author asserts the moral right to
be identified as the author of this work

ISBN 0 00 638251 7

Set in Sabon

Printed and bound in Great Britain by
Caledonian International Book Manufacturing Ltd, Glasgow

Grateful acknowledgements is made for permission to reprint the
following material:
Excerpt from *Pentimento: A Book of Portraits* by Lillian Hellman by
permission of Little, Brown and Co.
Excerpt from *Letters Home* by Sylvia Plath by permission of
Harper Row, Publishers, Inc.
Lines from 'Effort at Speech Between Two People' by Muriel Rukeyser:
reprinted from *Waterlily Fire* by Muriel Rukeyser: by permission of
Monica McCall, ICM. Copyright © by Muriel Rukeyser.
Lines from 'The Double Image' by Anne Sexton: reprinted from
To Bedlam and Part Way Back by Anne Sexton: by permission of
Houghton Mifflin Co.

When I stopped seeing my mother with the eyes of a child, I saw the woman who helped me give birth to myself.

This book is for Jane Colbert Friday Scott

Contents

Author's Acknowledgements

In 1973, I picked up a book that correlated women's orgasmic potential with the degree of security they once had with their fathers. I can remember the day, where I was sitting, the weight of the volume in my hands, and my instantaneous reaction: *what about mother?*

I had just written a book on women's sexual fantasies. It left no doubts in my mind where repression or sexual acceptance begins. Who first takes our hand way from our genitals, who implants pleasure or inhibition about our bodies, who lays down The Rules and with her own life, gives us an indelible model? That week I wrote an outline for a book entitled "Mothers and Daughters: The First Lie."

I thought myself a good candidate for this subject because although I would have told you I loved my mother, I also felt sufficient psychological space between us, a separation that would allow me to be fair and objective. As if any woman could. It took two years of research to get beyond the anger in that first title. Even to recognize how angry I was.

My intention was to do a series of interviews with mothers and daughters within a family, and where possible, with grandmothers too. In these last four years, I interviewed more than two hundred women across the United States. Most were mothers. All were daughters. On the most meaningful level, they were experts. But I quickly learned that a book of interviews would not be enough.

I had hoped to avoid the subjective through finding patterns that would hold for most women. By tracing these patterns through the generations, we could see the conscious and unconscious repetitions, correct for the best in our maternal inheritance, and get rid of the rest. If women's lives are going to change, we must have access to the formative strength of that relationship. We must get past the anger at lies told us 'for our own good', find what real love exists between mother and daughter – or be freed from the illusion of a love that never existed at all. I was looking for clarification. I discovered Rashomon. Mother: 'I very carefully prepared my daughter for menstruation.' Daughter: 'My mother told me nothing.' Two versions of the same story, different and yet the same. Neither woman thinks she is lying.

To understand contradictions like these I talked to psychiatrists, educators, doctors, lawyers, sociologists. I did not want textbook answers alone: of the twenty-one professional women quoted in this book, sixteen are mothers of daughters themselves. No woman gave more generously of her wit, wisdom, professional knowledge, and personal life than Dr Leah Schaefer; I will always be in her debt. What is most poignant to me is how often these highly trained people confess difficulties in applying what they intellectually knew to their own lives.

One of my earliest discards was the notion that I could learn all I needed from women. We can hop instead of walk, but why not use two legs? When Dr Sirgay Sanger telephoned in answer to my request to interview a certain eminent child psychiatrist – a woman – he informed me she was out of town. She had asked him to take my call. Rather impolitely, I said that since I believed women understood women best, I would wait for his female colleague to return. I am grateful to this day he did not hang up on me. Some of the possibilities of conduct and insights into behavior which I feel most rare and exhilarating in these pages come from him and other men. They have daughters too.

I first talked to Dr Richard Robertiello on an afternoon like any other. It was one of the shaping events of my career and began a series of conversations over the years without which this book would have been immeasurably poorer. As the reader follows the development of the argument. I hope it becomes clear that before I could explain the mother-daughter relationship to anyone else, I had to understand my own. Without Dr Robertiello's awesome knowledge, powers of analysis, original mind, and personal involvement (he is the father of three daughters), I would have given up long ago.

The authorities whose names appear below shared not just their learning but time and concern too. As I could not list their credentials within the text, I do so here with all my thanks:

Pauline B. Bart: associate professor of sociology in psychiatry, College of Medicine, University of Illinois; author of *The Student Sociologist's Handbook.*

Jessie Bernard: sociologist/scholar-in-residence at the U.S. Commission on Civil Rights; author of *Women, Wives, Mothers: Values and Options, The Future of Motherhood,* and *The Future of Marriage.*

Mary S. Calderone, M.D.: director of Sex Information and Education Council of the United States; author of *Release from Sexual Tensions.*

Sidney Q. Cohlan, M.D.: professor of pediatrics; associate director of pediatrics, University Hospital, New York University Medical Center.

Helene Deutsch, M.D.: psychoanalyst; author of *The Psychology of Women.*

Lilly Engler, M.D.: psychiatrist in private practice in New York City, consultant to various institutions here and abroad.

Cynthia Fuchs Epstein: professor of sociology, Queens College, City University of New York; project director, Bureau of Applied Research, Columbia University; author of *Woman's Place: Options and Limits in Professional Careers* and co-author, *The Other Half: Roads to Women's Equality.*

Aaron H. Esman, M.D.: chief psychiatrist of the Jewish Board of Guardians; member of the faculty of the New

York Psychoanalytic Institute; author of *New Frontiers in Child Guidance* and *The Psychology of Adolescence: Essential Readings*.

Mio Fredland, M.D.: assistant clinical professor of psychiatry, Cornell University Medical School.

Sonya Friedman: psychologist; marriage and divorce counselor; co-author of *I've Had It, You've Had It! Advice on Divorce from a Lawyer and a Psychologist*.

Emily Jane Goodman: attorney; co-author of *Women. Money and Power*.

Amy R. Hanan: personnel director, AT&T General Departments.

Elizabeth Hoppin Hauser; psychotherapist on the staff of the Long Island Consultation Center in Forest Hills.

Helen Kaplan, M.D., psychoanalyst and sex therapist; associate clinical professor of psychiatry, Cornell University Medical College; associate attending psychiatrist of the Payne Whitney Clinic of New York Hospital, author of *The New Sex Therapy*.

Sherwin A. Kaufman, M.D.: associated attending gynecologist and obstetrician, Lenox Hill Hospital, New York City; author of *Intimate Questions Women Ask*, *New Hope for the Childless Couple*, and *The Ageless Woman*.

Jeanne McFarland: professor, Economics Department, Smith College.

Gladys McKenney: teacher of marriage and family classes in a suburban high school in Michigan.

George L. Peabody, Ph.D.: applied behavioral science.

Vera Plaskon: family planning coordinator, Roosevelt Hospital, New York; clinical specialist in parent/child nursing.

Virginia E. Pomeranz, M.D.: associate clinical professor of pediatrics at Cornell University Medical College and associate attending pediatrician at The New York Hospital; author of *The First Five Years: A Relaxed Approach to Child Care* and co-author of *The Mothers' and Fathers' Medical Encyclopedia*.

Wardell B. Pomeroy, Ph.D.: sex researcher, Kinsey reports, *Sexual Behavior in the Human Male* and *Sexual Behavior in the Human Female*; author of *Boys and Sex* and *Girls and Sex*.

Jessie Potter: faculty member of human sexuality program, Northwestern University, School of Medicine; director of the National Institute for Human Relationships.

Helen Prentiss: professor of child psychology at a mid-western university. Her name is pseudonym since she asks to remain anonymous.

Ira L. Reiss: professor of sociology, University of Minnesota.

Richard C. Robertiello, M.D.: senior training consultant at the Long Island Institute for Mental Health; member of the executive board of the Society for the Scientific Study of Sex; supervising psychiatrist for the Community Guidance Service; author of *Hold Them Very Close, Then Let Them Go* and co-author of *Big You, Little You*.

Sirgay Sanger, M.D.: director, parent-child program, St Luke's Hospital; instructor, Columbia College of Physicians and Surgeons; author, *Emotional Care, Hospitalized Children*.

Leah Cahan Schaefer: psychotherapist; staff member of Community Guidance Service, New York City; executive board, Society for the Scientific Study of Sex; author of *Women and Sex*.

Joan Shapiro; professor of social work, Smith College.

Marcia Storch M.D.: head of adolescent gynecology and family planning clinic, child and youth division, Roosevelt Hospital; assistant clinical professor of obstetrics and gynecology, Columbia University College of Physicians and Surgeons, Roosevelt Hospital, New York City.

Betty L. Thompson: psychoanalyst in private practice.

Lionel Tiger: professor of anthropology at Rutgers University; author of *Men in Groups, The Imperial Animal,* and *Women in the Kibbutz*.

To those women whose names do not appear — both

mothers and daughters who gave me all they could, even if anonymously – my special thanks. They will recognize their words. I hope they will feel some of the added life I now have, knowing what this book, their lives, and my own have taught me.

Ideas on women's identity had been rolling in my mind for years. But I was a travel writer until I married. There are certain questions we do not dare to ask without the support of another person. In this book, as in my life, that person has been Bill Manville.

N.F.
New York City
April 1977

Introduction

Understanding what we have with our mothers is the beginning of understanding ourselves. How obvious that sounds today.

Any effort to change and shape our lives must begin with that first woman in whose image we live. We know this.

But we have not known it long.

Any woman reading these words remembers a time when emotions other than love and attachment between mother and daughter were denied. We denied them to our detriment, and in that denial lay the obstacle to real love – by which I mean love that acknowledges ambivalence, that we sometimes hate, fear the people we love most and envy the power they have over our lives. It is this essential ambivalence that characterizes the mother/daughter relationship more than any other relationship in human life.

'I raised my daughter exactly as I raised my son and love them equally,' a woman editor said, explaining her rejection of an early draft of *My Mother/My Self*. The sentiment sounds archaic, alien to our new wisdom. But we would be wise not to dismiss this mother's defense. Everything has not changed.

When the mother holds her child in her arms, whether it be her son or daughter, she feels many emotions. When that child is the same sex as she, she *sees* herself. She feels a tidal wave of every emotion she has ever felt – love, fear, anxiety, hate. It is not so much what a mother wants for a daughter that will determine how far a girl will go. More than anything, it is the mother's own self-esteem that will influence the daughter's emotional separation and independence.

Has our self esteem changed in recent years? I am not

referring to our brave new rhetoric and behavior. Self-esteem is not measured in words or dollars. It is a deep down good opinion of oneself which doesn't waver, and it is best given to a daughter by her mother.

Are we better mothers? As daughters, are we more responsible and autonomous?

When I began my research in the early 70s, there was nothing in the psychoanalytic library on the unique interaction between mother and daughter. Professionals in the behavioral world whom I consulted answered my questions not from any formed body of theory but from their own professional and personal experience. 'I have never understood what goes on between my wife and daughter,' mused one psychiatrist, 'and I do my best to stay out of it.'

Ordinary women whom I interviewed had no common shared wisdom on which to draw when describing the emotional bond with their mothers. Anger and guilt fought with love and attachment as if it were impossible, indeed dangerous and incomprehensible, to feel opposite emotions for a mother. As for their own daughters, when I mentioned the dreaded word 'separation', more than one drew back, saying she felt gooseflesh just hearing the word.

What was so frightening to women who had everything to gain for themselves and their daughters from an honest examination of the most important relationship in their lives? The answer lay not in the grown woman, intelligent, responsible for her work and family. To understand the terror of dead honesty between mother and daughter, the frightened child in each of us had to be faced.

As tiny children we had made a bargain with mother – as she had made with hers – never to question the bond between us. This bond was rooted in fear of loss of love, something she could not guarantee since unconditional love had never been given to her.

What changed this generational legacy of dependency that spread outwards from mother to undermine every intimate relationship a woman made, was the gradual awakening that began towards the end of the 60s. The women's movement, the sexual revolution, the new economics resulting from the entry of women into the work world, all combined could not forge us into the women we were striving to become so long as we perpetuated a bargain based on lies made by a frightened child. Something was missing and it was not in the world 'out there'. The work to be done was inside each of us.

It is easier to march as a group, arm-in-arm, opening doors previously closed to women, passing amendments, than it is to come to terms, alone, with mother. Neither her presence nor her knowledge is required. It is something a woman does by herself and it is very hard.

It is humiliating to accept that our mature relationships with men, our sexuality, our own roles as mothers, our ability to compete in a man's world and succeed with satisfaction are all rooted in what we had with her as children.

'Did you know that someone wanted to kill you last night?' a reader wrote to me shortly after *My Mother/My Self* was published. It was a reaction to which I would become accustomed and which never surprised me. Hadn't 'killing' emotions been my bed-fellows during four years of writing?

'I hurled your book across the room after twenty pages, then hid it on the top shelf of the upstairs closet,' another woman wrote. Six months later she climbed the stairs and finished the book. Just as I had returned, draft after draft, to finish writing it. Something stronger than anger and fear pulled us both back. It was in the air, this unspoken business beween us and our mothers. If it hadn't been my book, it would have been another woman's. We had to know.

Not that *My Mother/My Self* was an instant success. Sales were slow and steady as women hid and hurled the book. But as more and more got past those first twenty pages and reached the happy ending (nobody dies), women began telling other women – their friends, their daughters, their mothers – 'Read this!'

It is uncommon in the publishing business for a book to 'get its legs' – to start walking out of the book stores and become a best seller – six months after publication. But that is how long it took for women to give other women permission to read *My Mother/My Self*.

Women are the great permission givers. Women raise the children, giving or withholding love depending on women's ideas of what is right or wrong. No woman – or man – ever forgets the weight of mother/women's permission.

I had learned this with my earlier book on women's sexual fantasies. Until *My Secret Garden* was published in 1973, the behavioral world claimed that women did not have sexual fantasies. Indeed, women themselves denied their erotic reveries. 'What is a sexual fantasy?' women would ask during my research. 'I don't have fantasies, I love my husband!' was another typical defense of virtue.

It was only when women read other women's fantasies that they felt they too had permission to fantasize.

Today women's sexual fantasies are so much a part of our culture, our understanding and analysis of women, that we forget how recently women were universally suppressed. We must keep in mind this short time span.

Women's fantasies were bad, wrong, so forbidden to a Nice Girl that when finally made conscious, what emerged was scenario after scenario in which women made themselves helpless, passive victims, thus not responsible for going against mother/women's rules in the pursuit of sexual pleasure.

The fact is women still do not own their sexuality. The responsibility is not theirs. We see it in our real lives – in the epidemic number of unwanted pregnancies – and in the content of our erotic dreams. The so-called rape fantasy still prevails, the old traditional reverie in which the woman is neither hurt nor humiliated, but rather forced, *made* to enjoy the sex to which she still doesn't feel entitled.

Collective female wisdom once held that men made us sexual: 'Take me!', 'Give me an orgasm!' But men don't release women to orgasm. Once a woman's voice told us that Nice Girls Don't. If women are ever to become sexually responsive and responsible, it must be women's voices that say Nice Girls Do. And those voices must mean it from the cradle up.

It is women's voices – not men's – to which women listen. For how many centuries have men told their wives, 'You're just like your mother!'? The accusation was angrily denied. Only when women explained to other women *why* we become like our mothers was the truism accepted. We knew all along it was painfully so. We simply needed other women saying it. When women explained to others that one way we deny our rage is to become not like the mother we love, but the mother we hate, only then could we give ourselves permission to explore the other side of mother/daughter love.

Today, after countless films, books and television dramas on the mother/daughter theme, are we separate enough to see our mothers whole, people who are both good and bad? Are our lives monuments to the 'good mother'? Or do we still perpetuate the possessive, controlling, nagging, critical 'bad mother' we hated in the nursery?

It is ten years since I stood at my bedroom window, staring out at the park, knowing that writing a book had changed my life. I would never be the same. All my life I had shown the world an independent persona, a brave exterior which hid the frightened child within. This split in which I had lived had sapped my strength, leaving me divided against myself. The split had begun to heal when my writing forced me to recognize that my fears and angers were those of a child felt towards a mother of long ago who was also a woman, like myself.

In time I came to see this change as integration; the inner me was coming to resemble the brave, independent outer me. Energy that had been spent on denial was now mine. There was new room in my life in which to move as an adult, room which had been taken up by childish defenses against anger, competition and the host of other emotions denied to woman . . . *denied to women by other women*.

The process of integration, once begun, is lifelong. Mine is hardly complete. For instance, I am a professional person whose economic success leaves me dependent on no one. But at times I bitterly resent that I have outgrown my need to be taken care of. My only consolation is that I understand why it cannot be otherwise. Change takes time and not enough has elapsed in my life – or probably yours – to make my new attitudes and behavior resonate on the deepest level with what my mother taught me was right and wrong.

Our attitudes – what we think and say – change quickly. We read a book – or write one – sit next to an interesting, eloquent stranger at dinner and the next day we have a new way of looking at, thinking and speaking about the world. A change of attitude can be exhilarating, freeing. I think this is how many women, myself included, felt upon finishing *My Mother/My Self*.

Say we then move into the next level of change, behavior. We decide to put our new ideas into action. We have just read a *Cosmopolitan* report that says 48 per cent of married women have extra-marital affairs. Suddenly, we feel liberated from twenty, thirty years of sexual guilt. Though mother/society has raised us to believe adultery is wrong, we think *Cosmo* is right. Who thinks there is anything wrong with a little adultery? Not us.

We climb into bed with our new lover. But we wake up feeling bad, dirty, guilty.

What went wrong?

When change is at the speed of geometric progression, as it has been for the past twenty years, we often act on new attitudes that sound good but end up feeling very bad. Educated by books, feminist teachers, eloquent speakers, not to mention the full force of the media, we find ourselves caught in lives we have intellectually structured but don't totally approve of. We pursue careers, sleep in many beds, have babies without men through the service of sperm banks.

There may be nothing wrong with any of this if we understand the evolution of change in our lives, how we have come from being our mothers' daughters to making decisions so contrary to those mother made. If we do this consciously and honestly, we must deal with the third and last level of change that moves more slowly than attitude and behavior. It is how we feel deep down in our gut about what is right and wrong.

We get these deep, often unconscious feelings from our mothers, who got them from their mothers. When they change, if they change at all, they change between generations. If our mothers, grandmothers never worked outside the home, if they believed that sex before and/or outside of marriage was wrong, then that is our earliest picture of what a woman is. We may decide today that it is not how we want to be but we should recognize the internal ambivalence given this earliest, most primitive idea of womanliness.

'If only my mother weren't so passive! If only she'd stand up to my father!' a young woman cried out from the audience at a university where I was lecturing. Her lament had all the weight of a person caught between two worlds, trying desperately to be independent, fearing she would instead end up like her mother.

Her mistake was in thinking that if her mother changed, if she could *make* her change (sheer infantile omnipotence), then she too would be less passive, more independent. In fact, her energy would be better spent admitting anger that mother wasn't perfect. Only little girls need perfect mommies. Having found the target for her anger – the nursery – she could vent some of that anger in the appropriate place, rid herself of some childishness and be free to get on with changing her own life, grateful for whatever her mother was able to give her.

Traditionally we felt safety lay in being as closely tied to mother, as much like her as possible. We repeated her life out of fear that being different meant being separate, abandoned, the object of her disapproval and anger. Today we listen to our new voices, look at the visible differences between our lives and our mothers' and make the mistake of thinking we are New Women who have given birth to ourselves. It is practising deception on the maddest level. We think we are strong, big, putting our mothers far behind us, people of another place and time. It is a dangerous form of denial. In fact, real strength will come from an almost daily reminder of how much, on the deepest level, we are still our mothers' daughters.

If we are not conscious of this side of ourselves that is slowest to change and that most resembles our mothers, our decisions will be made out of frustration and denial. We will direct our anger at easy targets, blaming men, the system, anything or anyone but our own unresolved female world. Like the rebellious teenager who gets herself pregnant, what we do will be more in reaction to mother than an act consciously done for ourselves – a true act of autonomy.

We demand, for instance, that men and society treat us as equals. Our demand has the full force of our intellect and any standard of objective justice. But we are angry that men don't also take care of us. We have expectations based both on how we were raised – how our mother was with our father – and expectations arrived at intellectually, which is late in the developmental timetable.

Men too grow angry at our double message. Who raised them for a world in which women wanted their hearts and their jobs too? Their mothers didn't pursue careers, nor did their fathers help in the raising of the children. Women want it both ways, men say, and refuse our demands for love, for equal pay, for maternity leave, child custody payments or day care centers for our children that would make us better wage earners.

What man wants a woman who is a better competitor? A fair man wants as much for his wife as possible and recognizes the need for her paycheck. But should her paycheck grow too big, should she become too powerful, he is ambivalent, confused, envious. As I learned from research for my recent book *Jealousy*, men begin life fearing women's power. It is a fear they never forget. Why else would they construct a partriarchal society in which women felt dependent and powerless?

The fact is, most men still equate masculinity with being a good provider. If a woman is a good provider then what is he? Most men have not changed. Their attitudes and behavior are not integrated. As for how they feel on the deepest level about what is right and wrong, they are damned if they will relinquish the power handed down to them by their fathers, especially to women whose double messages leave them more confounded than ever over what women really want.

A study done by *Mademoiselle* five years ago left no doubt about what the New Woman really wants. Over half the respondents said they expected to make it to the top of their chosen career and to earn top dollar. An even greater percentage expected to find egalitarian husbands who would share in housekeeping and the raising of the children.

Where did these idealistic expections come from? Certainly not from men. How can these women not be angry today faced with a reality so far beneath their expectations? Towards whom will they direct their resentment and anger at not getting the exciting high-salaried jobs they'd anticipated? Today women earn 69 cents to a man's dollar. Surveys say that many women won't find a husband, let alone an egalitarian one. Half the marriages end in divorce. After divorce women with children can expect a 73 per cent decline in their standard of living, while men can expect a 42 per cent rise. More women live alone than even before in history. Despite the hype about sexual liberation, we still do not feel free to explore our sexuality without fear of repercussions from within or from without of being labelled 'bad'.

Women are not good at handling anger. We were not raised to acknowledge it opposite the first source of our earliest rages – mother. With no repeated practice in learning to express it safely, it nonetheless boils within, escaping when we cannot control it but avoiding the original source. If the extent of our anger at men is at times inappropriate, it is because they are getting more than their share: the full force of years of unexpressed, unacceptable rage at women.

We are one another's worst jailors and best liberators. If there is a sense of slipping back today, it is in part because we refuse to accept the power women have over one another. We deny the primitive ambivalence between women which begins in the earliest relationship with mother.

For instance, the women's movement and the sexual revolution went on simultaneously *but were not allies.* Early feminism had a decided asexual, anti-male tone. Men were the enemy. They kept women down, unequal and dependent, yes. But eliminating men – the earliest source of sexual competition between women – also hardened the denial of competition among women straight across the board.

Those women who wanted the new equality, but within a framework of a more liberated sexual life with men, felt they had to make a choice. Others who wanted family and children came to see feminism as a club from which they were excluded and to which they didn't want to belong. It was this exclusive, non-sexual, anti-family reputation of feminism that contributed directly to the defeat of the Equal Rights Amendment.

That the split in women's ranks was over sex is not surprising. The right to our sexuality, to our own bodies, is one of the most primitive, divisive issues between mother and daughter.

Ten years ago we read *My Mother/My Self* for our *selves.* Our mothers had not raised us to feel comfortable with autonomy, sexuality, a life different from theirs. In the struggle for independence we threw out everything associated with traditional womanliness – the pursuit of beauty was denigrated, having babies was unpopular.

Time has passed and as with all wars, women like men in centuries past are returning home. Glamour is back. Women want children, families, those things that along with independence, career make life worth living. Today more than ever we must remember, for our daughters' sake, how autonomy is achieved.

'That's what babies are giving women, as they no doubt gave them for centuries,' a woman wrote in last Sunday's paper, 'a love with no lines, with an intimacy that is easier and often sweeter than sex.'

Why did I feel a chilling sense of *déjà vu* in those words? If women are indeed having children out of 'a yearning for closeness that isn't always possible with a man, even a husband,' as this woman wrote, is our return to sweet mothering born in part out of a sense of our own loneliness and unfulfilment? We are not yet free of the need for symbiotic attachment had with our own mothers. My fear, I suppose, is that the cycle will repeat, that mothering will lead to regression, *unless we know our reasons absolutely*. It is the consciousness of decision I am stressing.

An infant needs all the love in the world, closeness, even the 'love with no lines' a mother herself seeks. But before the first year of life is over, a child begins to move away, to find her own life separate from mother, if mother will let her go.

We cannot teach separation to our daughters only celebrating love, denying its opposite – anger, envy, competition, resentment. These too are human emotions. By not learning to handle them among ourselves we have held one another back emotionally in a way that is far more destructive than any outer, physical restraints put on us by men.

If we are not good with competition, if we are uncomfortable with sex, if we have a sense of failure about our lives, then we must remember what we have learned these past ten years. We must do something terribly difficult but which is at the heart of mother love: we must help our daughters find other models, other sources of love, letting them know absolutely they are not betraying mother, losing her love. Having mother's permission to love and emulate others, a daughter will naturally seek people who will love her back. This is separation working at its best, the beginning of healthy self-esteem.

With more and more women working outside the home, mothers must accept they can't do everything. Mother never could be perfect. Today she doesn't have to be. One of our greatest resources is the number of admirable women in the world, more heroines and models for young girls than ever before.

Fathers too have so much to give their daughters. Only when women acknowledge the power of mothering will we share it with men. By denying it is the most powerful role in human life, we keep it for ourselves, possessing our children out of loneliness, fear of failure, need of confirmation of womanliness not found in men's world. Thus we bind our daughters to us more closely than our mothers held us.

Autonomy is best learned with mother in the first years of life. We had to learn it late and on our own. We must be our daughters' teachers. Whatever our accomplishments, whatever our failures, these are the gifts we have to give them. It is no time to be practising denial.

NANCY FRIDAY
Mother's Day, 1987

CHAPTER ONE

Mother Love

I have always lied to my mother. And she to me. How young was I when I learned her language, to call things by other names? Five, four – younger? Her denial of whatever she could not tell me, that her mother could not tell her, and about which society enjoined us both to keep silent, distorts our relationship still.

Sometimes I try to imagine a little scene that could have helped us both. In her kind, warm, shy, and self-deprecating way, mother calls me into the bedroom where she sleeps alone. She is not more than twenty-five. I am perhaps six. Putting her hands (which her father told her always to keep hidden because they were 'large and unattractive') on my shoulders, she looks me right through my steel-rimmed spectacles: 'Nancy, you know I'm not really good at this mothering business,' she says. 'You're a lovely child, the fault is not with you. But motherhood doesn't come easily to me. So when I don't seem like other people's mothers, try to understand that it isn't because I don't love you. I do. But I'm confused myself. There are some things I know about. I'll teach them to you. The other stuff – sex and all that – well, I just can't discuss them with you because I'm not sure where they fit into my own life. We'll try to find other people, other women who can talk to you and fill the gaps. You can't expect me to be all the mother you need. I feel closer to your age in some ways than I do my mother's. I don't feel that serene, divine, earth-mother certainty you're supposed to that she felt. I am unsure how to raise you. But you are intelligent and so am I. Your aunt loves you, your teachers already feel the need in you. With their help, with what I can give, we'll

27

see that you get the whole mother package – all the love in the world. It's just that you can't expect to get it all from me.'

A scene that could never have taken place.

For as long as I can remember, I did not want the kind of life my mother felt she could show me. Sometimes I think she did not want it either. The older I get, the further away she gets from my childhood, from her ironclad role as my mother – the more interesting a woman she becomes. Perhaps she should never have been a mother; certainly she was one too soon. I look at her today, and with all the love and anger in the world, I wish she had had a chance to live another life, mine perhaps. But hers was not an age in which women felt they had a choice.

I have no idea when I began to perceive with the monstrous selfishness that dependency lends to a child's eyes that my mother was not perfect: I was not her whole life. Was it at the same age that I began to make the terrible judgment that she was not the woman I wanted to be? It seems I have always known both. It accounts for my guilt at leaving her, and my anger that she let me go. But I am sure that she has always known, on a level her indoctrinated attitudes toward motherhood would never let her admit, that my sister and I were not enough. We had not brought the certification of womanhood that *her* mother had promised. That, once in her life, sex and a man had been more important than motherhood.

A more dutiful daughter than I, my mother wanted to accept the view of reality my grandmother taught her. She lied with the rest. She subverted herself, her genuine feelings, those burgeoning imitations of life's hope and adventure which she found in my father, and which induced her to elope with him against her family's wishes – all lost, in the name of being a good mother. Her mother's rules had the authority of the entire culture behind them. There was no such thing as a 'bad mother'; there were only bad women: they were the explicitly sexual ones, who lived out the notion that what went on between themselves and their husbands had at least as much right to life as their children. This is an illusion.

Mothers may love their children, but they sometimes do not like them. The same woman who may be willing to put her body between her child and a runaway truck will often resent the day-by-day sacrifice the child unknowingly demands of her time, sexuality, and self-development.

In our perception of our mother's inauthenticity – her own anxiety and lack of belief in over-idealized notions of womanhood/motherhood she is trying to teach us – anxieties about our own sexuality are born. There is the beginning of doubt that we will succeed as people with identities of our own, separate from her, established in ourselves as women before we are mothers. We try for autonomy, try for sexuality, but the unconscious, deepest feelings we have picked up from her will not rest: we will only feel at peace, sure of ourselves, when we have fulfilled the glorified 'instinct' we have been trained, through the image of her life, to repeat: you are not a full woman until you are a mother.

It is too late to ask my mother to go back and examine evasions she made as silently as any mother and to which I agreed for so long – if only because she doesn't want to. I am the one who wants to change certain dead-end patterns in my life. Patterns which, the older I get, seem all the more familiar: I've been here before.

The love between my mother and me is not so sacrosanct it cannot be questioned: if I lived with an illusion as to what is between us, I will have no firm resting place on which to build myself.

In my years of interviewing, how many women have repeatedly said to me, 'No, I can't think of anything significant I've inherited from my mother. We're completely different women . . .' This is usually said with an air of triumph – as if the speaker is acknowledging the enormous pull to model herself on her mother, but believes she has resisted. But in my interview with her daughter, she smiles ruefully. 'I'm always telling mom she treats me just the way she said grandma treated her . . . ways she didn't like!' In yet another interview, her husband says, 'The longer we're married, the more like her mother she becomes.'

To be fair, if my interviewees and I talked long enough, they themselves began to see the similarities with their mothers' lives. First the superficial, outward differences had to be worked through. Mother lived in a house, the woman I was talking to lived in an apartment. Mother never worked a day in her life, the daughter held down a job. We cling to these 'facts' as proof that we have created our own lives, different from hers. We overlook the more basic truth that we have taken on her anxieties, fears, angers; the way we weave the web of emotion between ourselves and others is patterned on what we had with her.

Whether we want our mother's life or not, we never escape the image of how she was. Nowhere is this more true than in our sexual lives. Without our own sexual identity, one we can put our full weight upon with as much certainty as once we enjoyed being 'mother's girl', we are unsure. We have spurts of sexual confidence, activity, exploration, but at the first rejection, hint of loss, of sexual censure or humiliation, we fall back on the safe and familiar: sex is bad. It was always a problem between mother and ourselves. When men seem bright and alluring, we momentarily ally with them against mother's antisexual rules. But men cannot be trusted. We say the fault is our own: we go from mother to men, with no self in between. Marriage, instead of ending our childish alliance with her, ironically becomes the biggest reunion of our lives. Once we wanted to be 'nice girls'. Now we are 'nice married ladies' – just like mother. Those quarrels with her over men are ended at last. The hardest thing to face in mother is her sexuality. She found it hardest to face in us.

Two women, each hiding from the other exactly that which defines her as a woman.

Unless we separate mother's love from her fear of sex, we will always see love and sex as opposites. The dichotomy will be passed on to our daughters. 'Mother *was* right,' we say, and the fervor with which we deny our daughter access to her own body is fired with all the anger, confusion, and self-abnegation we have experienced in giving up on our own sexuality.

'Believe that I love you, no matter what I say or do to you,' is the message behind the madonna. 'No one will ever love you as I do. Mother loves you best in all the world and I will always be there for you.' Many mothers offer this kind of impossible love because they are lonely and want to bind their daughters to them forever. All mothers imply it because they are in a trap too: to suggest less is to be 'a bad mother'. The real love she may have for us does not have the binding power of the idealized and perfect love we both need to believe in. It is a bargain none of us can refuse.

'If the mother has a genuine sexual relationship with her husband,' says psychotherapist Leah Schaefer, 'but pretends to her daughter that in some way all erotic life must be tied up with motherhood, the girl senses this. She gets the feeling she cannot trust her mother. In my psychoanalytic practice, *I have found again and again this is the basic lie*. Parents tell their kids, "No, no, you mustn't" – but the little girl senses that the mother herself is doing the forbidden. It makes a certain aspect of the mother's life and personality a big secret to the girl – and yet the mother always wants to know everything about the daughter. She pries into the girl's psyche, she's always telling her daughter they are friends, they must tell each other everything – but once more the girl knows mother is keeping one big secret from her, one part of herself is out of bounds. It is a one-way relationship, supposedly based on trust, but which the girl experiences as manipulative. She resents it.

'What makes the situation more difficult for the girl is when the mother is not conscious of telling this lie. She rationalizes: 'How can you tell a child *that*?' You may choose to withhold certain information, but this is not the right to tell your daughter a lie. Some women work their own minds around to where they themselves believe the only purpose of sex is motherhood. So they don't think they're lying at all.

They think they are safeguarding the girl's "morals". What they're doing is setting up a lifelong distrust on the girl's part, and also a feeling of isolation, of helplessness. Sex is very confusing to the daughter, but if she gets the feeling that her mother is lying about it – whom can the girl ever trust? And trust of yourself and the other person is the basis of life, marriage, and of sexual orgasm.'

Mother's difficulty is not necessarily that she is a liar or hypocrite. She says one thing, does another, and yet communicates on a profound level that she really feels something totally different. Most of us have learned to live with this tripartite split in the people we know and take each other as a whole. As daughters, however, we are so focused on our mothers that we take them literally and try to integrate all three warring aspects they present to us. Since this confusion permeates the mother-daughter relationship and will be seen again and again throughout this book, let me clearly separate the three ideas here:

1. Attitude. This is what we say, the outward impression we give people, and is the quickest aspect of ourselves to change. It is often a reflection of public opinion, books we've read, what our peers believe, etc. An example is the mother who decides that her daughter will not grow up in sexual ignorance, as she did; she buys the girl a copy of the latest book on sex education – like *Show Me.*¹

How she acts when the girl puts the book's precepts into use is the difference between attitude and:

2. Behavior. Mother finds her daughter touching and exploring her vagina, just like the photographs in the book. She grimaces and pushes the girl's hand away.

Behavior has changed greatly in recent years, but it is a mistake to believe how we act always correlates with our up-to-the-minute attitudes. Dr Wardell Pomeroy, Kinsey's foremost researcher, tells me that changes in behavior usually lag at least a generation behind changes in attitude. This conservatism is strongly influenced, if not determined, by our:

3. Deepest (often unconscious) feelings. These buried,

basic forces or motivations are usually learned from our parents. They are the most rigid aspects of ourselves, carry-overs from the past which often nullify the other two. They may be denied or 'forgotten' but will nevertheless often express themselves in irrational or distorted behavior. A mother tells (attitude) her daughter that sex is beautiful. In her behavior, she carefully does not 'know' that the girl has gone off for the weekend with a man. But her deepest feelings are betrayed when the daughter comes home on Monday to find mother resentful, worried, and angry for no reason she can name out loud.

Saying one thing about sex and motherhood, feeling contrary emotions about both at the same time, mother presents an enigmatic picture to her daughter. The first lie – the denial that a woman's sexuality may be in conflict with her role as a mother – is so upsetting to traditional ideas of femininity that it cannot be talked about. The girl is left with perception of a gap between what mother says, what mother does . . . and what the girl detects mother feels beneath it all. Nothing mother really feels ever escapes us. Our problem is that because we try to live out all parts of the split message she sent us, our behavior and lives all too often represent a jangled compromise. We don't know what to do. We un-button the top button on our dress and then button it back up again. That is a joke. But when we are in bed and feel the promise of orgasm, our unconscious and divided feelings assert their primacy, depriving us of satisfaction. That is no joke.

Our efforts to see mother clearly are frustrated by a kind of denial. It is one of our most primitive mechanisms of defense. Early on, children begin to avoid knowledge that mother is anything less than the 'good mother' she pretends to be. Very often this is done by splitting the idea of mother into *good* and *bad*. The bad mother is the other one, not the real one. She is the one who is cruel, has headaches, does not like us. She is temporary. Only the good one is real. We will wait for her return for years, always convinced that the woman before us, who makes us feel guilty, inadequate, and angry, is *not* mother. How many of us who live away from home, periodically go back to mother, perhaps at Christmas or on a birthday, hoping that this time 'Everything will be different'? Grown women ourselves, we are still looking for, still tied to the illusion of the all-loving, good mother.

Children think their parents are perfect, and if anything is wrong it's their fault. We have to think our parents are perfect because as children we are so totally dependent. We can't afford to hate mother, so what we do is turn our anger against ourselves. Instead of saying she is hateful, we say, 'I am hateful.' Mother *has* to be all wise and kind.

The most extreme example of our need to believe in the all-loving mother is found with battered children. Take a severely abused and physically mistreated child and put it with a loving foster mother. Again and again it is found that the child will prefer to go back to the original cruel mother. Stronger than the desire for cessation of beating and abuse, stronger than life itself, the child wants to perpetuate her illusion that she had a good mother.

The truth is that while the child *wants* to believe her mother loves her unequivocally, she can live with disappointment at finding out it is not so. What is most necessary is that the child feel her mother is for real, *authentic*. It is better to learn as early as possible that while mother loves us, it is not to the exclusion of everything and everyone else. If the child is encouraged to enter into collusion with mother, to pretend that the maternal instinct conquers all, both will be stuck ever after with mechanisms of denial and defense which cut them off from the reality of their mutual feelings; gone is any hope of a true relationship between them. The daughter will repeat this relationship with men and other women. The idea of mother and daughter lying to maintain a pastel-pretty fiction between them may sound touching. The reality is that the price paid for maintaining the lie is enormous. The cost to the battered little girl is to be beaten black and blue. Is that touching?

Little girls playing with their dolls give us an almost laboratory example of how the illusion of perfect maternal love is maintained. In his book *Playing and Reality*, the English child psychoanalyst D. W. Winnicott notes that children's play expresses a form of wish fulfillment. A little girl playing with her dolls acts in the way she hopes her mother will act toward her. The very act of playing this game out gives the illusion a form of substance.[2]

Where did the child of even a nonmaternal woman get this idea of perfect mother love? From what her mother says, if not from what mother does. Mother always presents herself as totally loving. Her verbal formulas tell the girl that there is no question of the ideal way she feels. The reason mother is so angry or upset or cold right now is that father has been awful, the groceries didn't arrive, there is little money in the house, or the girl herself has been bad. In the end, the child comes to understand that whatever it is, it is because *she* has been naughty. It is her fault the groceries are late, Daddy is awful, there is no money, etc., etc.

Primitive cavemen drew pictures of antelopes on the walls before the hunt to make the animals come forth. In the same magical way, little girls play the perfect mother with their dolls, hoping the incantation will bring forth the ideal mother hidden in the less-than-perfect woman who promises so much and delivers so little.

Playing with dolls, the little girl perpetuates the illusion. 'See how loving I am with my doll? It's so easy, it's so close, so near. Why aren't you like this with me?' It's been many years since I last played with dolls, but the hardest part of writing this book will be giving up the illusion that if I myself had just said or done or drawn the right magical thing, the illusion of perfect love between my mother and me would have been made real.

There *is* real love between most mothers and daughters. There is real love between my mother and me. But it is not that kind of love she always led me to believe she felt, which society told me she felt, and about which I have always been angry and guilty. Angry because I never really felt it, guilty because I thought the fault lay in me. If I were a better daughter I would be able to take in this nourishing love she had always told me was there. I have recently found I could get angry with mother and that it would not destroy her or me. The anger that separated me from her also put me in touch with the real love I have for her. Anger broke the pane of glass between us.

I have heard daughters say that they do not love their mothers. I have *never* heard a mother say she does not love her daughter. Psychoanalysts have told me that a woman patient would rather consider herself 'crazy' than admit that she simply does not like her daughter. She can be honest about anything else, but the myth that mothers always love their children is so controlling that even the daughter who can admit disliking her mother, when her own time comes, will deny all but positive emotions toward her children.

Difficulties begin with the word *love* itself. Literature and daily human intercourse might have been better off if the word were never used. It is too ambiguous; we recognize this in our most intense relationships when we become aware of the mystery that always surrounds its meaning. But we cherish it for its very ambiguity, which allows it to say anything we want. No wonder so many people say they don't know what it means.

'I love you, it's for your own good,' mother says when she forbids us to play with a friend. 'If I didn't love you so much, I wouldn't fuss so about your wearing galoshes.' 'Of course I love you, but that's why I want you to go to camp. I want you with me always, but it's better for you to enjoy a summer of fresh air.' All these explanations seem reasonable on the surface. We want to believe that love is the motivation for everything mother does. Often it is not love, but, respectively, possessiveness, anxiety, and outright rejection that is being expressed in sentences like these. We cannot afford to believe this on a cognitive level. Way down deep we feel it.

To take mother's words about love at face value is to

distort the rest of our lives in an effort to find again this ideal relationship. 'Love is not an indivisible emotion,' says psychoanalyst Richard Robertiello. 'Our job as adults is to separate out the elements in this big package we got from mother which she called love, and to take in what she did give us, and to look in the real world for those other aspects we did not get from her.'

We learn our deepest ways of intimacy with mother; automatically we repeat the pattern with everyone else with whom we become close. Either we play out the role of the child we were with mother, and make the other person into the mother figure, or we reverse: playing mother to the other person's 'child'. 'All too often,' says Leah Schaefer, 'what we play out with this other person has little to do with them or who we are today.' This is why arguments or frictions between some people can never be resolved: they are not reacting to what is going on between them, but to old, unhealed hurts and rejections suffered in the past.

Intimacy is just an old record we replay. 'First,' says Richard Robertiello, 'we *introject* – take into ourselves – mother's tangled-up notion of what love is. Then we *project* it upon our lovers, husbands, and our own daughter.'

Perhaps mother was very possessive and tried to live through us, but at the same time did give us a lot of cuddling, satisfying physical contact, and affection. It is all too easy for us forever afterward to buy the whole package – clutching dependency and physical warmth are both tied into an inextricable knot and labelled *love*. Our husband may be physically affectionate, but unless he is possessive too, we decide he doesn't 'really' love us, something is missing from the perfect love he is supposed to feel for us.

Another example is the mother who tells her daughter she loves her, but is always sending her away to stay with grandmother, leaving her in the care of nurses, or packing her off to boarding school. Is it surprising that a girl like this will often grow up convinced that the only people who love her are the ones who don't want her around? Rejection and affection have become inextricably mixed.

Sometimes we are so hurt by mother's ambivalences that we reject the entire package – throwing out the good, positive aspects mother presented to us, along with the painful ones. It is not useful to merely say, 'Mama never loved me, she didn't do this or that for me!' This is to refuse, in our childish anger, to acknowledge what love there was.

Says Dr Robertiello: 'What we must do is break down the specific components of mother's love – analyze exactly the ways she did not love us, but also the ways in which she did. Did mother give you a kind of basic security – a structure of stability, shelter, nurturing? Did she give you admiration – a genuine feeling that you were worth plenty in your own right? Did she give you warmth and physical affection, cuddle, hold and kiss you? Did she really care what happened to you and accept you – my daughter right or wrong? These are some of the components of real love.'

No mother can score 100 in all of them. Perhaps your mother was good about admiring and praising you, giving you a feeling of value – but what she also called love was her need for someone to mother *her*. If so, you may have few problems of self-esteem, but often feel you cannot get enough closeness, intimacy with others. People always let you down. Here is just such a woman, twenty-seven years old, and on the ladder of a career.

'My mother always told me,' she says, '"Aim high! Dare to be different!" She was the rare kind of wonderful mother you can talk to about your sex life, but since I was six or seven, I've felt very protective of her. I knew I was stronger than she. She used to confide in me about her troubles with my domineering father. Even when I was growing up, I'd stand up to him for her, as if she were a child. My mother's emotional support helped me a lot. I've made myself up. But I don't trust men. They can't understand what a woman needs. They won't support you emotionally, but want it for themselves instead. I need a man who's as self-confident as I am, a man I can lean on. That's why I don't sleep with any of the men I know nowadays. There's not much a man can do for me other than give me enormous emotional or financial support, but I haven't found the strong partner who can, or is willing to, do that. Everything else, I can do for myself, but I know that a one-to-one relationship with a man is the most important thing in my life.' She tries to make up for the maternal protection and solicitude she didn't get from her mother by extracting it from men. Her emotional politics are that men must take care of her as if she were a child, while she withholds the sexuality they expect from a woman.

I've heard many a grown woman still lament the fact that mother wasn't home when she returned from school in the afternoon. Forget that mother may have been a terrific role model as a professional working woman – the role model the daughter may have patterned her own career upon. Until she accepts that mother didn't have to be perfect, her childish anger will inhibit the full use of the admirable traits her mother did have. Very often for women like these, their very success in work will bring with it associations of the 'bad' mother they do not wish to grow into. They marry suddenly, giving up their career with a sigh of relief. But the marriage doesn't work out either: the wife tries to turn her husband into the all-caring, protective mother she never had.

Mother may have felt she had to present an image of perfect love. As adults we have to accept that we can live without it. We must give up our resentment that she wasn't ideal so that we can take in what she was good at; it will enhance our lives.

Spontaneous and honest love admits errors, hesitations, and human failings; it can be tested and repaired. Idealized love ties us because we already intuit that it is unreal and are afraid to face this truth.

'I only tell my mother what she wants to hear,' women say. The inference is that the lie is an outgrowth of love; the daughter is merely translating into action her desire to protect her mother. The fact is we become our mother's protectors not because we are such good daughters but to protect ourselves. In some part of our psyche we are still children who are afraid to risk losing mother's unbroken love even for the short space in time of an argument. Telling the truth is a test; it lays bare what in fact goes on between two people.

'I have a wonderful relationship with my mother,' a thirty-eight-year-old woman says, 'but why do I start climbing the walls if I'm around her for more than a few hours? The awful thing is I can see my daughter is already becoming that way with me.' Fantasies of perfect understanding are hard to maintain when you are face to face with reality. It is easier to do when you are apart.

Our mutual refusal to show our true selves, good and bad, to each other does not allow either woman to explore her separate life, her own identity. The unspoken fear is that if one partner leaves, if either questions the perfection of mother-daughter love by being 'different', we are both destroyed. How many grown women dread the idea of living alone, being alone? There is only one thing in this world that approaches the pain of letting go of our mothers, more wrenching than giving up the illusion that she loves us unambivalently. It is separating from – letting go of – our daughters.

'I needed and loved my mother so intensely at times,' says a young mother of a five-year-old daughter, 'that I remember saying to her when I was eight, "I will never love my child as much as you love me." Now I know that I meant *smother*, not love. So many harmful ideas are hidden by the word love. My mother seemed so selfless, so giving. I remember dreading the thought of my mother dying. But I didn't want her to live for me. It piled too much guilt on me. And yet, I didn't dare ask for any space. It would have made me guilty. When I was seventeen I couldn't wait to get away from home. When I married and had a daughter of my own, I became just as possessive of her as my mother was of me. I was a working mother, and thought that meant I was giving my daughter the space I never had. But I used to telephone home all the time from work, and when I got home, guiltily made up for being away by smothering her. Just like my mother, I called every possessive, overprotective thing I did "love".'

The maternal instinct says we are all born mothers, that once we are mothers we will automatically and naturally love our children and always do what is best for them. If you believe in the maternal instinct and fail at mother love, you fail as a woman. It is a controlling idea that holds us in an iron grip.

I propose to use 'maternal instinct' as it is emotionally experienced by most women. For us it does not necessarily have the same meaning as it does for biologists, ethologists, or sociologists. The concept has as many meanings as there are scientists, and many will tell you the maternal instinct doesn't exist at all. Anthropologist Lionel Tiger advised me to avoid using the phrase even in quotes. He felt no matter how I qualified the term, I would be jumped on. It is outside the purpose of this book to prove or disprove the reality of the maternal instinct. But I don't think any woman interested in the forces or choices that shape her life can avoid thinking about what these words mean, not genetically, but imaginatively.

Whether you call it 'instinct' or not, most women enjoy having children, want to, and do. For this majority, the trouble begins not with being mothers, but with the emotional propositions contained in the notion of maternal instinct – that being a good mother is as natural and undifferentiated to humans as it is to a she-wolf with her cubs.

Those who like to make this argument from nature forget that while a she-wolf does care for her cubs instinctively, guards them with her life, and teaches them to hunt, the same instinct leads her to abandon them without a backward glance as soon as they are able to fend for themselves. Other instincts may well lead her to mate, in season, with her son.

Nor does mother love in humans spontaneously well up the moment a child is born. 'I tell mothers on the first day,' says pediatrician Dr Sidney Q. Cohlan, 'it's not having the baby that makes the relationship, it's the day by day living and caring for the infant that makes the relationship. You can't love your baby twenty-four hours a day, seven days a week. Taking care of a baby in the first few months can be hard work and at times a monumental bore. The rewards begin to come after the mother and infant have lived through a period of adjustment and responsiveness to each other's needs. But she has read all the poetry in the magazines and expects "instant motherhood", and thinks there is something wrong with her if she doesn't respond at first sight to her new baby in picture-book fashion. Maybe she doesn't deserve to be a mother? How can she explain even a fleeting negative emotion? Her society won't allow her to verbalize this – so there is a good deal of lying that goes on subconsciously when you ask a new mother about her feelings of fulfillment. They often tell you what they want to believe themselves.'

Says psychiatrist Mio Fredland, who is the mother of a three-year-old daughter: 'I've seen many mothers who were rapturous at the birth of their child, and others who were profoundly depressed. This implies they were in love with a fantasy. In fact mothers often feel extremely guilty and depressed because they don't love their babies at first. The baby looks like a stranger. Yes, we build up some Gerber baby-food fantasy, the great American myth that all mothers love their babies. I've heard women say it can take them two or three weeks before they really begin to "care" for the child. There is that moment of shock when you first see your baby. You don't love her automatically at all.'

This is the tyranny of the notion of maternal instinct. It idealizes motherhood beyond human capacity. A dangerous gap is set up. Mother *feels* the mixture of love and resentment, affection and anger she has for her child, but she cannot afford to *know* it.

The split between what mother says, the way she behaves with her baby – *and what she unconsciously feels on the deepest level* – leaves her unsure of herself. Says Dr

Robertiello: 'Women walk around feeling they have something to hide, that they are secretly "unnatural" or "bad mothers". The act of giving birth does not set up an ability in you to be a mother, you will not necessarily feel this marvelous "maternal instinct" welling up in you, telling you what to do with your baby at every moment. Women must have this myth taken off their backs. It puts them at the mercy of a male chauvinistic society. Men are "sure" that women are meant to be mothers. But each woman in her heart, when she has a baby, is not so "sure". She becomes paralyzed, looking to other people to tell her what to do. Male supremacy uses the myth of the maternal instinct to reinforce its power position.'

If we are going to give women emotionally – on the deepest level – all the alternatives and options of contemporary life, we must enable both sexes to believe that some of us, male and female, have the desire to take care of small creatures like babies, *and that this has nothing to do with one's sexual identity*. Nor need it be instinctual. We may or may not be born with the reflex to pick up and comfort a crying baby, but we can be taught. 'A lot of people, and this includes men,' says Leah Schaefer, 'do like to take care of small, dependent people. In my clinical practice, I've come to believe what is ordinarily called "the maternal instinct" is just this simple liking to "take care of" smaller creatures. Some human beings do not like it at all. It is not some great biological imperative, which if frustrated will ruin or impoverish a woman's life. Mother love may once have been an instinct in humans,' continues Dr Schaefer, who is the mother of a teen-age girl, 'but civilization bred it out of us. I doubt that any woman is born more "maternal" than any other. I wouldn't be surprised if men were born with about the same capacity as women to care for and nurture children – except for the obvious biological differences.'

A human baby's needs are greater than an infant wolf's. The skills we must learn are too complex to be left to animal instinct alone. Human childhood goes on far longer than any other creature's. And so while we may say, if we like, that maternal instinct plays a role in mothering a human child, it is clear that instinct alone could never do the whole job. It has to be supplemented by skills, arts, emotions, and desires humans have learned from other humans. Professionals who work in children's shelters find that mothers who themselves never received adequate mothering when little do not know how to mother, and show little interest in learning. 'The battered-child pattern usually runs in families,' says Dr Lionel Tiger. 'There's a very strong correlation between battering your baby, and having been one yourself.'

'My mother didn't know how to give love,' says a forty-year-old lawyer, 'so when I had a daughter, I didn't know how to do it either. Where was I going to learn how to give love? I'd never known it as a child myself. You can't learn it from books. You cannot grow up in a home where there is hostility and not reflect it later. Maybe I shouldn't have been a mother . . . No, I take that back. I should have been a parent because I want to and can give everything a child needs. But my daughter turns away from my efforts to give her love. Maybe I'm doing it wrong. I should have been taught, there should be some form of education, how to convey love to children. I didn't know how to get love as a child so I don't know how to give it . . . beginning with giving it to myself.'

Says child psychologist Dr Aaron Esman: 'To give good mothering, you have to have received it.'

It is commonplace that the notion of 'the teen-ager' did not exist before the present century. Similarly, the idealization of motherhood, of infancy and childhood, is also an invention of modern times. Recent books suggest that only when the desperate struggle for existence had been won on a broad enough scale could society afford to apportion sufficient amounts of time, emotion, and money to the care of babies. 'Maternal infanticide was "the most common crime in Western Europe from the Middle Ages down to the end of the eighteenth century",' writes Adrienne Rich.[3] Says Edward Shorter, ". . . traditional mothers were not monsters . . . If they lacked an articulate sense of maternal love, it was because they were forced by material circumstances and community attitudes to subordinate infant welfare to other objectives, such as keeping the farm going or helping their husbands weave cloth . . . Good mothering is an invention of modernization.'[4]

'Why do so many women rush into motherhood?' says Dr Esman. 'It surely isn't out of "maternal instinct". Not if they are hoping to get a lot of the experience out of identification with their own children that they didn't get themselves. Or if the reason they have a child is to hang on to their husband, to save the marriage – that's a terrible reason. People say, "Well, maybe we should have a child," when a marriage is going badly, which is the worst advice. Again and again I see women whose own childhoods were deprived, who have the fantasy that they are going to do for their baby what their mother didn't do for them. They are going to relive their childhood through their baby, and that baby is going to be given all the things they didn't get . . . Or else. Maternal instinct? We have no evidence of it. Women want to become mothers for lots of reasons; it's part of their biological condition, having the equipment for it, one of the things being a woman is about, but I wouldn't call this "instinct", not in the terms in which I define the word. Also there are social expectations; all her life a woman has been expected to grow up, marry and have babies, it's been drummed into her all along, so that her whole orientation is geared toward these expectations from others. But this is not "maternal instinct". Reasonably healthy women want to have children because of what I would describe as wanting to nurture somebody, to get pleasure out of feeding and caring for a child, to do for somebody else what was done to them by their mother, and to share a particular type of experience with their husband. This is a growth, developmental experience.'

The first thing it can be said a mother honestly feels in relation to her child is a kind of self-love. The child is essentially a narcissistic extension of herself. The child used to be a part of her, inside her. It is now external but is still closely connected with her own body. Whatever investment she has in her body is continued in the child. If the infant is all she hoped it would be, she may more easily live up to society's injunction that she love the child more than herself. But if there is something about the baby – if it's a boy instead of a girl, too fat, too thin, too lethargic – that makes her feel less than the exaltation she has been led to expect, she must deny it. Any wound to her narcissism – that tidal basin out of which all maternal emotions flow – must go unacknowledged, repressed, unfelt. I suspect that when post-partum depression enters, it begins in the silence she must maintain if her child does not fulfil her fantasy of perfect maternal bliss.

The glorification of motherhood demands that when her child is born, autonomy over her own emotions must end. Like most unnatural madonnas in early Christian art, she is supposed to focus only on the infant. Little emblazoned letters follow the golden beam from her one eye to the child: love. The four letters cancel her emotional past, command her to unlearn a whole life's way of thinking and feeling about people. She must ignore her own subjectivity, her real pleasure in physical beauty if her child is not pretty, her boredom with stupidity if the child is slow. Above all, she must not let the sex of her child make any difference to her. She must shut her eyes to the very first item of information we take in about any new person we meet, and which colors every single transaction we have with them thereafter. The day the baby's pram is bought, we decorate it in pink or blue, signaling to the outside world what it wants to know. Only to the mother is it not supposed to matter if her child has a penis or a vagina.

And yet the truth is that when one woman gives birth to another, to someone who is like her, they are linked together for life in a very special way. Mother is the prime love object, the first attachment for both male and female infants. But it is their sex, their sameness that distinguishes what a mother has with her daughter. No two people have such an opportunity for support and identification, and yet no human relationship is so mutually limiting. If a mother suggests to her daughter that motherhood was not the glorious culmination she had been promised, that life had not opened out for her but been somehow diminished instead, this is saying to the girl: I should not have had you.

A woman without a daughter may try to explore life's infinite possibilities. Her own mother left out so much. But when a daughter is born, fears she thought she had conquered long ago are re-aroused. Now there is another person, not simply dependent on her, but *like* her, and therefore subject to all the dangers she has fought all her life. The mother's progress into a larger sexuality is halted. Ground gained that she could have held alone is abandoned. She retreats and entrenches herself in the cramped female stance of security and defense. The position is fondly hailed as mother protector. It is the position of fear. She may be only half alive but she is safe, and so is her daughter. She now defines herself not as a woman but primarily as a mother. Sex is left out, hidden from the girl who must never think of her mother in danger: in sex. It is only with the greatest effort that the girl will be able to think of herself that way.

'I think what frightens me most is my daughter's vulnerability,' says a mother of a six-year-old. 'It's my own fear that I would be exploited sexually. I know I overprotect her. But I'm so afraid she'll be hurt, taken advantage of. She's so naturally unguarded.' How is she going to protect this pitifully vulnerable female infant until she reaches the safe haven of marriage? The mother just doesn't know. What she does know is that for a little girl – as opposed to a little boy – sex is a danger. It must be denied, suppressed. Her daughter will not be raised a sexy hussy, but 'a lady'. No erotic stimuli must intrude into the little girl's consciousness, no dirty jokes, no daring clothes, no indication that the mother's own body responds sexually. If mother doesn't mention it or think about it or respond to anything herself, it will go away. In order to keep the child's attention from turning to the anxious-making topic of sex, the mother goes the final step and desexualizes herself.

'A couple of months after my daughter was born,' says a twenty-eight-year-old woman, 'I had lunch with a man I'd known for years. "Well," he said, "how does it feel not to be a sexy woman any longer?"' Society gives mother all the unsolicited help she needs in her desexualization. The week before Mother's Day recently, this banner headline ran in a full-page newspaper ad for a famous designer's seductive at-home wear for women: '. . . before she was a mother, she was a woman.'

From the girl's earliest years, her emergent sexuality will be a cause of anxiety, seeming to make her not more like her mother, but unlike her. If mother denies her own sexuality, and reacts to mine with such shame or fright, how big an asset is it? How difficult it is to be a woman! Better to remain a child, a good little girl.

By trying to protect her daughter from sexual hazads which, imagined or not, lie far in the future, the mother begins, from the daughter's birth, to withhold the model of herself as a woman who takes pleasure and pride in sexuality. The daughter is deprived of the identification she needs most. Every effort on the daughter's part to feel good about herself as a woman will be an uphill struggle – if not betrayal – against this sexless image of her mother. The lifelong puzzle between mother and daughter has begun. Is it any wonder that mothers and daughters scan each other like unfinished murder mysteries, unable to let one another go?

When I was an art history student at college, I used to yawn over the great masters' efforts to explain the greatest miracle of them all: The Virgin Birth. I blamed my boredom on an aesthetic ennui with all that sweetness and symmetry beloved of the Renaissance. I know now that what we call boredom is often a defense against anxiety, and what was making me anxious was the Mystery embodied by the Immaculate Conception: how to have sex and remain a virgin at the same time? Eventually I lost my virginity, but I never learned how Mary did not. Any girl who ever uncrossed her legs and prayed may be interested in one explanation I recently heard.

Mary and Joseph *did* have sexual intercourse. What kept Mary chaste was that she wasn't thinking about it. She was pure of mind and with God. Therefore, it didn't count.

Sometimes I wonder what kind of model Mary makes for our daughters, but it can't be far from how we perceive the sexual image of our mothers: certainly she did it with our father, but from what we know of her, we can't imagine for a minute that she enjoyed it.

'Close your eyes and think of England,' Victorian mothers told their daughters on their wedding night. Today we laugh at the joke. But one of the growth industries in our culture is the sex clinics whose job with women is to put them in touch with their sex, to get them to think about the unthinkable, and push past the sexless image of their mothers.

When women's lives were more predictable, we could more easily afford this enigmatic picture of womanhood. When we had no alternative but to repeat our mother's life, our mistakes and disappointments were pretty much confined to her space, her margin of error and unhappiness. I do believe our grandmothers, even our mothers, were happier; not knowing as much as we do and not having our options, there was less to be unhappy about. A woman might give up her sexuality, hate being a housewife, not like children, but if every other woman was doing it, how could she articulate her frustration? She could feel it certainly, but you can't want what you don't know about. Television, for instance, gave them no sense of thwarted expectations. Today women's lives are changing at a rate and by a necessity we couldn't control if we wanted to; we need all the energy that suppression consumes. If we are going to fill more than women's traditional role, we can't afford the exhaustion that goes with constant emotional denial. There are pressures on women other than the 'maternal instinct'. They are the new economic and social demands. Even if we decide to lead our mothers' lives, the fact is that our daughter may not. We may continue, through denial and repression, to keep alive the idealization of motherhood for another generation, but where will that leave her?

If women are going to be lawyers as well as mothers, they must differentiate between the two, and then differentiate once again about their sexuality. That is the third – and *not* mutually exclusive – option. As the world changes, and women's place in it, mothers must consciously present this choice to their daughters. A woman may incorporate all three choices within herself – and even more – but at any given moment she must be able to say to herself and her daughter, 'I chose to have you because. I wanted to be a mother. I chose to work – to have a career, to be in politics, to play the piano – because that gives me a different feeling of value about myself, a value that is not greater nor lesser than motherhood, only different. Whether you choose to work or not, to be a mother or not, it will have nothing to do with your sexuality. Sexuality is the third option – as meaningful as either of the other two.'

'If a mother has a life of her own,' says Dr Robertiello, 'the daughter will love her more, will want to be around her more. She must not define herself as "a mother", she's got to see herself as a person, a person with work to do, a sexual person, a woman. It isn't necessary to have a profession. She doesn't have to have a high IQ or be president of the PTA to have this added life. So long as she isn't just sitting home, chauffeuring the kids, and baking cookies, giving her children and herself the feeling that their life is hers. Of course the best thing the mother can do is try to have her main connection with her husband instead of her daughter.'

The truth is that the woman and the mother are often at war with one another – in the same body. Dr Helene Deutsch, in *The Psychology of Women*, takes the classical Freudian view on the 'passivity' of women, one in which many analysts today do not join (nor do I myself), but I think she gives us an important clue here: 'The origin of this longing in primitive, unsublimated instinctual drives,' she says, 'manifests itself in various ways. Ardent wishes to be desired, strong aspirations to exclusive egoistic possession, a normally completely passive attitude with regard to the first attack . . . are characteristic attributes of feminine sexuality. They are so fundamentally different from the emotional manifestations of motherhood that we are compelled to accept the opposition of sexuality and eroticism on one hand and reproduction instinct and motherhood on the other.'[5]

Like so many women since the world began, my mother could not believe in this opposition of the two desires. Tradition, society, her patients, religion itself told her that there was no conflict; that motherhood was the logical and natural end product of sex. Instead of believing what every woman's body tells every woman's mind, that as Dr Deutsch states, sexuality and eroticism are a 'fundamentally different' and 'opposite' drive to motherhood, my mother accepted the lie. She took as her act of faith the proposition that if she were a real woman, she would be a good mother and I would grow up the same. If I repeated her path and pattern of mother-hood, it would show I did not blame her for her choice. It would justify and place the final stamp of value on what she had done. It would say her attitude, behavior, and deepest feelings were not split, but were in fact in harmony, a woman in unison with nature.

Some women do make this choice gladly. They may be the majority, but my mother was not one of them. As I am not – her daughter in this too. Even in a good marriage, many women resent the matronly, nonsexual role their children force them to play. My mother didn't even have a good marriage; she was a young widow.

Frightened as she was, as much in need of my father as my sister and I were of her, mother had no choice but to pretend that my sister and I were the most important part of her life; that neither fear, youth and inexperience, loss, loneliness or her own needs could shake the unqualified and invincible love she felt for us. My mother had no body of woman-to-woman honesty and shared experience to use in her fight against the folk wisdom that said just being a woman carried all the inherent wisdom needed to be a mother – that it was either 'natural' to her, or she was a failure as a woman.

In all the years we lived together, it is a shame we never talked honestly about our feelings. What neither of us knew then was that I could have stood honesty, no matter how frightening. Her angers, disillusionments, fears of failure, rage – emotions I seldom saw – I could have come to terms with them if she had been able to speak to me. I would have grown used to the idea that while mother loved me, at times other emotions impaired that love, and developed trust that in time her love for me would always return. Instead, I was left trying to believe in some perfect love she said she had for me, but in which I could not believe. I did not understand why I couldn't feel it no matter what her words said. I grew to believe that love itself, from her or anybody else, was a will-o'-the-wisp, coming or going for reasons I could not control. Never knowing when or why I was loved, I grew afraid to depend on it.

The older I get, the more of my mother I see in myself. The more opposite my life and my thinking grow from hers, the more of her I hear in my voice, see in my facial expression, feel in the emotional reactions I have come to recognize as my own. It is almost as if in extending myself, the circle closes in to completion. She was my first and most lasting model. To say her image is not still a touchstone in my life – and mine in hers – would be another lie. I am tired of lies. They have stood in the way of my understanding myself all my life. I have always known that what my husband loves most in me is that I have my own life. I have always felt that I had partially deceived him in this; I am very clever at pretense. My work, my marriage, and my new relationships with other women are beginning to make his assumptions about me true – that I am an independent, separate individual. They have allowed me to respect myself, and admire my own sex. What still stands between me and the person I would like to be is this illusion of perfect love between my mother and me. It is a lie I can no longer afford.

CHAPTER TWO

A Time to be Close

I grew up in a house of women. It's a different way to begin
life, but I didn't allow myself to feel the loss of the father
everyone else had. I would later theorize that perhaps my
kind of childhood had its advantages: not having seen a man
diminished by women's impossible demands on him, I grew
up believing all things were possible between a man and a
woman. Of course I missed him.

In our house there were always four women: my mother,
my older sister Susie, and myself; at first, the other woman
was my nurse Anna. I loved Anna so much I let her slip out of
my life as painlessly as my father. The day she left I told
myself I felt nothing. I had learned everything about love and
separation in the first years of my life.

Anna was fearless, and she loved me in a way I can still feel.
She was as tough and dependable as my mother was timid
and out of her depth. 'My poor mother'; why do I think of
her that way even today, with my stepfather and a world of
friends around her? I suppose in the same way that she still
sees me as a child, I still see her at twenty, a widow with two
baby girls. But what did I feel then? With the terrible injustice
of children who know that to be fair can cost them their lives,
I always wanted her complete and unswerving love and
attention; all she had to offer was her vulnerability and
sadness.

In the space between what I demanded and she could give, I
lived. From there it was not a far step for a child to decide my
demands were what made her unhappy. That in some way I
was the cause of her unhappiness. It's why I hated her to
braid my hair: I could hear her sighing behind me. Her

sadness was my guilt. Whenever she talks about her own mother, whom I never knew, that look comes over her face. It's worse when she talks about my father. She only does when I ask, and I was twenty-two before I dared. Can you stand your mother's sadness? We believe that if we had been better children, or even right now could do or say the right thing, we could make it go away. I cannot bear to be in the same room when my mother's face changes from the look I love to that maddening unhappiness. My intellect tells me the guilt I feel whenever I say good-bye to her has nothing to do with what I did or didn't do. My mother is a reasonably happy woman, other people would say. I've been a reasonably good daughter, my mother would say. But until I understand my guilt, I will not be free of her.

'Oh, Nancy,' she'll begin, 'I wish you had known Mama. She was such a wonderful woman . . .' and her voice will drift away to some distant image which she sees beyond me, and we'll talk about something else. I'd like to see that image, to share anything that may tell me more about my grandmother – and so about my mother, and so about me. But the stories my mother tells about her mother, lovely as they are, much as I like to hear them again and again, are as diffused with sentiment as the faded, misty Bachrach photos in the leather volumes at my grandfather's house that I have pored over every summer of my life, looking . . . for what? My mother is the oldest child, but in all the photos even the sister eleven years younger looks more self-assured than she. How dizzying it must have been to be picked at seventeen by my handsome father, she the thorn among the roses in her father's stern eyes. She eloped with him against that father's wishes, though sometimes I wonder if even her elopement itself didn't express her silent dutifulness as a daughter: if she did not find favor in her father's eyes, she was prepared to go away. How unprepared she must have been for motherhood a year later, and two years after that for my father's death. So much loss for a person who never had a sense of self.

As we both grow older I see how suited she was to be a

wife, how gracefully she moves now that she has a second chance and my sister and I are grown, leaving her role as our mother almost negligible beside her life as a woman. I am sure much of her talent as a wife comes from her mother, as does mine; again and again she tells me what a strong influence her mother was on all her children – this woman who has taken on almost mythic magnitude in my imagination. But my grandmother died suddenly and mysteriously of an incurable disease called sleeping sickness when my mother was sixteen. *Sleeping sickness.* All my life it has seemed the appropriate and romantic end for this fairy-tale woman. 'I can remember coming home from school, running into the house and calling, "Mama, Mama,"' my mother says, 'and then realizing she wasn't there any more.'

As much as I want my mother to go beyond the pretty pictures of her mother ('so beautiful, so kind'), and of my father ('so handsome, so charming'), I have come to realize she needs her own protection against loss and pain. She will see in those early years only what she can afford to live with.

Nowadays my mother and I talk more than we used to. It began with my marriage, an alliance that has always seemed to have strengthened her as well as me. It has been gradual, this unravelling of the unspoken between us, but I think she is as eager as I now to talk. Suppression eats up her energy too. I am not the only one who is guilty. Several years ago my husband, Bill, and I were visiting her and my stepfather, Scotty. We'd just come down to the library for our welcome-home martini when she handed me a faded letter. It was almost as if she'd been waiting to give it to me, unable to take it in until I too had read it.

It was a letter written to her when she was fourteen by her mother. My grandmother had just left my grandfather, and gone to Florida with the youngest of their five children. It was a stunning thing to do in that era. I've often stared at her self-portrait that now hangs in my living room and wondered, angry as she was with my grandfather, how she could have left her children – none of whom to this day can speak of her without a kind of adoration and longing. But then, given my grandfather, I would probably have married and left him too. In the portraits of him which she painted, he looks like the young F. Scott Fitzgerald. He was easily twice as difficult. They met at an amateur theatrical, and she flatly refused to play opposite a man with red hair. She had red hair herself. They did the play, and though I'm told he never loved any woman as he loved her, they never stopped arguing.

My grandfather made his fortune in steel alloys in Pittsburgh, lost it in the Depression and made it all back again. He loved power, horses, trophies, and beautiful women. He never forgave my mother for not being one. She grew into beauty too late. As a little girl I would stand in the room with the silver cups, the red and blue ribbons, the stuffed swordfish, the photos of yachts and fox hunts, and I would imagine myself beautiful and winning them all for him. On those evenings when my grandfather dined out with the Mellons and the Carnegies, I'm told my grandmother cooked spaghetti for her arty friends in her studio at the top of the house.

My mother, her three sisters, and brother loved and feared my grandfather until his death a few years ago. Their feelings about their mother are totally unambivalent. I have seen each of them turn at different moments to one of us grandchildren and say, 'For a moment there, you looked just like Mama . . .' It has always been the highest compliment. It promised more than beauty, some inner secret that would make people love you forever as they did her. From their stories I have a picture of a woman who was every child's dream, a beauty with large eyes and dark hair who wrote plays for her children, who dressed up with them and was as capable of entering their world as she was of taking care of them. She was as romantic and sensitive to life as my grandfather was ambitious and incapable of demonstrating the love he felt for his children. The reason I love the paintings that fill my house is that she painted them.

When my grandmother wrote this letter, I doubt that she

intended to return to my grandfather. I don't think her leaving him was a false gesture, but a desperate last alternative. She saw only separation ahead and clearly wanted to give her eldest daughter something to help fill the void. Of all the memorabilia that came out of my grandfather's files after his death, this is what my mother wanted me to see. It was a message to her from her mother, of course, but I think it was also her own silent way of saying something to me:

My darling Jane:
    When you read this I want you to do it with an open heart. Forget the things that have been said – the thoughts you may have had, and try to remember only the better, more beautiful phase of life. When I am not there with you, it is going to be your task to try to help the little ones to see things. Try to guide them in the right way. This is your work and your duty.
    To me motherhood has been the most beautiful thing in my life. The wonder of it never ceases for me – to see you all developing from tiny helpless babies into big strong girls and boys, to see your minds changing with your years and to remember that some day you will be grown men and women. It is overwhelming.
    All my life as a child I looked forward to the time when I would have children of my own – and in spite of my so-called talents or urges toward other things, underneath was that spark which had to burst into flames sometime. And when I held you, Jane – my first baby – in my arms, I had the greatest thrill I have ever experienced. I felt almost saintly, as if I had really entered heaven, and now I know that every time a mother receives a new baby she really does enter heaven. There is nothing else in life like it. And anyone who receives such a blessing should be eternally grateful.
    I am telling you this, Jane, just so you will understand my love and feeling for you. Always remember this and

as you grow older, think of me sometime and try to understand what I am trying to convey to you.

My heart is full, but I could not write the things I feel in a thousand years. Love each other and be good to daddy and he will take care of you. This is the hardest, bitterest moment of my life, leaving you, but I cannot do anything else. I cannot see through my tears. God bless you all,

Mama

I believe my grandmother did feel close to heaven when she first held my mother, but I feel that what makes this letter most valuable to my mother is that her mother could feel other emotions too. My mother doesn't remember reading the letter when she was fourteen. Perhaps her father kept it from her. But however he explained his wife's departure, her leaving could only be felt as loss, the kind of intolerable pain no one can admit to. Perhaps this letter confirmed for my mother what she always wanted to feel, not so much that her mother deeply loved her, but that her mother's act of leaving my grandfather when she felt his imperiousness too denigrating was proof that while she was a mother, she was a woman first. She would not go through all her short life celebrating only self-abnegation and the maternal emotions. She loved other ideas and people besides her children. She was their mother, but would not be their martyr – which is one reason they loved her so. I have never heard one word from my mother, aunts, or uncle of any guilt she ever made them feel. If they have idealized her to disguise the pain and anger they felt at the loss of her, surely this letter confirmed, at least for my mother, what she needed to know, not just as her mother's child, but as a parent with children of her own. In showing it to me she was saying, 'See, if I wasn't as present, as close, maternal, and mothering as other mothers were to their children, it wasn't because I didn't love you. My mother loved me, but she was absent too.'

My mother's life doesn't look like her mother's, but the

emotions beneath the surface are hauntingly familiar. My mother too chose a man who could not give her the emotional security she desperately needed. She too found that her life as a woman created demands opposed to her role as a mother; she abandoned that role as her mother did, separated herself from her children emotionally because without my father, in the midst of bitter deprivation of her own, she had little left to give my sister and me. In her letter, my grandmother tried to face her children's inevitable anger and loss by speaking to them of the perfect love for them by the part of herself which was their mother. Unable to speak to me herself, but resonating in her depths to my sense that I too had somehow been deserted when I was little just as she had been, my mother used her adored mother's own words to tell me she recognized my anger, to say that she had always loved me even if imperfectly, and to ask me to forgive her, just as she had forgiven her mother.

We are the loving sex; people count on us for comfort, nurturing warmth. We hold the world together with the constant availability of our love when men would tear it apart with their needs for power. We feel incomplete, alone, inadequate without a man, devalued outside marriage, defensive without children. We are raised for love, but when love comes to us, sweet as it is, somehow it is not as ultimately satisfying as we dreamed. We are being loved for being a part of a relationship, for our function – not for ourselves.

He asks us out for dinner, and even as we hang up the phone, hot with pleasure, we wonder who else he asked before us. As he holds us in his arms, we are already half afraid he will forget us tomorrow. On the day he marries us, we ask him yet another time: 'Do you really love me?'

Men don't say to us, 'Climb the highest mountain, catch me a star, prove you love me so I can believe it.' If we are so loving, why are we not lovable in ourselves? When our children are born we believe at last in love, our own and theirs too. These people, our children, will never stop loving us, ever. Love. It's all we know, but we do not trust it.

The seed of our disbelief goes back to our first love, a time we can't remember. The lessons learned from mother in the way she loved us and the way she loved herself stay with us for life.

All my life I've resented the tyranny of infancy, the notion that my adult behavior was determined by a stage of life that I couldn't remember, that was past, and therefore beyond change, regret, or control. Sentences filled with psychiatric rhetoric of 'oral rage,' 'infantile omnipotence,' and 'penis envy' irritated me almost to anger. What did all that mumbo jumbo have to do with my life? I believed in learning from experience, that we could make ourselves up out of whatever material had been handed us; that we could change our lives if we were strong enough. Didn't I know my own fears and anxieties? Hadn't I learned to keep them in check? I was proud of my self-discipline, resentful of the very idea of a doctor rummaging around in my neat emotional closets.

Strong – the very word has always been glamorous but mystifying to me. Surely if it means anything, it is the ability to be effective, do something by and for one's self, using one's own inner resources and leaning on no one? The puzzle has always been then – why did one person have this inner strength and someone else not? To say someone is 'strong' is only to give that person a name or adjective; it is merely labeling. It gives no clue to where strength comes from.

If I am 'strong,' why is there so much anxiety in my life? Why am I so haunted by fear that my work isn't good enough? Yesterday's triumphs have little meaning; tomorrow 'reality' will take over again and I will fail or be found out. Above all, why can't I enjoy what my husband and friends tell me – that they love me? Why do I dream at night and worry by day about the loss of others? Ever since I can remember, I have been, outwardly at least, a winner – good in school, good at sports, people liked me, I did accomplished work. Why then do I still feel insecure?

How often I've heard my own rationalizations and defenses in the voices of other women I have interviewed. How stubbornly most of us resist what now seems to me to be common sense; over the years the 'mumbo jumbo' of the psychiatrists whose names fill this book took on a power I could no longer deny: in our beginnings is our essence.

We get our courage, our sense of self, the ability to believe we have value even when alone, to do our work, to love others, and to feel ourselves lovable from the 'strength' of mother's love for us when we were infants – just as every single dyne of energy on earth originally came from the sun.

Most of you will never be psychoanalyzed. I have not been myself. Like me, you may have a built-in resistance to going back to where lack of belief in yourself began. First impressions of life cut the deepest. They form the grooves of character through which experience comes to us; and if this or that groove becomes distorted, this or that emotion becomes blocked or twisted. We can understand it intellectually. We can never 'take it in.' Certain patterns that come heavy-laden with ambivalence, rejection, and humiliation from the past have us in their grip. The maturation process demands that we understand our history before the energy bound up in repression can be released. Self-deception begins with boredom or cleverness: 'Oh, I know all about my mother and me,' you may say. 'All that business with my mother was over years ago.' You don't and it wasn't.

There is a great deal of data that says an unresolved relationship with her mother sets a woman's mind in certain nonautonomous patterns, encloses her in fear of certain experiences, often stops her from going after what she wants in life, or, when she finds what she wants, keeps her from taking from it the gratification she needs.

If as a tiny child we didn't get the kind of satisfying closeness and love that gives an infant the strength to grow on, we do not evolve emotionally. We become older but a part of us remains infants, looking for this nurturing closeness, never believing that we have it, or that if we do, soon it will be taken away.

Freud, Horney, Bowlby, Erikson, Sullivan, Winnicott, Mahler – the great interpreters of human behavior – may disagree profoundly in some ways but are as one about beginnings: you cannot leave home, cannot grow up whole, separate, and self-reliant, unless someone loved you enough to give you a self first, and then let you go. It begins with our mother's touch, our mother's smile and eye: there is someone out there whom she likes to touch, there is someone out there she likes to see. That's me. And I'm OK!

It used to be thought that if you loved a child too much, you would spoil her. We know now you cannot be loved too much – not in the first years of life. In the depths of that first closeness to our mothers is built the bedrock of self-esteem on which we will erect our good feelings about ourselves for the rest of our lives. An infant needs an almost suffocating kind of closeness to the body whose womb it so recently and reluctantly left. The technical word for this closeness is *symbiosis*.

It is especially important for women to understand the meaning of this word because for so many of us, it becomes our lifelong way of relating. Very early on, the young boy is trained to make it on his own. To be independent. As young girls, we are trained to see our value in the partnerships we form. To symbiose.

At the beginning of life, symbiosis is of prime, positive importance to both sexes. It begins as a growth process, freeing the infant of the fear of being vulnerable and alone, giving her the courage to develop. If we get enough symbiosis in the beginning, we will later remember its pleasures and be able to look for it in others; to accept and immerse ourselves in it when we find it, and *move out of it again* when we are sated, knowing that we will always be able to re-establish it. We will trust and enjoy love, take it as part of life's feast – not feel we must devour every crumb because it may never come again. If we do not experience this first symbiosis, we look for it the rest of our lives, but even if we do find it, we will not trust it – hanging on so desperately that we will suffocate the other person, boring him to death with our cries of, 'You don't love me!' until, in fact, we have made it come true.

The first meaning of symbiosis is found in botany, where it means two organisms, a host and parasite, who cannot live without each other. In the animal world, it often means a slightly different relationship, one of mutual help; the bird that wins its food by obligingly picking the hippopotamus's teeth clean is a partner in symbiosis. In human terms, the meaning shifts a little once again. The most classical symbiosis is the fetus in the womb. Here we have an illustration of two different kinds of symbiosis.

The fetus is in *physical* symbiosis with the mother; literally, it cannot live without her. The mother (most of the time) is in *psychological* symbiosis with the unborn baby. She can live without it, but pregnancy gives her the feeling of more abundant life. In this way, the fetus nourishes her. In our earliest symbiosis with mother, both partners win.

At birth we don't know there is anything outside of ourselves. Our unfocused eyes cannot differentiate shapes, we don't know where mother ends and we begin. When we reach out our hand, she is there to touch. When we cry, we are fed or picked up. We rule the world! No wonder we are so reluctant to give up mother; she sustains this wonderful feeling of total power, 'infantile omnipotence'. In a sense we continue to be physically connected to her, just as mother psychologically still experiences us as almost a part of her body, her own narcissistic extension. The symbiosis is mutual, complete, and satisfying.

Gradually, our eyes begin to be able to focus. Things, people, are near or far. We become aware that another person is there – mother – but she is so close that we still see her as merged with us, not separate. She is different from anybody else, anything else. She is still us, we are her.

In this early stage of symbiosis, the good mother sees her needs as entirely secondary to her infant's. This is to mutual advantage: the infant is enabled with gradual comfort to get used to the idea of powerlessness; nor is it presented as very terrible anyway: mother is always near to fix things. As for the mother, knowing what the child wants, feeling with her baby's skin, sensing with her tiny daughter's eyes or ears or stomach, gives her an almost mystic feeling of union and being needed. It is an experience of transcendence.

In the next stage, we may begin to distinguish our body from mother's, but can't separate our thoughts from hers. When we are wet, she changes us. Hungry? She knows it almost as quickly as we do, and food arrives. But now anxiety begins to enter. When mother is not around, the blanket isn't pulled up, the breast or bottle isn't offered. Our power has begun to erode. Anxiously we keep watch for her. If she's around, everything is OK. If she's not, we can die. When mother's love is steady and uninterrupted, we gradually come to be able to do without having her around for longer and longer periods of time. Trust is being born.

Instead of clutching at mother in fear that she will leave, the infant lets her go, secure in the knowledge that she always comes back when needed; meanwhile, there are these colored toys to play with. But if the fear should ever strike that mother may not come back, that she may be inattentive to our needs, that she does not care about us, growth stops. Interest in bright lights or playing with crib toys disappears. The self has been swallowed by fear. The baby can think of nothing else in the world but that mother must never go away again. We must not be left alone. The foundations of a lifetime of uncertainty have been laid.

The word for the next stage of development is *separation*. The child, more or less secure in the symbiotic love of her mother, begins to feel she can do with a bit less of it. She wants to venture out into a larger world. As important as it was for the mother to symbiose with her infant when that was all baby could understand, it is equally important now for her to begin to let her child go, to let the daughter proceed into her own life according to her inner, psychic timetable.

The long march toward individuality and self-reliance has begun.

Symbiosis and the early beginnings of separation do not proceed on one long, smooth, upwardly inclined plane. There are ups and downs, of course. Nor does any single absence of mother when we want her mean that traumatic damage will inevitably result. *Mother doesn't have to be perfect.* She merely has to be a 'good enough mother', in words of the English psychoanalyst, D. W. Winnicott,[1] to give the growing child a feeling of 'basic trust'[2] – that on the whole people and things, life itself, are more to be trusted than not. We all know how quickly children recover from this or that emotional upset, if the upsetting event doesn't go on too long, or occur too frequently.

In the normal course of events, a sense of self begins to emerge at about three months; the child shows she is reacting to specific events or faces: she smiles. Around eight months, the child can tell the difference between mother and a stranger. At the age of one and a half (give or take), the growth process away from mother picks up momentum. We start to separate from her more and more, *to want to separate*. It's a beautiful exciting world, and there are so many things other than mother to bite, touch, taste, see. The self is becoming more and more conscious.

The fascinating process of growing away from mother and becoming our own person is crucial between eighteen months and three years – a period of life to which Dr Margaret Mahler has given the name 'Separation –Individuation.'[3] By age three or three and a half, if we are lucky and mother has been loving, we emerge with a sense of ourselves as separate people – still loved by mother, but with a life of our own that is not hers. All those hours and hours of attention she has paid us, the sacrifice of her sleep and most of her waking hours, have become part of us. Memory has developed, and we can feel her tender concern follow us around like a supporting arm on our shoulders.

'The first demonstration of social trust in the baby,' says

Erik Erikson in *Childhood and Society*, 'is the ease of his feeling, the depth of his sleep, the relaxation of his bowels.'[4] The child has begun to trust his mother, to relax; he doesn't have to keep awake or sleep with one ear open for fear she will go away. 'The infant's first social achievement, then,' Dr Erikson goes on, 'is his willingness to let the mother out of sight without undue anxiety or rage, because she has become an inner certainty . . .'[5]

This need to feel a basic trust of life is essential for both males and females. But because of the inevitable modeling relationship between mother and daughter, we are not just stuck for life with the sense of basic trust she did or didn't give us. We are also stuck with the image of her as a woman, *her* sense of basic trust that *her* mother gave her. A boy will grow up, and following his father's lead, leave home, support himself, start a family. He may or may not be successful. Much of his success will depend upon the basic sense of trust his mother gave him; but he will not identify with his mother. He will not base all his relationships on what he had with her (unless he is a certain kind of homosexual).

But a girl who did not get this sense of basic trust, though she may leave her mother's house, get a job, marry and have children, will never really feel comfortable on her own, in control of her own life. Part of her is still anxiously tied to her mother. She doesn't trust herself and others. She cannot believe there is another way to be because this is how her mother was. It is also how most other women are. If our mothers are not separate people themselves, we cannot help but take in their anxiety and fear, their need to be symbiosed with someone. If we do not see them involved in their own work, or enjoying something just for themselves, we too do not believe in accomplishment or pleasure outside of a partnership. We denigrate anything that we alone experience; we say, 'It's more fun when there's someone else along.' The fact is we're afraid to go anyplace alone. How many adult women have you heard joke, 'I haven't decided what I'm going to be when I grow up . . .'? How many women call their husbands Daddy or Pappa, and think of their children as '*my* daughter', instead of Betsy or Jane?

Emotionally unseparated from mother, just as afraid as she was, we repeat the process with our own daughter. An unfortunate history, a way of growing up female that our society has amazingly left unchallenged. Being cute and helpless, clinging, clutching, holding on for dear life, becomes our method for survival – and ultimate defeat.

It is important to understand it is not the mere number of hours that mother spends that assures the child of those early, satisfying, symbiotic feelings of warmth and life assurance she needs. 'It is better,' says Dr Robertiello, 'that the child doesn't get her mother's full attention than a charade of a mother who would rather be at her office or out having lunch with her friends. Inauthentic behavior, especially when it comes disguised as love, creates the worst problems.' A lifetime pattern is set up in which the person feels that love is faked, easily distracted, or at best, grudgingly given.

It is the *quality* of attention we get from mother that counts. If we, as infants, are cold or hungry and she doesn't notice; if when she looks at us she is thinking of something else and so we do not see on her face a smile of love, we are deprived. A shadow on the sun. 'I was always thinking about so many things, I had so many ideas and ambitions when my child was little,' Dr Helene Deutsch told me, 'that when my little son was with me, he would take hold of my chin with his hands and focus my attention on him. He knew I was thinking about something else.'

Incomplete, unsatisfying, or interrupted symbiosis stamps a woman for life. We missed something from our mothers; despaired; grew guarded – and learned early a cramped line of defense: not to expect too much from the world. Even as our lovers hold us we cannot believe they will not leave. Our husbands complain that we are suffocating them: 'What more do you want of me?' they cry. We cannot give it a name but we feel a distance is there. As mothers, we turn and cling to our own daughter. 'Call me when you get there, no matter what time it is.'

Life for the woman who did not get enough symbiotic closeness as a child becomes a problem of juggling security *v.* satisfaction. We marry the first man who asks, afraid we may not be asked again; we take a safe civil service job instead of braving the risks of an independent career. 'Unless the little girl has had a successful symbiotic period with her mother,' says Dr Robertiello, 'she is still fixed on that warmth she missed. In babies we see this in the fact that they don't have the energy available over and beyond this craving to explore the sound and meaning of the words mother speaks, or the amount of new space she gives the infant to crawl in. In grown people, unsatisfied symbiosis is often expressed in terms of low energy too. They are too tired for this, not interested in that, never believe in themselves enough to try all out for any of the fascinating and novel aspects of life that present themselves. But if they are able to attain separation through therapy, we see a dramatic difference. There is a sudden burst of energy, of creativity. We see this in their lives, their work, their sexuality.'

Each of us knows people, on the other hand, who obviously were emotionally deprived in their first years, but who are successful enough in their adult lives. All is not lost if we missed out on early symbiosis. But it is unlikely – most psychiatrists would say impossible – for these people to enjoy fully their success or be emotionally secure in what success brings. These are people who say, 'I have all this or I have accomplished all that, but what does it all mean?' Emotionally impoverished as infants, they are emotionally impoverished still amid all their worldly success.

Society plays us a dirty trick by calling us the loving sex. The flattery is meant to make us proud of our weakness, our inability to be independent, our imperative need to belong to someone. We are limited to need and nurture, leaving erotic love to men. A 'lovesick' man makes people uncomfortable because the condition weakens him, jeopardizes his manhood, cuts down his productivity. But a woman who can't think clearly, who dreams over her law books, loses weight, and walks into brick walls arouses warm feelings in everybody. Men and women both know how good it feels to be knocked out by love, but someone has to mind the store. Since women haven't got anywhere to go anyway, and a needy woman makes a man work harder in order to provide for two, romance itself becomes fuel for the economic mill.

He will make love to us in the moonlight to the sound of violins, but in the morning he will shower, shave, put on his clothes, and go to the office in pursuit of his 'real' interests. In almost every novel you read or film you see, love is a disaster for the female protagonist, depriving her of initiative, courage, or sense of order, sending her down into masochism and loss of self.

Modern corporations, hiring Ph.D.'s in psychology to set employment policies, take advantage of female fears as standard business practice. Often mistakenly called 'paternal' organizations because they are run by men, they are psychologically much more like giant mothers, havens of symbiosis which await us: secretaries, clerks, office managers, assistants, women who will work loyally, part of the 'great corporate family' for twenty-five years in dull, safe, routine jobs — willing victims of shrewd personnel people who know we would rather have the cozy joys of the Widget Division Glee Club, and going on the Annual Company Picnic, than striking out alone (leaving mother) to get higher pay. Thousands, millions of women never leave the boss who 'needs' them, and happily work overtime for him because they symbiotically feel his career is theirs, they are part of him. Nevertheless when his raise comes, it is not divided into two shares. In sex or in business, the cost of symbiosis comes high.

A good mother finds it very hard to let her baby fall on its face the first time it takes a few steps, but she knows that is the way you learn. A little boy will crawl away, try to maneuver the stairs, even push his mama away when she interferes because the impulse to grow is so strong. She is afraid for him but knows she must train him in courage. Before they have left for kindergarten little boys have learned to push away little girls who want a kiss. Mom has already begun to teach him not to cling to her, much as they both may still want it. 'Don't baby him,' her husband says. 'Let him go,' the culture warns. The boy is emerging from symbiosis into the pleasures of separation. The world opens before him. Through experience, practice, and repetition the boy learns that accidents happen but are not fatal, rejections are lived through, the self goes on.

Little girls, on the other hand, get the opposite training. The great, crippling imperative is Nothing Must Ever Hurt My Little Girl. She is denied any but the most wrapped-in-cellophane experiences. When a little girl ventures into the backyard and hurts herself, mother doesn't encourage her daughter to try again, as she would her son. She holds the girl tighter, fearing for them both because she's been there; she has been hurt, anxious, and afraid much of her life. 'I knew this would happen,' mother says, repeating to her daughter a life-long warning to herself, implanting the notion that women are tender, fragile, easily and irremediably hurt by life.

Other elements of the mother-daughter relationship inhibit the little girl's sense of adventure: she seeks kisses but expects rejection. In mother's earliest and usually unconscious efforts to handle feelings of competition with her daughter, she teaches the little girl not to expect too much physical attention from daddy. 'Come away. Daddy has important papers to go over.' Mother is teaching us that men don't have 'our' need for love.

The message to the little girl is clear: there is only one person who will never leave her, who always has time for her. Even if there should be an absence of mother's kisses, it is not due to mother's lack of love. If only the little girl were more obedient, if only mother had more time, if, if, if . . .

We forget the faulty performance. The promise that love

will be available next time has seduced us. Brothers, sisters, friends – they are all unreliable. Only mother will be ever constant.

'You can see why a little girl may cling to her mother through fear of the threatening outside world,' says Dr Robertiello, 'but what must be realized is that mother isn't an ogre, keeping the girl locked up for spite. Mother has real fears and needs too, which seem to be met by symbiosis with her daughter. Too often, the mother never separated from *her* mother, and as the grandmother gets older and mama begins to feel the loss of that secure tie, she substitutes a bond to her daughter. She fears more than anything that she may end up alone, with no one to tell her what to do. She wants to be "a prisoner of love".

'Because of this primary, unconscious tie to her own mother, the wife/mother was never free to give her first loyalty to anyone new, including her husband. Oh, she may have had a sudden spurt of separation on getting married, a fine new flush of sexuality for a while. But all too often, when her daughter was born, she settled back into that less exciting, but known-and-safe feeling she had with her mother . . . only doing it this time with her daughter. She cuts off her independence, diminishes her sexuality, her intellect; she is no longer a young woman but a "matron" instead; a mother. Now she's safe forever. She's got a guarantee against ever being alone again for the rest of her life because her daughter is going to outlive her.'

No wonder partings between mothers and daughters at airports and railroad stations are so packed with guilt.

To explain separation, how we build an identity, we must go back once more to symbiosis, just as the tiny child who is learning to be on her own keeps going back to mother. The urge that brings baby, in panic at being alone, suddenly crawling back, to see that mother is 'there', that 'everything is all right', is as inevitable as the Second Law of Thermodynamics.

Technically, this is called 'the rapprochement stage', but I prefer a more familiar term child psychologists use: 'refueling'. Having touched base with mommy, thus refueled, the child is confident and ready to venture out again. The good mother understands the frightened return, but does not use it as a warning not to leave again; in fact, once she sees the child is refueled, she encourages it to go off again. The clinging mother magnifies the child's fears: 'Ah, poor baby. It's so scary out there. Don't ever go out again unless I come with you.'

A mother like this is so unseparated from her daughter that she cannot figure out if the anxiety is her own or her child's. In the end, it doesn't matter: the girl will pick up the mother's fear and make it her own. The outside world comes to seem threatening, forbidding. When she grows up and is away from home, she worries that the gas was left on, that somebody is sick or dying. Above all, she does not like to do anything alone. She wants to feel *connected* at all times, at any cost.

There is a phrase a woman I once knew used to use at the end of an evening. She had been a Martha Graham dancer and had had a successful life of her own. By the time I met her, she was married and the mother of two. 'Gee, it's been a great night,' someone would say. 'Let's find a place to have ham and eggs and Irish coffee.' My friend would always demur. 'Well,' she would say to her husband, 'we've been all around Robin Hood's barn, it's time to touch home base.' They would leave. Childhood phrases, childhood emotions. I think this story is a metaphor for her whole life – beginning with her decision, made years before, to give up dancing because the road trips made her 'too nervous'. Her need to touch home base – not to be separated from some idealized notion of security – always brought her running home when most people would have gone on.

In explaining how a daughter's sense of adventurousness can be nipped in the bud, Dr Robertiello speaks of the mother's anxiety: 'She is the first one afraid when she realizes *she* is alone, without her child. So she decides her child needs her, or is in danger. She goes running after the little girl. The daughter may be sitting safe in the backyard playing with the daisies, but here is mother, alarmed, worried, calling her home, retrieving the little girl *before* the girl feels the need to return, to refuel. So the daughter develops a sense that even if you are having a good time, something may be going wrong back home.'

However, every action has an equal and opposite reaction. Beginning around fourteen to eighteen months and continuing to about the third year, the child begins to experiment with resistance to mother's demands on her. This try at self-assertion is marked by the almost constant use of the word *NO*.

This is a very important experience for the child, separating out what she wants to do – even if it is not to make up her mind yet – and what mother wants her to do. '*We* want to go to the park, don't *we?*' says mother, using the symbiotic pronoun as imperiously as any queen. 'No,' says the little boy, asserting an early step toward individuality and separation. '*I* don't want it.' Everyone who hears him applauds – even mother. 'What a little man he is! He knows his own mind, just like his father.' Girls get the opposite treatment.

Says child psychiatrist Sirgay Sanger: 'Boys have an easier time in this period because mother thinks, 'Well, I don't know enough about boys. I'd better leave him alone.' There is also a cultural bias against mothers who keep their sons tied to them. But if her child is a girl? Well, she knows all about girls. She's the expert. So she gives her daughter less latitude, less chance for growth. She rides like a steamroller over her girl's individuality. 'Come on,' mother will say to the little girl. 'You always like to go shopping with me, so we're going to do that now.' Right away the little girl becomes less assertive. She loses a lot of her gumption. This starts as early as the time between the first and second year.'

Separation, outgrowing the need for degrees of symbiosis inappropriate to the present stage of development, is not a case of black or white. Theoretically, separation from mother should be completed by age three or three and a half, 'but I think it goes on as long as we live,' says Dr Robertiello. 'I've never met anyone yet for whom it had ended, man or woman. We are all very much connected to our mothers or some substitute. I think it's especially acute with women because the girl has that constant image of her mother from which she never escapes.' Vital as it is in our first year of life, the only way to describe symbiosis between mother and daughter after age three is unhealthy. It is a sticky issue because our culture confuses symbiosis and love; *but when we are grown, symbiosis and real love are mutually exclusive.* Love implies a separation. 'I love you,' can only have meaning if there is an 'I' to love 'you'.

In a symbiotic relationship, there is no real concern for the other person. There is just a need, a craving to be connected, no matter how destructive. Marriage is often seen as releasing the daughter from her symbiotic tie to her mother. In fact, it may be merely a switch to her husband. Now he must support her, supply her with life, make her feel good about herself. Unless we have separated from mother long before marriage, it is almost impossible to set up a healthy relationship with a man.

The best definition of love I know is psychoanalyst Harry Stack Sullivan's: love means you care almost as much about the other person's safety, security, and satisfaction as you do about your own. I feel this is a realistic definition; you *can't* love somebody else more than yourself. The truly loving mother is one whose interest and happiness is in seeing her daughter as a person, not just a possession. It is a process of being so generous and loving that she will forgo some of her own pleasure and security to add to her daughter's development. If she does this in a genuine way, she really does end up with that Love Insurance Policy. The mother will have someone who cares about her forever – not a guilty, resentful love, but a daughter who gives her love freely.

'Genuine mother-daughter love?' said psychiatrist Mio Fredland when I first interviewed her in April 1974. 'I think it implies a recognition on the part of each of the separateness of the other, and a respect for the other. In the case of the daughter, she has to first love her mother so that she can love herself as a woman; then she can love her mother back when she is more mature. But she must first 'take in' the good mother while she is still an infant; then she will emerge from infancy as a separate person.

'How do I feel about my daughter? I think she's heavenly. I was just waiting for her. In fact, I had dreams about her when I was pregnant, and she's just exactly the way she was in my dreams. I wanted a daughter for many reasons. One of them was that I wanted to make up in my relationship with my daughter, for what I had missed in my relationship with my own mother. My mother wasn't really there. She loved me and did her best to be a good mother, but she was so frightened of so many things. My daughter is exactly what I wanted all my life.'

It is interesting to note how Dr Fredland's feelings about her daughter had changed by the time I interviewed her again, one year later in April 1975:

'How do I avoid seeing my daughter as a narcissistic extension? My training helps me to see her objectively, of course, but I also think my attitude has changed since we talked last year. As she has become older and more her own person, I feel more detached from her, which doesn't mean I love her less . . . but I love her in a different way. I see her as quite separate from myself. I see what her talents are, what her interests are, and what her shortcomings are. If you allow the child to detach herself from you, *she* will draw the limits, *she* will tell you what she insists on for her living space.'

I like these two statements by Mio Fredland. They show real growth in mother-daughter love. Dr Fredland's first comments were made at a time when she still felt her daughter to be a kind of narcissistic extension of herself. One year later, the mother's focus has turned outward upon the girl, *her* separation and growth.

*   *   *

Most of the time it is too difficult to examine what we really have with mother because there is not enough distance between us. Is she a 'bad mother'? Are we 'bad daughters'? Either proposition is so emotionally loaded, so *hot*, that we cannot reply sensibly. I would also suggest that another reason they are so difficult is that they are put as moralistic propositions. We are asking the wrong questions. The real question is, Have the two of us loved each other in the early years and separated in the later so that we allow each other room enough, air enough, freedom enough to continue that love?

Those telephone calls to mother, are they done out of real love or a need to maintain symbiosis? If we call her happily, voluntarily, because we get a lift out of talking to her – that is love. If we move to the phone – though it be daily – with a heavy feeling of constraint and duty, with an anxious need that these calls never seem to fill, if they leave us in tears, angry, defensive, or guilty, then, though the culture may call ours a loving mother-daughter relationship if only for the sheer size of our telephone bill, I would not.

Another place to look for clues as to whether we may still be overly tied to mother is in our relationship to men, to other women, and in our approach to work. The need to cling, fear of loss, the inability to push forward and/or complete – these are not patterns of behavior picked up after we got on that plane and left home. They are patterns of action and reaction learned at home during our formative years with mother.

I have known women whose mothers loved them for themselves and then let them go. Their hallmark is a consistency of behavior; they do not play the chameleon, changing to suit every new personality or situation they encounter. When they talk to their mothers they remain grown women – and do not relapse into childish voices, querulous tones, and evasive answers. When asked what they think, they give a straight answer. They are not afraid the other person will become angry at their candor. Faced with a difficult emotional situation, they may not be able to resolve it right away, but their first impulse is not to try to spy out the response expected of them by others. The question they ask is, What do I want, how do I feel about this? They have a certainty about themselves.

On the other hand, uncertain people often make their fears come true. A woman tells me: 'Right from the start, I knew it wouldn't last. You know what he said when he walked out on me? "I'm sick and tired of you asking if I love you and then not believing it when I say I do."' Insecurity often masks itself as its opposite. It does not surprise us, for instance, that the macho stud often has doubts about his virility. In the same way, women are accused of being vain, of being caught up in self-admiration. The truth is we have no certainty at all about the way we look.

A woman friend with a beautiful figure constantly complains about her 'huge' hips. She tells me how lucky I am not to have to worry about such things. She is my height. Finally I ask what her hips measure. I tell her mine are two inches bigger. 'But they can't be!' she cries. 'You have a great figure, your hips can't be bigger than mine!' We refuse the facts today because the image was set at a time we can no longer remember by someone who knew everything. We do not spend all those hours in front of the mirror because of vanity, because we are in love with ourselves. It is because of anxiety. Something is wrong with our basic narcissism.

Until recently, narcissism was thought to be a kind of pathological development – a dirty word to the psychiatrist and general public alike. Freud thought of it as regression, a withdrawal of interest from other people and reality, a morbid concentration of the libido (energy) on the self. Today, we make a sharp distinction between this faulty sense of self, which is called 'secondary narcissism', and healthy, primary narcissism.[6]

Secondary narcissism is pathological because it attempts to fill the void in the healthy self-image with an intense preoccupation with the self. This can be expressed through an excessive focus on appearance, or physical and emotional symptoms (hypochondria). A person like this is trying to make up for a lack of attention in childhood – most especially in the first year of life – by paying the same kind of exaggerated attention to herself that she needed from her mother but did not get at that stage of development. Secondary narcissism is marked by anxious repetition; since it is an ineffective substitute, we can never let it rest. The irony is that these are the women who are usually called vain because they can never stop praising themselves, never cease trying to attract attention or get compliments.

They are a splendid example – if only in reverse – of how not too much but too little admiration 'spoils' children. All the praise in the world cannot help them, nourish them, once they've missed out at the appropriate time. Compliments fly right past as though meant for someone standing behind them.

Usually it is easy for mother to gratify our narcissistic needs when we are first born. In the early stages of symbiosis, we are still so meshed, so undifferentiated from her, that to love us is to love herself. But as we grow away from her it takes an informed, mature kind of selfless love for her to accept that baby's needs are not always her needs. Mother must grow herself, to give the child room and space to gratify its desires even if they are in conflict with, outrage, or disappoint, hers. In early stages of toilet training, for instance, the baby may be proud of her first productions, pick them up and offer them to mother as tokens of love. If this conflicts with mother's image of us as nice little girls made of pink ribbons, serious trouble can ensue. She must let us be separate enough from her so that we can develop at our own pace, not hers. She must love us for what we do and need, not just when we coincide with her fantasy image of the perfect baby.

'The first time I saw my newborn daughter, Katie,' says Dr Leah Schaefer, 'she was immense – edemic, water-logged. "Oh, God," I thought, "don't tell me she is going to be one of those fat kids?" I had this sudden fantasy of me as this trim, chic, *Ladies' Home Journal* mother dragging this eight-year-old into Best and Company, hoping against hope I'd be able to find something to cover all that fat. On the third day, I was combing my hair in a mirror and it occurred to me: maybe she isn't going to like having a mother who is older than her friends' mothers. Maybe she's going to want a park mother instead of a professional mother. *Maybe she won't like me!* Just to have said that to myself was the most freeing thing I could have done for her. Just as I had given myself freedom to think it was possible she wouldn't be the child of my dreams, I had also given her the freedom not to have to approve of me. It was an extraordinary experience, fundamental to everything in our relationship.'

What mother hasn't dreamed that her baby will be some ideal creature? Side by side, intertwined with, and the very first cause of mother's symbiotic love for us is her own self love. She begins by loving us because we are her own body and spirit made flesh – a narcissistic extension of herself. We are going to be everything she wanted out of life.

'But the dream doesn't last more than a few months,' says Dr Sanger. 'The baby can't give what Mother wants – she is asking that it make *her* dreams come true. Reality quickly steps in. The baby lets mother know it is not going to fulfill her every fantasy. It is colicky. It cries and vomits. It lets mother know that it has a real life of its own.' It is a first hint of separation; some mothers become displeased at these signs of the child's self struggling to be born. They are hurt or disappointed. The adoration turns off. When the baby looks into mother's face, she no longer sees herself in a loving, kind mirror; no longer is the little girl 'the fairest of them all'. 'Mother's adoring looks may stop,' continues Dr Sanger, 'because she feels the baby is not responding to her enough. She takes this as an accusation. She has a very strong and self-reverent ideal of how baby should be toward her and it is not being satisfied. Very simply, once more the mother turns off.' Mother's inability to allow her baby an authentic, separate life of its own has disrupted the relationship between them right from the start.

Healthy, primary narcissism is rooted in infancy. Mother is the first 'objective' voice we hear; her face is our first mirror. When we are born, she cannot hear enough wonderful things being said about us. She absolutely absorbs the praise of friends and relatives as they coo and gurgle about our beauty, size, and amazing agility. She transfers it to us like heat. At this stage she is rightly so tied to us that she doesn't know where praise for us leaves off and admiration for her giving birth to such a miraculous baby begins. We feed her narcissism and she feeds ours. It is the height of symbiosis at its best, primary narcissism functioning as it should. Our ego is being born.

All this is grist for the mill of identity. Out of this experience will come a person who is going to have a good image of herself. Someone who will be able to walk into rooms without undue shyness, believe that other people like her, accept praise for her work as her due, and smile at the nice reflection of herself in other people's eyes just as she smiles back at what she sees in the mirror. When a man says, 'I love you,' she is pleased, not gripped by disbelief and fear.

Does this describe you, or women you know? What happened? What becomes twisted, even when life begins with strong primary narcissistic gratification? Why do we either not continue to seek it in later life, or, if we do, cannot enjoy it – take no nourishment from it to feed our self-esteem?

'Five years ago,' says Dr Robertiello, 'we didn't know what narcissism was all about. Now we know that healthy narcissism is a normal and necessary part of growth. Today we try to get people in touch with their needs. For instance, in group therapy, I'll have people stand up, show off, give a speech about themselves as though they've just died and have to give a eulogy. Even with this explicit permission – even an order – to say something nice about themselves, this is the hardest thing in the world for people to do. They'd rather take their clothes off.

'The reason they are so upset at seeking praise, getting a good feeling about themselves from others, is that as infants they didn't get enough adulation from their mothers. This kind of mother is usually someone who is very condemnatory of being "conceited". So that when the child, in a normal, healthy way, does make some attempt to get this, the mother not only squashes her but humiliates her too for showing off. Eventually babies like this grow into people who either can't seek praise or are unable to believe it when they do get it. Today we are trying to get people past this feeling of being ashamed of their needs. We encourage them to go out and find people to give them the praise they need in a very open, direct way.'

Take this as a familiar enough occurrence: a mother who could not hear enough praise for her infant, suddenly begins to say to admiring friends when the girl is three or four, 'Now, that's enough. She gets enough praise from her daddy. We don't want a conceited little girl on our hands.' Primary narcissistic gratification stops.

What has happened to turn mother off praise and begin to make the little girl self-conscious about getting it – and unable to take it in when she does – is that the mother has begun to project upon the child her own fear of seeming irrationally conceited. Now that we are no longer infants – little mute, passive, adorable receptacles for admiration – but have become active people instead, mother identifies with us. She knows how she would feel if she were getting this extravagant praise. *She projects herself into our minds because she is not separate* – and brings with her *her* own damaged narcissism, *her* inability to believe compliments, *her* fear that if she let herself think they might be true for one moment, *she* would get a swelled head. When we were infants, she shared the warm praise we got. Now that we are people – her own image – she projects her shame onto us. This is the way in which *her* mother began to undermine and make her feel embarrassed about her own healthy narcissism. Now she is doing it to us.

This is the essence of the chain of low self-esteem and ego-abnegation that binds women through the generations: unless the mother can grant her child her own identity, *unless she is separated,* she will not be able to contain her anxiety at the compliments being showered on a child. Have you ever watched an untalented friend get up and sing at a party? Remember how your skin crawled in embarrassment for her? You felt in yourself her naked hunger for attention and approbation; you felt in yourself in advance the humiliation she would feel when she did not get it. In this experience you have identified yourself with your friend. How much more deeply a mother feels for her daughter, when the little girl, with the trusting, naive innocence of children, hurries forward to a stranger, seeking a rewarding smile; mother blushes, embarrassed, and snatches the baby from its path.

The seed has been planted: if we do not learn to reject these compliments ourselves, we are not good little girls. We are bad daughters, unlike mother. Mother must be aware of flaws in us we do not suspect and which the stranger will detect in a moment. We blush at our stupidity in thinking we were so lovable.

Mother's shame for us is the expression of her effort to protect us. Picking up her anxiety, we reject the stranger's smile – the approval of the outside world – and turn in toward mother. Mutual lack of separation is reinforced. The very thing – admiration and praise from others – that would give us the courage to grow into ourselves, to fix a clear line between activities that might embarrass mother but have a totally different and positive effect on us, has been erased.

Giving a baby too much praise, love, or adoration is impossible – *just as long as it begins to be accompanied by separation.* If mother didn't let me go, doesn't let me be myself, if she and I continue to be merged in symbiosis, then all the praise in the world isn't going to help – because there isn't any me. There isn't any self-image. There is only 'we', and anything good said about me merely because I am an extension of her will make me uncomfortable. It says I am praiseworthy only as part of her; by myself, I barely exist at all.

How many mothers have you heard say to their daughters (of any age), 'You look absolutely wonderful!' – without any howevers, buts, or qualifiers like, ' – but must you wear so much eye shadow?' When did your mother last say to you, 'You did that perfectly, darling!' with the absolute certainty of one individual admiring another?

Says Dr Sanger: 'Almost from birth, we see mothers conveying to their daughters that they aren't good enough as is. Mom doesn't fuss much with her son, but she is constantly adjusting, fixing, trying to perfect this little female picture of herself in the same way she fiddles with her own never-perfect appearance. She can't keep her nagging hands off the girl. We even hear it as the mother hangs over the cradle. 'Now, let's fix this little piece of hair . . .' In time the daughter learns that this kind of attention is a knock. She thought she looked OK, but the instant her mother lays eyes on her, she knows she was wrong.'

In time the daughter may learn to shrink from her mother's nagging eye or hands. She may go so far away geographically that mother can't reach her. Or she may become tied to mother in a sullen, half-shrinking, half dependent relationship, constantly looking and hoping for her mother's promised – but never *felt* – unqualified love. Either way, the mother who never gave us her total approval binds us to her forever. We keep trying for mother's praise because we never outgrow the child's belief that maybe, just once, if we do it right, she will admire us totally in that pure, unqualified way we always wanted.

But mother cannot do it. Since she does not feel separated from us, every tiny failure of ours is *her* failure. When something goes wrong, she says, 'How could you do this to me? What will the neighbors say?' Our desires, feelings, actions – even our failures – are not our own.

If a mother experiences herself as unattractive or unsuccessful, she may easily project these negative feelings onto her daughter and make her feel she is a failure too. She may feel competitive with the daughter or push the girl to be the beautiful person she would like to be herself. The combinations and permutations are endless: two people with two sets of physical, intellectual, emotional, and temperamental histories, constantly interacting. A mother can say about a boy, 'My son, the doctor.' He may be annoyed, but he is not an extension of her. Psychiatrists call this 'child wearing' – mother wears the child like an ornament.

A twenty-eight-year-old woman tells me: 'When my child was born and the doctor held it up, I started to scream. I thought I saw a penis. Then, thank God, I realized it was a girl.' Does the intensity of this mother's wish for a female child fill you with high hopes for the girl's future? I feel a certain foreboding. A mother who wants a daughter that much has such expectations that her girl may never live up to them – never get away from the mother for whom she is such a pleasure-giving service. As long as she is mother's little girl, the praise will not stop. If she tries to grow up and grow away, the approval, which has come to mean life itself, will stop. *Narcissistic gratification without separation is a trap*. Praise for yourself alone is lovely. Praise because what you do makes me look good – that denies you count for yourself at all.

Daughters with mothers like this often grow up in a paradox: 'My mother loves me, she has given me everything. She is concerned for me, is interested in everything I do. We write often, we talk often, we visit often, and if I ever need someone to talk to, I know I can count on her . . . but why do I feel something is missing in my life?' Daughters who have tried to live out their mothers' dreams end up with a diminished self. Little is ever felt – success, beauty, marriage, wealth – because the daughter has always been her mother's extension and not her own person.

To one degree or another this describes most of us. We go through life wondering after the fact: why didn't I let myself love that terrific man, grab that opportunity, do that exciting thing? We didn't because mother wouldn't have. We cut the self-actualizing, individuating things out of our lives because that's what she would have done, though *to have done them anyway, in spite of her, would have strengthened our separation.*

'The cause of most of the indignities that are labeled "female" usually begins at birth,' says Dr Sanger, citing mother/infant studies going on now at St Luke's Hospital in New York. 'The subtle deprivation of physical demonstrations of affection that little girls often suffer from their mothers makes women more vulnerable to fear and the loss of attachment; they were never sure of it to begin with. It makes women greedy to hold on even to men who treat them badly, more possessive and competitive for whatever crumbs of love may be available to them.

'This deprivation that little girls suffer begins very early, and there need not be any conscious prejudice or bias on the mother's part. If a little boy does something cute or winning, he will be rewarded by mother with a fond pat, a touch, a physical expression of approval he cannot misunderstand. On the other hand, if a little girl infant performs the same action, we notice that she will often be rewarded only with a smile on her mother's lips, or a verbal compliment. Neither baby of course is capable of making any comparison; both children would be said to have an approving, accepting mother. But in the strong feeling of physical approval he is getting from his mother, the boy unconsciously – even before he is able to speak – begins to build his bank account of life-long self-acceptance. For the girl, the absence of physicality – which is the most direct communication of security and approval a mother can give an infant – means she will not be nearly as rich in autonomy and self-esteem.'

Dr Sanger concludes: 'In time, the little girl may come to feel that mother doesn't fondle her enough because she isn't good enough, not valuable enough. Very often, what makes things worse is that the kind of touching she does get from mother – primping, adjusting, fiddling, fixing – is a negative kind. It tells the girl there *is* something about her that is not right, missing, not good enough.'

Though Dr Sanger's studies are documented with filmed, objective evidence, most mothers with whom I've discussed these findings deny any degree of difference in the physicality they show their daughters as opposed to that they show their sons. The idea is deeply threatening. A woman will smile fondly at the old saw about mothers being fond of their sons while fathers prefer daughters; but when you try to translate the idea into personal terms – that maybe she kissed and hugged her son more than she did her daughter – she is offended. But no great psychological mystery is being presented here. Simple common sense and experience tell us that women kiss, touch, and find it more 'natural' to hug men than women.

Great consequences follow for the psychological life of women from this everyday fact. 'It's like the sapling,' says Dr Robertiello. 'If you make a small scratch on its bark, when it grows into a big tree, it will have a big cut in it. The earlier something happens, the bigger the impact. These things aren't irreversible, but they are time-specific. If you didn't have that mother who absolutely adored you and whose face and whole body manner showed it during that first year, a mother who loved you enough for yourself to let you go by the end of the third year, it's awfully hard, no matter what happens from then on, to make up for it later.'

In fact, after the child is eighteen months old or so, it is usually destructive to try to make up for the kind of closeness that should have been there from birth. Here's how one thirty-seven-year-old remembers what happened when her mother tried to give her the kind of love as a little girl that she had really needed as an infant:

'I have a photo of me being held up in my christening dress by two enormous nursemaids. Years later I asked my mother why she wasn't in the picture. "Oh," she said, "I was out antiquing." Before I was three, I was sent to nursery school. I remember not liking it, but my mother said I went off with a bottle under one arm, some extra diapers under the other, and I waved the bottle and said, "Hi, kids." She thought that was a wonderful adjustment. Then my younger sister died – I was five – and that changed everything. My mother became tremendously possessive of me. Of course I responded to all that love she offered – I was a very needy little five-year-old – but it crippled me for years. I may have been insecure, but I had worked out ways of dealing with that situation. When my mother moved in with all that suffocating love, it just took away all the security I'd won on my own. I can remember that my fears and insecurities really began about that age. I'd have been better off if she'd continued to just let me alone.'

The primary rule is always that a mother can't go wrong, *ever*, by encouraging her child after age one and a half to be as individuated and separated as possible. If she was not as good a mother before as she would like to have been, she must get over her guilty desires to overcompensate, and place herself on the side of the child's developing ego. The symbiotic train has left.

In the name of fairness, and reality too, let me add an important postscript which is true not only for this chapter but of this whole book: looking over our shoulders at what mother may or may not have done so many years ago locks us into the past. 'She did it. There is nothing I can do about it.' *Blaming mother keeps us passive, tied to her*. It helps us avoid taking responsibility for ourselves.

All any mother can do is her best. She doesn't have to be perfect – just a 'good enough' mother. Unfortunately, children are more single-minded than adults in their standards. 'Children are so dependent on their parents,' says Dr Sanger, 'that any flaw or imperfection seems to the child to threaten her/his existence. "If mother is forgetful or careless about this little matter, maybe next time she won't be able to take care of me at all." It is directly tied with the nurturance, the sustenance of life.'

Perhaps it is too much to ask of children that they appreciate complexities, but is it too much to ask now that we are grown? Mother seems so godlike to children that they forget she too is subject to the vicissitudes of life. Perhaps the family was poor. Maybe father drank or ran after other women. Perhaps the child herself brought certain temperamental traits into life which made her develop in a manner no mother could have helped.

'One of the major resistances in analytic work,' says child psychiatrist Aaron Esman, 'is the notion, "It was my mother's fault." Patients don't want to see their own responsibility, so they blame mother. In our post-Freudian world, it's very fashionable, but to blame mother means one doesn't have to examine one's self, to face one's own problems. Parent-baiting, mother-baiting uses up energy that might better go into examining the wrong choices one has made oneself.' Brooding over past injustices, we have little emotion left over to create a better future.

Those of us who had rejecting mothers are often drawn to men with the same cold temperaments. We try to manipulate warmth from them. This is merely to repeat the past. We would be better off giving up the sour comfort of recriminations and finding someone who doesn't have to be cajoled but gives warmth easily and gladly. Our job as adults is to understand the past, learn its lessons, and then let it go. Blaming mother is just a negative way of clinging to her still.

CHAPTER THREE

A Time to Let Go

Over the years I've collected from family attics a sepia-toned history of my mother's youth. My grandfather photographed everything. The pictures hang in their original ornate frames in a hallway in my house where guests invariably stop. 'Who's this?' They point to a young woman bent low over the neck of a horse in mid-air. 'My mother at the Pittsburgh Steeplechase,' I say. 'And these people?' they ask. I tell them that the woman seated at the grand piano is my mother once again, and the others are her sisters and brother. Most of my friends don't know my mother's family, of course; but they stare as though they did. Old family photos, even other people's, fascinate — we're all looking for clues.

The expression on my mother's face is always the same: concern. Whether at the peak of a six-foot hurdle or seated placidly at the piano, hands in her lap, the anxious face seems to be waiting for her father to tell her — what? To hide her unattractive hands? But how do you play the piano and hide your hands? And how did my mother, who today will not drive a car over forty miles per hour, jump those horses? I remember as a small child asking her, 'Can't I see you jump a horse like in those pictures?' 'Oh, Nancy,' she would say with a nervous laugh, 'that was years ago.' At most it had been six or seven, but I could see even then that all the tea in China wouldn't get my mother back on a horse now that she had left her father's house. I've never seen her ride.

Several years later, in my perpetual attic rummaging, I came across steamer trunks filled with all the riding and hunting regalia of the photos I so loved. I put on my mother's boots, but my feet were already bigger than hers. The heavy riding habits were too uncomfortable even for an eight-year-old in search of a way to be. Luckily I'd had another model of courage from the day I was born. They tell me I was put in my nurse Anna's arms the day I was brought home from the hospital.

Anna lived on Camel cigarettes and murder mysteries. Like me, she preferred horror films and Westerns to the romantic movies my sister, Susie, begged to see. She preferred me to my sister. I don't know why Anna favored me; perhaps she saw the bond between my mother and sister; maybe it was our similar temperament, but no doubt about it, I was Anna's girl. I grew strong on the toast dunked in her coffee and milk. My home was her kitchen, my security her lap, my days began with her rough hands that braided my hair. She made the best meatloaf in the world, and would give it to me raw, seasoned with onions and green peppers, from the bowl. When it was time for the State Fair she made sandwiches out of ground ham and pickle and I remember the aroma and Anna talking of the joys of the roller coaster, as we drove to the fair grounds. I was four and I loved the roller coaster because she was beside me.

When Susie heard footsteps coming and tried to hide the forbidden candle behind the window shade, thus setting the bedroom on fire, it was Anna who pushed aside the other squealing women and extinguished the blaze. Before I went to kindergarten Anna and I made a pact: when I grew up she and I would go West and put Dale Evans out of the horse business. Meanwhile, we settled for protecting the home front, meaning my mother. Mostly, this amounted to avoidance.

From my earliest years I learned from Anna not to tell my mother anything that would cause her anxiety. I don't remember much of my mother from those years. I never got on with my sister when we were little. It seems I was always angry with Susie, ready for a fight. Even as a little girl she was sweet-natured. I considered her 'soft', a loser at all the games we played. 'Leave me alone,' I'd tell her when she tried to

cuddle me, 'I don't like all that mushy stuff.' I didn't mind it
with Anna. With her I was allied to a winner, and the first
time I left the earth in a plane, along with the thrill of speed
and power, I felt *the safety* I'd known when I was four and
Anna took me on the roller coaster.

And yet I am my mother's daughter still. In her life I see an
eerie and yet comforting precursor of my own. She jumped
her father's horses at fourteen, daredevil enough to win silver
cups – yet it took my marriage in Rome to get her into an
airplane. That reckless physical courage I had as a child – no
tree too high or dangerous to climb – had diminished now
that I am grown. I will take the cable car to the highest
mountain, but I will ski down carefully, always in control.
Today I prefer trains and boats to flying. The fear in the house
in which I grew up left me when I left that house, but it did
not go away. It seemed to have waited its time and I
sometimes feel it stirring within me now that I have a house of
my own. I wonder how much more of my mother's anxiety I
would feel if I had a daughter. If I close my eyes and imagine
me with a little girl in my arms, I know the answer too well:
too much.

Anna had a boyfriend named Shorty. He used to drive his
beat-up Chevrolet behind the house where Anna had taught
me to dig to China – my earliest effort to leave home. Shorty
would stand just inside the screen door of our linoleum-
floored kitchen, as if he wasn't sure Anna was going to let him
stay or throw him out. After dinner, the two of them would
smoke countless Camel cigarettes that stained their fingers the
same brown and yellow as the Camel pack itself.

My mother smoked Chesterfields from a cool gold and
white pack, and her fingers were never stained at all. I knew
the man who brought her the delicious chocolate butter
creams loved her more than she loved him. Sunday evenings
he would take us to a restaurant where they played Jack
Benny on the radio and served a children's ice cream dessert
surrounded by marching animal crackers. The ice cream
made us shiver when we went outside and he would wrap us

in soft blankets in the back seat of his big car. I don't know what love meant, but I felt sorry for him; he gave the most beautiful wrapped presents I'd ever seen.

Once Shorty drove Anna, my sister, and me to visit some people in the country. I don't know if they were Anna's or Shorty's friends, but they were different from us. Their whole house was covered in linoleum. And all the children were bathed in a big metal tub in the middle of the kitchen. I'd never seen so many naked people. I don't remember any shame. I can still see the steam and feel the thrill of being part of all that good-humored nakedness. At home we may have been a house of women; that didn't mean you left the bathroom door open. I undress without hesitation among friends, but to this day I am modest around my mother. I worry if other people's bathroom doors don't lock properly, even if I've only gone in to comb my hair. I imagine their embarrassment at walking in on me. But I have the clearest recollection of Anna on the toilet, smoking cigarettes and reading *The Return of the Grave Snatchers*.

There was no worrying about doors during that visit with Anna's friends. There were no doors. There were no bathrooms. On the landing at the top of the stairs there was a bucket, a communal chamber pot in which everyone peed in the night. I don't know where we went during the day, but in my memory the time is night and that bucket is full to the brim, with a puddle around it on the linoleum floor. A nasty place to have to tiptoe in the dark. It is a persistent memory filled with chords of fear and excitement. What made it all OK was that Anna took me there.

I recently told this story to a psychiatrist I was interviewing. 'You were probably lucky to have had someone like Anna,' he said. 'Because she was "lower class" and physical, it helped you accept your sexuality.' It sounds so simplistic, but the minute he told me I knew he was right. I have always known that I owed Anna. I don't like his words 'lower class' applied to someone I loved, but I know that sex is different from love, and if I am able to enjoy them both today it is because of Anna, who loved me and let me go. Of one thing I am positive: we never told my mother about those Breughel baths in the kitchen or the bucket of pee. I am her daughter and Anna's too; I carefully wipe out the wash basin with a Kleenex when I have finished my make-up, but I can stand up and pee without wetting my shoes as neatly today as when I was five.

The first trip away from home gave me a taste for other people's houses. I knew our neighbors' homes as well as my own and the sidewalks of Pittsburgh lay before me like an invitation. I wasn't yet in school when I picked up my first nice old couple. They were walking their dog, and when I followed them home they served me cream of tomato soup and peanut butter sandwiches. I learned the traveler's wisdom that things taste better in other people's houses. I also learned that there was always another place at the table for a kid who knew how to turn on the charm. Eventually Anna stopped calling the police because I always came home. I had to. I didn't know how to braid my hair.

Four years later I still hadn't learned and was puzzled, even embarrassed because I couldn't, nor could I answer my mother when she asked why I didn't want Anna to teach me. A big girl like me who wasn't afraid of anything? But Anna knew: every morning I'd go to her with my comb and every night she would take off the rubber bands without pulling my hair while we sat on her bed and listened to 'The Lone Ranger.' I don't think I ever did learn to braid my hair.

When I was five we moved from Pittsburgh to Charleston, South Carolina. Anna came with us, but she didn't like the South. Maybe she missed Shorty. When I was nine, she left us to go back up north. I don't remember saying good-bye, cannot even recall my last image of her, but I do remember the night, remember the anxiety of the others surrounding me like a protective circle. I was put to bed in my mother's room, something that had never happened before. But I didn't cry. I don't even remember missing Anna in the days that followed. There's such an absence of feeling around her departure that I must have done what children automatically do when the pain is too unbearable: I blanked out everything, Anna and her love, along with her leaving.

There were some Bobbsey Twins books that arrived on later birthdays, but strict as my mother was about thank-you notes, I don't think I wrote Anna back. Many years later an aunt told me she thought she had seen Anna scrubbing floors in the Pittsburgh railroad station. I changed the subject. I could no more accept the guilt that somehow I'd abandoned her to scrubbing floors than I'd been able to accept the rejection of her leaving me. Until I married, I could only think about winning love, prizes, silver cups – winning, winning, *winning* – winning something the world did not easily give.

It was only at night when I closed my eyes that the old separation and guilt came to haunt me. They still do.

In an interview with a young mother in Detroit which lasts five hours, she smiles and talks easily about how she is raising her daughter to be 'an individual person'. She never uses the word *separation*, and I am not sure if she understands what I mean, or if she is simply light years ahead of me in acceptance of the idea. 'You don't think then that mothers have problems separating from their daughters?' I ask as we are parting. She laughs nervously: 'When you first said that word, I felt goose flesh up and down my arms.' Separation – the word sounds so final, fraught with loss, abandonment, and guilt that mothers don't want to talk about it.

Nor can we as daughters easily contemplate an act so desperate *vis-a-vis* our mothers. We sidestep the issue, taking the word not in its emotional sense but in a cooler, more pragmatic way: separation is so simple *we* don't have the problem at all. 'Oh, I've been separated from my mother ever since I left home and came to Chicago five years ago,' a woman tells me. No need to face the emotional turbulence of the issue. The problem is solved with an airplane ticket.

It's not us; mother is the one with the problem. 'I love my

mother,' a young woman says, 'but she can't seem to understand I'm an adult. She still treats me as if I were twelve.' The slightest hint that this kind of attention is not wholly unwelcome, that it still carries ambivalent notions of security and connection, is denied. To buttress the argument that we have outgrown the need for mother, many of us smile and say we have reversed the roles – mother is now the 'child' in the relationship. *This ignores the fact that the tie, the link through dependency, is still there.* Just because we're now mother's protector doesn't mean we're separate. Until research for this book forced me beyond superficial meanings of the idea, I would have told you I was well and truly separated from my mother. I have since learned that my ties to my mother permeate every aspect of my life as a woman in ways as numerous and mysterious as the ways of love.

'Letting go' is perhaps a friendlier way to put it. It implies generosity, a talent a good mother needs in abundance. Separation is not loss, it is not cutting yourself off from someone you love. It is giving freedom to the other person to be herself before she becomes resentful, stunted, and suffocated by being tied too close. Separation is not the end of love. It creates love.

It is hard for women to let go. We are born collectors. We live in the treasured bits and pieces of past life. Mothers collect the memorabilia of their children's past, shoes from the time they possessed baby most totally. Grown women collect match covers and menus from nights when a man held us close, when we felt most possessed, and we count the hours dead until he calls and brings us back to life. A woman and a man exchange Valentine cards; he opens his, smiles, kisses her and then throws the card away. 'You're not going to keep it?' she cries. She's saved every card since she was thirteen. But men don't need our collections; their future may be uncertain, but they feel they have a hand in its creation. They are not dependent on the past. When we cut our hair, mother cries, 'You've changed!' It is not a compliment to growth but a fear of disloyalty and separation. 'You're leaving me!'

When a mother refuses to let her daughter grow up, she is retarding her own growth as well; in overlong symbiosis, both partners suffer. Speaking of various disguises symbiosis can take, Dr Fredland names what has been traditionally called 'school phobia'. The child isn't phobic to school,' she says, 'the little girl is phobic to leaving the side of her mother.' She has been conditioned to think leaving mother is to leave love. 'I don't want to go to school today,' the child says. 'I have a cold,' or, 'the other children play too rough.' The mother who is lonely, who fears separation as much as her daughter, takes these excuses at face value. By ignoring reality and going along with her daughter's fictions, she turns the child into a jailer. Being a 'good mother' is her excuse for not doing anything with her own life.

Motherhood is also a good excuse for giving up sex. Mother has 'more important' things to worry about than the ambivalent emotion which has tempted but troubled her all her life long; she stops thinking of herself as a sexual woman. 'This is usually unconscious,' says educator Jessie Potter, married thirty-four years and mother of two daughters. 'She may in fact have been an interesting sexual partner until her child was born, but now she is too tired, too busy, she says the children take up too much of her attention. It's all culturally induced, but the result is that she goes underground sexually until the kids are grown. As for the daughter, she grows up seeing a mother who has no sexual life at all.'

Little wonder that physical love comes to seem frightening to young girls. 'If mother has given up on sexual life,' says Dr Fredland, 'she will send the little girl bad vibrations. When the daughter asks questions, as four- and five-year-olds do, the mother will denigrate the subject or communicate her embarrassment. The daughter soon comes to think her own sexual feelings and fantasies are bad.'

Nobody knows a mother like her daughter. Mother says sex is beautiful. When her words go in one direction, but the music is going in another, the daughter listens to the music. 'It is extremely important,' says Wardell Pomeroy, 'that the five-year-old girl be enabled to recognize that mother has something very warm and special with daddy. Studies show that teenagers overwhelmingly complain, not that their parents did not give them the technical facts but that they never presented their children with an image of physical affection between mother and father.' The girl develops an image of sex, not as something to grow up to and hope for but as something to fear.

When mother's silent and threatening disapproval adds dark colors to the girl's emergent sexuality, this fear becomes eroticized in such strange forms as masochism, love of the brute, rape fantasies – the thrill of whatever is most forbidden. But it is not the rapist, not the man who will impregnate us and run away whom we fear – though in our efforts to give flesh to our dread fantasies we may say it is. In reality we can learn to protect ourselves against men like these, but even after years of psychoanalysis, doctors find that women cannot or dare not mention the real root of their sexual anxiety. To name her would be to have to face our anger at her, and to lose her – the mother who first planted fear in us.

The emergence of our sexuality arouses in mother all the pride she ever felt about her body and her sex . . . but all the shame, fear, guilt, disgust, dirtiness, and rejection too. Grown women, we ask ourselves why instead of our putting his hand on our vagina or guiding his mouth there, we feel an almost instantaneous reflex of rigidity when he touches us. We want to enjoy sex; our mind tells us we are free to. We examine and re-examine our anxieties, wondering if the inhibition is in us, in him – is the fault in our social system that sets the sexes at war with each other? The truth is you cannot be sexual with another person until you accept yourself. Another person doesn't make you sexual. Often with the best intentions in the world – to protect us – mother denies our sexuality, loading sex with a fear that makes us want to cling to her all the more. Only in partnerships, in mergers, in marriages like hers – runs the silent message – can we be safe? Masochism? Rape? Like sex itself, the beginnings and fascination of these ideas lie more between the ears than between the legs.

'When I look at my daughter, I feel all the fears and anxieties that have dogged me all my life,' says a mother of five-year-old twins, a boy and a girl. 'I treat my son as I would a man, and my daughter as I would a woman. No – as I would treat myself. I know I do this; I have since her birth. For instance, I'll let him go to the corner store alone, but I wouldn't trust her for a minute. She'd get lost or forget what she went for. I treat them this way in all things even while I realize I'm projecting all my fears onto her.' Raising a daughter to be an autonomous person with a sexual identity is a job for which few women are equipped because they never succeeded in doing it in their own lives; it is why the business between a mother and daughter is never finished. 'Now there's a real woman,' a man says, and every woman in earshot turns to glean what a 'real' woman is.

Sexuality is one of the first forces to forge our identity. At four, five, six, children go through a big spurt of sexual growth and separation. 'But they're practically babes in arms!' is the outcry. There is an unconscious logic to the adult denial of the sexual component of these oedipal years: intuitively we know that without separation there is no true sexuality.

'A kind of inborn timetable,' says Dr Aaron Esman, 'brings children to a sexual polarization around five or six. Little boys talk about wanting to marry mother. Little girls can become extremely feminine and seductive with their fathers.' But while mother may fondly recognize and even enjoy her son's 'romance' with her, she will deny the little girl's open flirtation with her father. The denial may take the form of, 'Stop bothering your daddy!' Other mothers practice avoidance, ignoring what the little girl is doing even as she parades naked in front of daddy, dances for him, or falls into the flirtatious poses she's picked up from watching TV or mommy herself.

This early interest in daddy is a childish but meaningful rehearsal; it is practice opposite the one man who loves us enough to applaud what we are becoming. That's all we want at this stage; we may come on as if to steal him away from mommy, but we'll happily settle for his smile, his fond kiss, his lighthearted acknowledgement that we're just about the prettiest little girl he's ever seen. But if he ignores our gleeful dance-of-the-seven-veils, or worse yet, dismisses us with embarrassment, the rehearsal ends prematurely. The show never opens. A fearful, frigid personality is being born. 'This kind of woman often marries early,' says Dr Sanger. 'Having been oedipally rejected by her father, she is afraid to take risks. She marries the first man who asks.'

It is important that the daughter feel there is room for privacy from her mother by the time the oedipal stage is reached. The little girl needs a psychic place of her own to get used to the turbulent desires, fantasies, fears and unaccustomed body signals welling up from within. But while she wants to feel she can shut the door on mother, she also has the seemingly contradictory wish that from the other side of that closed door mother approves. She doesn't want any detailed talk with mother right now; she hasn't sorted out her emotions yet. To have to put them into words makes them too real, too concrete and frightening. This is why children so often 'forget' answers to sexual questions they have asked.

The girl wants to feel that mother acknowledges and approves whatever signs of sexuality she may show. If she can react to her experience, life, and body without guilt, she can learn to enjoy and be proud of her sexual self. But the symbiotically tied girl picks up on her mother's fear or dislike of sex. She is afraid to enjoy these new feelings; they would mark her as *different* from mother, separating her from the only source of love she has been taught she can depend on.

Afraid of losing mother by seeming to prefer expression of the burgeoning new feelings she has for daddy, many a little girl ignores him instead. Even if there is no man in the house – mother may be divorced or widowed – there are still a hundred ways a daughter will try to get acceptance and acknowledge- ment of her sexuality. If mother ignores or calls it by other names, the girl retreats. A pact is set up: 'It's you and me against the world, mummy darling!'

It is a triumph of the human spirit that in spite of all our fears we don't give up on sex. It is as if nature, knowing how seductive and powerful is the pull of symbiosis, creates in sex a counterforce more powerful still.

Ever since we were four months old we knew there was a wonderful sensation if we rubbed ourselves between the legs. When mother changes her baby's diaper and inadvertently touches its genitals, the infant, male or female, feels pleasure. The tiny hand naturally goes to the source of that pleasure; mother automatically pushes the hand away. She does this whether the baby is male or female, but the way she does it – her deepest, perhaps unconscious feelings behind the gesture – will already be different depending on the sex of the child.

Four years later her boy's sexual awareness may worry or frighten her, but what does she know about male sexuality? She is reluctant to meddle in male business, maybe to set up inhibitions in him as a grown man. In her hesitation, she gives him space. She may even feel an unacknowledged thrill, sensing the emergence of the man who is so unlike her, but is the product of her body. Unconsciously sensed by the little boy, this adds to an early basis of his pride in being male.

She feels no such hesitation conveying her feelings to her daughter. Without mother having said a word, by the time we are four we know that touching ourselves makes her angry. 'Women say to me, "But I never masturbated,"' says Dr Fredland. 'We know from clinical experience that a child's natural impulse *is* to masturbate. 'Can you remember why you didn't?' I ask. 'Were you told not to or were you punished for it?' The standard response is, 'Oh, nothing was ever said to me.'

'Of course it *was*,' says Dr Fredland, 'but it has been repressed. Maybe something as mild as, "Ladies don't do that," which is quite enough, if they're afraid of losing their mother's love – enough for them to feel humiliated, frightened.'

I hear this story at a Parent/Teacher workshop: A mother takes her baby to the pediatrician. The baby is only six or seven months old and the mother holds him on her lap. When the baby begins to play with his penis, the mother takes the child's hand and holds it for the rest of the interview. At the end of the interview the doctor says, 'And what do you do when your baby plays with himself?' The mother looks him in the eye and says, 'My baby never plays with himself, Doctor.' All the mothers in the room smile nervously at the story; their own children are anywhere from five to eight years. They begin tentatively to discuss problems of masturbation they have with their own sons. *Daughters are never mentioned.*

'Mothers' expectations of boys,' the teacher who is leading the group explains to me, 'are quite different from girls. Girls are expected to be neater, quieter, better behaved, do better scholastically. They are good, and good little girls don't masturbate. These expectations are almost wish fulfilling.'

Little girls can be furtive about masturbation; we soon learn to be furtive about everything sexual. A little girl can rock back and forth in her chair watching TV, masturbating under everybody's nose. While she gets away with it, it is a small triumph. Her sexuality comes to seem too unimportant to notice. The problem, like our anatomy, is buried. What nature has begun – hiding our clitoris so well that many of us never find it – repression finishes.

'Whether she did or did not masturbate,' says Dr Schaefer, 'everyone in my study on women and sex was anxious about the subject. Some women masturbated but didn't know that is what they were doing. When they heard the word for it, they stopped.'

Where does guilt come from? We aren't born with it. Guilt is the result of introjection, the taking in of the critical parent we can't afford to leave 'out there,' to hate, be angry with, and possibly lose. Instead, we introject the critical mother inside ourselves and carry her around in the form of her restrictive rules for the rest of our lives. We turn the anger at her against our self. It no longer is mother who denies us this, says no to that. We do it to ourselves, and if we break any of her rules, even if she does not know it, our overly strict conscience punishes us for her with feelings of guilt.

The mother of a six-year-old tells me how determined she is

to raise her daughter without these overwhelming feelings of guilt so recognizable in women. 'It frightens me,' she says, 'the power I have over my daughter.' Several hours later in the interview, she tells me that the previous summer her daughter had one of her little friends sleeping over. Around midnight the mother had gone into the room to see that everything was all right. 'I found both girls with their pajama bottoms off, under the covers,' she says. 'I was too tired and irritated to act the way the books tell you. I just said, "OK, put your pants on and get into your own beds." I made them sleep in different rooms, though I didn't say they had done anything dirty. And now in the past year, when I call my daughter, she comes running out of her room with this frightened, guilty look as if she *knows* I'm going to scream at her. It makes me cry that she thinks of me this way.'

In her own mind, this mother has never said anything to her daughter to make her feel guilty about sex. She's never called it dirty. But the girl has read her mother's emotional message anyway – one that fills her with fear, that makes her come guiltily rushing out of her room as if mother could know what she was doing in there. Of course mother cannot. 'But the girl has introjected her no-saying mother,' explains Dr Robertiello. 'The antisexual mother *is* in the room, in the girl's conscience; so she does know what the girl is doing or thinking of doing. This mother must have been angry at *her* mother for being sexually repressive. Instead of overtly experiencing the anger, she took her critical mother into herself, as a part of her conscience. Now she is playing the same model to her own daughter.' From the daughter's guilty reactions where there was no realistic way for anyone to know what she was doing or thinking, it is clear that the girl has dutifully introjected her mother's guilt too. Is there any doubt that she will probably pass it on in time to her daughter.

'The taboo against looking at and touching yourself,' says Dr Schaefer, 'is directly associated with the taboo on masturbation, on self-pleasure. Young girls are taught that pleasure for pleasure's sake is bad. When you masturbate you can't elaborate or embroider what you're doing into an idea that you love somebody madly, or that you're doing this because you want to be a good wife or mother. You have to face it: you are doing it for yourself, with no other goal but your own pleasure. Most people can't face it. Do you know that until I was twenty-seven I didn't know women *could* masturbate?'

Because sex is so visible today, so talked about, we tend to assume 'everything is different'. We confuse our new liberal attitudes with our deepest, often unconscious feelings. National surveys indicate people today are far more liberal in their sexual attitudes than they used to be. Liberal about *other* people. 'The most interesting thing I've learned,' says Dr Schaefer, 'is that people's attitudes about sex *outside* the family are exceptions to what they feel about sex within the family.'

A mother can read a book and intellectually accept masturbation, but when her own little girl locks the bedroom door, mother is in agony as to what's happening on the other side. We think it very sweet to watch romance bloom between an older couple in a film, but when it's our own seventy-five-year-old mother, we are dismayed. 'Imagine, at their age!' People aren't even necessarily aware that they have these two sets of attitudes.

Mother has an uncanny way of thinking that if she doesn't tell us about something we will never find out, that she is our only source of knowledge. The extension of this crippling, symbiotic way of thinking is the older woman's assumption that *her* feelings of shame and embarrassment are what we feel. It is a self-fulfilling prophecy: the daughter who goes against her mother and does the forbidden does so with her mother's anxious feelings. When I masturbate today, my fantasies deal with the thrill of the forbidden, of being discovered, an anxiety my mother didn't have to voice. Psychiatrists have told me that one of the common fantasies women have while they masturbate is of their mother walking in on them.

Sexual self-discovery is the only self-discovery that is not celebrated in infancy and childhood. The day the child learns to eat with a spoon, everyone says, 'Isn't she wonderful? Isn't that great? Someone get the Polaroid!' But the day she discovers her vagina, nobody says, 'It's six months earlier than it should have been, isn't she the precocious darling!'

In her research Dr Schaefer found that even mothers who masturbated, who enjoyed it and said they wanted their daughters to enjoy it too – sexually oriented, college-educated women – nevertheless could not discuss the subject with their girls. 'How can you talk to a child about such a thing?' they say. 'How can you not?' replies Dr Schaefer, who is the mother of a thirteen-year-old girl. It is as though there are two kinds of honesty: one for adults, the other for children.

'There used to be a widely held theory among psycho-analysts,' says Dr Sanger, 'that during the Latency Period – from about eight to ten – a child's sexual impulses disappeared to reappear again only in adolescence. In the last twenty years, we've come to realize that the sexual impulse goes up, up, up all the way along. What happens is that by the time a little girl is seven or eight, she has become socialized enough to learn to keep it quiet, to be afraid of it and not let mother know because it would upset her.'

To grow into a sexual woman we must fight the person closest to us. A blade of grass will crack through cement to reach the sun. We too must go on blind, uninstructed energy. Even when we make it, and emerge sexual women at last, how many of us are not crippled by the struggle?

When you teach a girl not to touch herself, you make her passive, someone who will look to others not just to arouse her but also to take care of her. By keeping us ignorant (the usual word is 'innocent'), we are kept from learning sexual responsibility. We resist an intelligent understanding of how we are built, we keep the truth of our vagina a dirty secret. We do not contracept and become pregnant. We learn duplicity with ourselves long before it becomes our standard behavior with men – to say No when we mean Yes, to feign what we don't feel, to fake orgasm, to tease him and ourselves, not because we don't want it but because we don't know what it is we want.

When we get a scratchy feeling in our throat, the most natural thing in the world is to drink water. When a boy is sexually aroused – even if his mind does not know that is what it is – his body gives him a signal as real as the thirsty person's scratchy throat: an erection. And so sexual excitement comes to him as 'natural.' He didn't do it. It just happened to him. He moves to satisfy this new desire his body has informed him of.

A young girl's anatomy doesn't tell her she has a sexual life. When she reads a book, has a fantasy, sees an exciting movie or a picture of a naked man, there is no physical signal by which she can connect the inchoate feelings in her mind to the life of her body. 'Oh, it's so romantic,' she says, having no words for it, no sign of her desire, wanting to keep what is happening to her safely in the mind, cordoned off from the body she has been taught to keep her hands off.

The idea that she might stimulate herself, give physical expression to her inner feelings, is too threatening. Mother would never do a thing like that. Sex becomes not the 'natural' expression of her body's life but a statement of her will. If she wants to connect what is in her mind to her sexuality, she must perform the action, overcome the safety of passivity, take responsibility, give up the great childhood excuse, 'It's not my fault, I didn't do it!' It is too much for us. We make up a set of yearning fantasies instead. They express what we expect of men, and what we think they want of us; the erotic becomes so connected with the forbidden that sex, fear, and protection are merged together and fused.

During adolescence when sex with a partner – intercourse – enters our lives, the picture becomes more muddled than ever. Men are not raised with our fears. Sex does not present them with the idea of losing mother. When we are in his arms, he feels no need to stop. We must put on the brakes not for us only but for him too. So there we are: young boys applauded for their sexual adventurousness, young girls filled with the romantic fluff they've been taught by magazines and films to feel is somehow 'better,' more refined – certainly more acceptable to mother – than sex.

Had we learned the ABCs of masturbation before boys entered our lives, we might have explored our sexuality and our fantasies, and gotten used to this erotic new world. We might have learned there are different things you can have with men, some of them sexual, some of them romantic, some warm and friendly, etc. We might have learned to trust and follow our feelings so that we knew when it was sex we wanted – to be fucked – or when it was romance and loving comfort – to be held. There is a difference between love and sex; it is nice when they are combined, but they needn't be. You can have and enjoy one without the other.

Nor is our command over reality, our feelings of sexual identity, strengthened by the ambiguous code language in which we are trained to speak about sex or emotions. We lose power over our lives when we can't call things by their real names. (No wonder we have been the silent sex for so long.) If you cannot call a vagina a vagina, you are in trouble with your own body. We find that menstruation is called the curse, passivity is lauded as feminine while autonomy is masculine; competition, possessiveness, and anger are called signs of love, and lust is pronounced romance. Is it any wonder we have not been able to answer Freud's, 'What do women want?'

We ask mother, 'Can I go out?' 'No,' she says. We are made to feel that it is for our own good, while in fact her real reason for not letting us go is that she is lonely, afraid, irritated at father. No is easier than Yes. 'Why?' we ask, when she tells us that certain words aren't 'nice' to use. If she tells us what she wants us to believe and not what she really feels, we too learn to give people double messages. 'Don't,' we say when a boy touches us; we mean 'Do,' but he is meant to make it happen against our will or in spite of us, and we lose faith in him when he doesn't understand our code.

'A lady never talks about money,' mother says. How do you do *that*? one part of us questions, but the part tied to her dutifully suppresses any hint that cash concerns us. We twist our minds to please her. From this, how far a step is it to learn to twist others? These misnomers and crosscurrents of mother's anxiety leave us uncertain of a foothold in any reality but hers. 'But *why* do you love me?' we ask her as children. We need a specific answer to help us know who we are. Says Leah Schaefer: 'When I say in a burst of feeling to my daughter, "Katie, I just love you!" she always asks me why, just like she asks why I'm angry. I don't think it's enough to say, "I love you because you're my daughter." It says no one else can love you but your mother. But if I say I love you because you're bright or fun to be with and we had a terrific afternoon, then she *knows*. It is a kind of power. She knows she can be that way to someone else and arouse love in them . . . she's an effective person at getting love and it's not only because she's my daughter. I don't ever remember asking my mother why she loved me or why she was angry. It was some mysterious gift my mother could give or withdraw.'

To protect us against real dangers, and the imaginary ones she fears even more, mother makes it understood that she knows everything. 'The maddening thing is that everything seems out of your control,' a mother tells me. 'There is the fear always: can I cope or can't I?' Since she cannot control the world so that nothing bad happens to her little girl, mother manipulates the girl into the only security she knows: the false security of symbiosis. The bargain is, if we stay close and listen to her, do as she says, she will love us always. It is a very attractive bargain because her love is what we want more than anything. More than love, more than control, this is manipulation.

'Right from the start,' says Dr Sanger, 'mothers teach daughters to be followers, good dancing partners. They tell us, "I know the kind of girl I want you to be. I'm going to show you, just leave your arms there and I'll move them." Like a puppet on a string. Mother feels entitled to manipulate her daughter because she, the mother, is a woman. She knows the way. She's the expert on women. The daughter only has to do what she is told. When the girl grows up, she turns to a man and says, "now move my arms, tell me what I should do, how to be."' It's a transference expectation on to men that started when mother was only too willing to give us a total map.

'What irony!' says Dr Sanger. 'That the woman asks a man to show her how to be a woman, and after marriage resents his not being able to do this. This may explain the attraction for older men, who may be better instructors, or at least favor the child in the woman. If he can't make her feel like a woman, at least she feels like a pampered child.'

Mother's manipulative love doesn't give us the security we need. It keeps us anxious and drives the real self down deeper into shadows and secrecy. If she knew our 'secret selves,' our fantasies, desires, the things we do, think, and hide from her, she would no longer love us. The ironic lesson is that to keep mother's love, we learn to manipulate her.

The lesson is carried on throughout life. Through manipulation, we may get our way this time, win mother, keep the friendship, get the job, fascinate the man. But we can't be sure of tomorrow. The victory doesn't warm us. Are we really the femme fatale in the slinky black dress we put on because we heard that's the type he likes? What will we do tomorrow when he finds out that's not really us? Play the helpless little cuddly thing and hope that'll hold him for a while? What if he sees us without our false eyelashes, our fall, our bra . . . should we undress in the dark? We don't know what he loves us for because we have no idea who we are.

We manipulate to keep him with us through guilt, if nothing else – convinced we would die on our own. Just as mother convinced us she would die if we left her. If in the end he does go, it hurts, but we are not surprised: knowing we tricked and duped him into loving some persona that is not ourselves, how can we believe his love would last?

Sometimes at the great crises of our lives, when these manipulative methods for getting what we want have not worked out, we look back to mother in anger and in tears. 'My daughter is suddenly bringing up all this business from the past,' a mother exclaims. 'The last time we met, she practically accused me, 'But why did you and daddy go to Europe when I was four?' Imagine! Why, she's thirty-eight.'

Sometimes we make the journey back over thousands of miles, and a lifetime of physical separation. 'I telephoned my mother in Wisconsin last night,' a woman tells me. She is the mother of three daughters and we are sitting in an outdoor restaurant in southern Florida. 'Why did you call her?' I ask, surprised. She has repeatedly told me how she never got along with her mother. From the day she was fourteen and lost her virginity, she'd made it a point to get as far away as possible. 'Because – ' begins this fifty-three-year-old woman who prides herself on having 'fucked' while her mother only had sexual intercourse, 'because I wanted her to tell me what this goddam womanhood business was all about!'

While these journeys back to mother are often disastrous, the instinct is correct. Before we can understand the fears that plague us today, we have to find where they began for us as children. We must distinguish which of our fears are real, and which are only carry-overs of mother's long-ago fear for her vulnerable little girl.

In the beginning, a mother cannot but fear for her child. The girl is a projection of herself, she loves her as she loves herself. And so she sees all her own fears magnified in her daughter. It follows therefore that the quality of a mother's protection will be determined by the value she puts on what she is protecting. In the end, for any woman, this is her sexuality.

This opens something of a paradox, a double bind. We have been raised to think sex is wrong, dangerous, and dirty, but also that it is our prime bargaining exchange. We protect what is between our legs but keep our own distance from it, we don't like it, we don't have an easy, affectionate name for it; and yet 'everything' depends on it. It is a mysterious, poisoned jewel but the game is on: we must get men to believe 'it' is life's golden chalice. We can't bear to touch it but must pretend to him its possession is worth his giving up other women and working his ass off in our lifelong support. Sex is offered on condition. Manipulation again.

We offer men our bodies if they will marry us; afterward, we are mystified because we are less interested in sex now he is 'ours.' What we wanted all along wasn't sex, but closeness. *Mother most rewarded us with symbiotic love when we denied our sexuality*. Sex, even with its infinite pleasures, becomes merely a means to an end; nothing is sweeter than symbiosis. Grown women, we find we have manipulated ourselves out of our own sexuality.

Besides the awakening of sexual identity in the oedipal years, there is also an increase in all kinds of across-the-board assertiveness; great progress in separation and individuation. We want to know about sex and where babies come from, but also want to explore the world in general. The exhibitionism and seductiveness of a four-year-old is as much an assertion of self – 'Here I am, world!' – as it is a come-on with daddy.

Overworked, anxious, fearful herself, mother sees too much life in her children, coupled with too little caution; little wonder vitality is seen as dangerous. A mother may accept an overactive little boy. 'That's how boys are.' But girls are different. 'Even before the little girl is old enough to know what is being done to her,' says Dr Sanger, 'her mother begins to put the brakes on. She limits the girl: "Don't get too excited, don't get too full, don't run so fast, don't overdo it, don't get too tired!" What I would prefer to see is a mother who encourages her girl to feel that accomplishment can lead to even greater levels of energy. It is marvelous for a girl when her mother can be seen as someone who gets turned on, who says, "Now that I've sent out all the Christmas cards I really feel good. Now I'm going to do something I enjoy. Let's go ice skating in the park!" just because a certain level of satisfaction is reached, it doesn't mean you have to relax and recover – you can go on to even greater excitement. I like mothers to show their daughters that they are exhausted with excitement, not to just talk about doing something, but *do it*, right then and there. So what if there's school tomorrow?

Once in a while it's not going to kill the girl to lose an hour of sleep.'

Another factor works to make women more docile and compliant than men. As Dr Sanger's studies at St Luke's Hospital show, boy babies more often get direct physical expression of love and approval from their mothers, while girl babies get it in words and smiles. The important gulf that opens here is that a physical caress needs no interpretation, and carries no conditions. It is spontaneously offered, spontaneously accepted, almost without going through the cognitive centers of the brain. But a smile, a kind word has to be interpreted . . . thought about. Verbal signals and facial expressions carry under- and over-tones, perhaps shades of ambivalence. From her earliest days, the little girl thus learns she must interpret what somebody else wants of her before she gets approval – and even that approval cannot be accepted at immediate face value. That is her first lesson in compliance. 'The physical thing with a little boy is easier, more natural than with my daughter,' a mother tells me. 'In a way, I'm closer to my daughter, but I'm not as physical with her.'

In kindergarten, teacher knows the best way to handle an excited little boy. 'A touch calms them down,' says Dr Sanger. But while the little girl next to that excited boy may be as starved for touching, holding, and hugging as he is, she has already learned to respond to other, more verbal signals. And that's what she gets. Ironically, it is because of this deprivation little girls go through that they are so often better students than little boys. 'Their distance perceptors,' says Dr Sanger ' – eyes, ears – have been better exercised. Little girls aren't born "brighter" and more verbal than little boys, any more than they are born more passive.' We have been socialized that way at a certain psychic cost.

In nursery school, the first structures little girls build are enclosures, and the boys' first are towers. You may interpret these along strictly Freudian lines, but it is not necessary to do so to understand what is being expressed. An enclosure stands for something safe, cozy, protective. A tower assaults the heavens, and stands for effort and adventure. In a free, nonsexist society, one might expect that since both these ideas are legitimate to children, there would be some little girls who might build towers, some little boys who construct low houses. But the normative pressures in our society are so terrific that the rigid demarcation along sexual lines continues. It isn't just mommy who praises us for staying with enclosures, for playing quietly with dolls, who lets us see she is displeased if we imitate fire engines or make raucous noises: 'Now, dear, don't do that with your mouth.' 'What's my little snooksie-poopsie doing?' says daddy. 'Playing like a rough Indian?'

Passivity isn't always a mask, hiding a more active – often angry – and assertive person. Questions of temperament enter. Quietness, passivity may be genetic for some. Many little girls are simply born with lethargic dispositions. 'There is nothing wrong,' says Dr Sanger. 'The girl is just relaxed and nonassertive. But there are so many others who, underneath that passivity, are just seething. There's a beautiful person just waiting to come out, but she won't emerge. She's waiting, always waiting to be spoken to before speaking, waiting to be asked, waiting for the ice cream to be passed to her, waiting, waiting, waiting. If the waiter forgets her portion of ice cream, she just doesn't get it.' A little girl goes to school and sits quietly, like a robot. Nobody thinks it matters because at least she isn't throwing bricks through the window like the little boy. But her inner disturbance can be just as great, the problem underlying the behavior may be the same.

'There's a crucial growth period from five to ten,' says Dr Sanger, 'When little girls' passivity and under-achievement is too often accepted as normal. They are losing essential technical knowledge because these years are vital to developing life patterns. I see ten boys professionally for every girl in this age group. Little girls aren't less troubled than little boys, but mothers are more willing to admit they have a problem, maybe made a mistake, with a boy than a girl. The most "aggressive" behavior little girls show at this age is they become very bitchy, competitive with other little girls.

With everyone else, they behave in a passive manner.'

The term 'passive' has been used as much an all-embracing label for women that it has become almost a definition for feminity itself. And yet the meaning is always at least slightly pejorative. The problem is compounded further by the fact that it is not always easy to separate what is active from what is passive.

In sexual terms, for instance, it is usually thought the woman is passive because the man is on top, with most of the 'doing' left to him. But even in the missionary position, the woman may be far from motionless. She can be even more active than he. Many women have told me that far from finding any truth in the *Playboy* joke that the big male turn-on is the 'nymphomaniac whose father owns a liquor store,' they have found a more seductive image to be the woman half asleep. The man stays up late, ostensibly to do some work. When he comes to bed, he finds her passive, drowsy, not asking/expecting anything. Thus he feels safe in expressing his sexual needs. Indeed, he feels aroused because she seems less active, less powerful, unthreatening. The contact of their bodies helps, but equally important is her pose of symbolic passivity.

The sexual act may then take place. But who is the active partner? Who is the passive? Who has initiated it? Or let us say that we ask him to perform certain sexual acts. While we may lie back and enjoy them, we are not the passive partner. We have initiated the event.

This is not just playing with terms. If you and I use different words to describe the same thing, we will place different values on what is happening. For instance, mother says to us, 'I want you to grow up to be a woman with a personality of your own, to know what you want and take care of yourself.' But when we try to be that way with her, she criticizes us for being willful. We tell our lover, 'I want you to be very aggressive sexually,' but at the same time say, 'I get scared when men come on to me.' This puts him in a double bind, just as mother did with us. Two contradictory and mutually exclusive demands are being made simultaneously, paralyzing him. He is the one who must decide what to do. But it is we who have determined the quality of the relationship.

In even this simple analysis, we can see that the words *active* and *passive* are overly rigid and emotionally loaded. In our society men need us to seem passive if they are to assert their 'manhood'. If we want to change these traditionally limiting ideas of masculinity and femininity, we must give up the ambiguous advantages of passivity. Says Dr Sanger: 'Women have to learn to say, "I re   like this part of my body, and, god damn it, I'm going to get it taken care of. I like my clitoris, I like my breasts to be played with. I really want it, and now it's your turn to do it!" If she finds her partner won't, she should find someone who will.'

There are men who like sexually active, autonomous women. Women tend to say such men are hard to find. We have to ask ourselves if the fault is not half in us. We ask him to let us get on top, to fondle our breasts, adore our clitoris – *taking the initiative* – but still holding on to the image of ourselves as people who need others to take care of us, who are vulnerable, little, perishable, and passive. Confused, the man turns away, to seek a more traditional, even if more inhibited, partner. Both sexes have lost, the crippling game of role-playing perpetuated.

The girl of four or five is facing two rough separations. She's physically leaving home for the first time – going to school. She is also facing the difficult need to separate psychologically from her mother, to work out her oedipal rivalries and compromises; mother can't help her in this.

Nor does she get much help or encouragement from daddy. 'Most men in our culture,' says Dr Robertiello, 'may be flattered by their little girl's attention, but they have such an incest taboo built into them that they ignore the little girl's sexuality.'

The daughter is left with feelings of unfinished competition with mother. But right along with her wishes to replace her is the accompanying anxiety about retribution from mommy for having these jealous feelings. None of this gets expressed, most of it is unconscious. How can the little girl get angry if mother is pretending that nothing has happened? But somewhere in her soul, the little girl has shifted; mother has become the enemy, and all that tamping down, all mother's pacification, are now seen differently by the girl. Under the aegis of the competitive oedipal situation, the former relationship with mother is now seen to have been something less than perfect sweetness and light.

When someone teaches us to sit on our hands, modulate our voice, control our temper, check our enthusiasm, bite our tongue, control, control, control every spark of spontaneity – unless we are born that way, unless we are temperamentally, constitutionally, genetically a quiet, compliant person – we are going to be angry at the inhibitor. Even though we cannot afford to show that anger out of fear of loss, even if the anger is denied, it is still there. One of the earliest ways a child may handle her anger against the dominating mother is to develop certain romantic fantasies. When we meet other little girls' less manipulative mothers, we decide, I was not born to my mother, there was this changeling thing that went on in the incubator. *I don't want this mother*, the daughter is saying, she is just a baby-sitter who stole me from my real mother.

Rage is a human emotion. Male or female, we all have known it, felt it first as infants when we realized we could not control mother, that she was *not* us, but in fact could go away and leave us. The pioneering work of child psychiatrists like John Bowlby[2] and Margaret Mahler[3] tells us that these first signs of anger occur around age eight months and are a normal part of development no matter how well loved we are.

It is the fear of loss that makes babies bite and pull mother's hair. This fear is 'normal,' even a part of growth. Unless mother raises us to feel secure in ourselves, to have an identity and feeling of value separate from her, we will always be terrified of anger at her. It means we might lose her, and we need her still.

And yet it is only by learning we can show mother our anger, and that she will not stop loving us, that we can begin to accept our furies enough to handle them. It is a noble role that mother must play here – the target of all our storms, but one strong enough not to storm back. If she cannot allow us to go through this process, if the loving contact with her is not there, if the formation of our separate identity doesn't take place, then we are forever left in the position of frightened infants, never secure, always open to rage that shakes us with unexpected furies.

Frightened by these rages against a mother we cannot afford to lose, we enter what is usually called *latency*, hiding our oedipal competition from mother and ourselves. Often we root out our old baby dolls at this period, throwing ourselves back to a simpler time, calling a truce to the sexual wars, becoming close to mother again. But this denial of our bodies, desires, and independence is not based on love for mother. It is a reaction formation in which we disguise what we really feel and act out its opposite. It is a form of 'protesting too much': 'Oh, no, I'm not mad at mommy for keeping daddy away from me, and telling me there's something wrong and dangerous about what I feel in my body. In fact, mother is the one I want to be close to all my life long.' Competition and anger have not been resolved, only denied and repressed.

Very often this state – at age seven or eight – is marked by a passing focus on the little boy who sits next to us in school. But we quickly learn that this arouses antagonism in the other little girls; they have given up their own oedipal strivings and want to present a united front, solidarity with mother – with men left out. So out of fear of retribution from the other girls – ostracism – we give up on little Johnny too.

Our anger at being kept compliant, at not being able to express our anger, may never come out. 'When my friends criticize my mother for being so strict,' says an eight-year-old, 'I won't listen to them. When they want to go somewhere, and I know my mother won't let me go, I don't say my mother won't let me. I say that I'm the one who doesn't want to go. I can't bear it when anyone says anything against my mother.'

Reaction formation again: hearing any negative remarks about her stern mother arouses such guilt in this girl that she won't let them be spoken. In her depths she realizes they name out loud the angers she herself feels but is afraid to let flare up.

Hidden angers may boil like Vesuvius just under the surface, or pop up in distorted, disguised forms. A year ago a woman called me from California; I had interviewed her for this book six months earlier. She is twenty-seven, one of the sweetest-natured women I've ever met, with a responsible position in a bank. 'Ever since you and I talked,' she said, 'I've been thinking about your questions: How was I like my mother, what had I learned from her? Six months ago, I told you I couldn't think of any way I was like her. And that seemed strange to me too. But recently I developed stomach pains, and my doctor said it was an ulcer. He asked if I was aware of bottling up any of my angers. Trying to answer his questions made me aware that what I had learned from my mother is that you don't ever express negative emotions. You are polite, never angry. I never saw my mother angry at my father. She played the martyr, and I grew up believing my father was an ogre. Now I've come to see this blameless-victim role she played—that's what made him seem to me to be such a difficult man. Thinking about this brought back another memory whose importance I never realized before. I must have been five, because my mother and I were in the grocery store around the corner from where we lived. They had those big old-fashioned glass cookie jars, and the counter-man offered me a cookie. My mother said, 'No,' and I hit her. I've remembered that all my life and felt guilty about it. It was the only time I've ever struck out at my mother . . . or anyone.'

These unspeakable furies are the source of countless physical and psychological problems women have. 'Often, part of the anger a little girl of eight or nine feels is a realization that all the ciriticism, the manipulation, the intrusion from mother wasn't because she loved me for my *self*,' says Dr Sanger, 'it's because she loves me to be a little mommy, an image of her. "Boy, I'm going to let her have it!" may be the girl's reaction. There is the fight, a postponed individuality struggle. It is the same fight between them twenty years later. Angry as the daughter is, she keeps going back, though all they ever do is argue. She's still looking for those crumbs of mother's affection.'

The oedipal stage, adolescence, love affairs, our first job, marriage, the birth of our own children . . . these are rites of passage, marking important stages of our lives. Why are they so often accompanied by fear, anxiety, or depression – women's disguise for anger? The moments are incomplete, we find ourselves unable to live up to them because something is missing: a feeling of self with emotions we can trust. 'It was my birthday . . . and I was told to be happy,' are lines from a poem by Muriel Rukeyser.[4] I do not believe it is an accident that this poem about the alienation of a child's emotions, the injunction to pretend to be happy when she's not, was written by a woman.

In his book *The Female Orgasm*, psychologist Seymour Fisher states he finds orgasmic difficulties in women correlate with the fear of desertion by the men. Little importance is attached to erotic technique. The woman's inability to 'let go' can be traced back to her feelings about her father. If she 'trusted' him not to leave her, she will be able to trust the man in bed with her and have an orgasm.[5]

Without doubt the relationship with father is enormously important. He was our first model of what to expect of men. If he was accepting, happy to see us – we expect other men to be. If he ignored our sexuality – we became insecure about it ourselves. But who put on the sexual brakes to begin with? Who pushed away the tiny hand long before we became oedipally interested in daddy, who invaded our privacy? Above all, who, with her own body, in what she said and didn't say, provided our most enduring image of how to be a woman? Who says, 'Nice girls don't'? I agree with Dr Fisher that trust is the basis for letting go, for orgasm, for love and life itself, but who, more than father, earlier than anyone else, inhibits our ability to trust ourselves?

'Why are you so critical?' we ask, and mother's reply is that we wear too much lipstick.

CHAPTER FOUR

Body Image and Menstruation

It was a decision of Daddy Colbert's (he was young and
didn't like to be called grandfather) that my mother should
move from Pittsburgh south to Charleston, where he was
building a steel alloys plant on the banks of the Ashley River.
He was a patriarch and liked his family near him; he also
thought it would be a good place for my mother to raise my
sister and me. He was right.

Our house was tall and pink with pale blue shutters and a
wrought-iron balcony. I remember my first walk, and the
stillness of those narrow streets. Had I turned left, I would
have come to the bay and seen Fort Sumter. I turned right
instead and eventually found what I was looking for – a
grocery store where I bought a box of Mallomars with coins
taken from the pocket of a coat in the hall closet. The shabby
grocery was on the corner of what Gershwin had named
Catfish Row, and a few years later I was to get my first job
there, paying $2.50 a week. Mother only found out about it
when one of her friends saw me sweeping the doorstep in my
Girl Scout uniform. I never told her about that first walk
either, or that I'd got lost and frightened. I was five, but I
knew the mother-daughter bargain: if you don't stay close,
it's not fair running back for consolation.

I'd had only two near misses with danger. Both had happened in Pittsburgh. I remember a man and woman in a car calling to me from across the street to come ride with them; then
there was the newspaper boy who unzipped his fly and showed
me the most amazing thing. Each time I'd run like crazy. But
Charleston was safe for all of us. I'm sure my mother found a
kind of haven there after the unhappy years in Pittsburgh.

The people in my dreams are the people with whom I grew up in Charleston. The houses there were four-storied, and had their elegant shoulders to the street; the verandas ran back at right angles. All my life I've judged the beauty of other cities by Charleston, where you cannot see the gardens from the street. You have to be invited in.

Our own house leaned slightly to the right. When you sat in the drawing room, your head automatically tilted in line with the sloping walls. There were metal poles running just under the ceiling. 'In case of late summer hurricanes,' someone told me. But nothing ever fell down in Charleston. And nobody ever left. I grew up surrounded by permanence, a world that was warm and generous and promised to go on forever.

I wanted desperately to belong to that world. Society was defined very strictly. It meant living 'below Broad Street,' having a deep Southern accent and generations of kinfolk just around the corner. Our address was right, I learned to say mirruh instead of mirror, but neither my grandfather's money nor the private girl's school I attended could change the fact we were Yankees. There wasn't a house in which I was not welcome, not a time when I didn't feel loved by the extra mothers I found all over town; but I knew we didn't belong. Even my name – Friday – was different. Later I grew to love its uniqueness just as I grew to love being tall, but when I was ten and people asked my name I would slouch and say, Nancy.

Had I not grown up at this tiny angle of divergence from the inbred security of Charleston and the strict rules that such closed societies lay down, I'm sure I would be different today. Perhaps I would never have married Bill or written books on women's sexuality. My life would have been a straight, strengthening line, one solid note; the life of a woman who never questioned her convictions. But I wasn't cut out for a straight line anyway, or I would not have taken so many walks. I would have stayed forever below Broad Street. I would rather live with my old anxiety about feeling left out than to have been merged so completely that I never left Charleston at all. But I know that my ability to live different lives today, to deal with abstractions, to change and accept consequences rests on what I found in Charleston. As I place one foot forward into the unknown, I have one foot in the secure past.

Today my mother lives a thousand miles away from Charleston, where she has roots and friendships as deep as the old ones. She puzzles at my disinterest in 'settling down', but we share a deep nostalgia for those years when we almost could believe we belonged to a community that held to the preservation of anything beautiful – old houses, eighteenth-century hymns, and, above all, family. I don't have to know where I will be next year, but I have my own need for permanence. I find it in people, not houses. What luck I have finding it comes from a basic trust I learned in Charleston: that if I expose my need for love, I may find it in others. It's only in my dreams that they still reject me.

There was a girl named Sophie who moved onto our street when I was ten. Her family came from 'above Broad Street,' which made her more foreign than a Yankee. It wasn't because she was a year older that I became her slave. Until Sophie, I'd been used to taking the lead. When a friend slept over, it was I who insisted we have a string between the twin beds, tied to each of our big toes, so that any movement during the night would be sure to awaken us. Quietly, we would get up, dress, and slip down the three flights of stairs past my sleeping mother and out onto the dark streets of Charleston. It was I who insisted we play in the forbidden warehouses on the waterfront, sneak aboard the ships in the harbor, and ride with the black delivery men on the horsedrawn ice wagons that still serviced that part of town. But I never questioned Sophie's leadership.

She had the mysteriousness of someone from the moon. She had lived the déclassé life 'above Broad,' which fascinated me almost as much as the Saint Cecilia Society, for which I would never be eligible due to my Yankee birth. It was Sophie who told me where babies came from; never mind that she was incorrect. I'd never even known one could have such a conversation. There was, in fact, an amazing level of sexual ignorance in my 'group' that stayed with us throughout our teens. In all those years of heated dreams and steamed-over car windows, no one talked of sex. We spoke of love.

Even Sophie's house was different. Charleston homes were kept immaculate by maids who had been with the family forever; the disarray at Sophie's said there were more important things in life than the genteel hush of beautiful rooms. Ashtrays spilled onto the carpet, the morning coffee cups glued to the slopped-over coffee, still on the table at noon, the heavy, awkwardly placed furniture – all were exciting, half-revealing, half-concealing clues to another, secret, and exuberant sense of life more enticing to Sophie's family than neatness.

There were no scheduled meals at Sophie's, no time to be home, no rules; when a grownup entered the room I was the only one who shot to her feet. Upstairs deepened the mystery. There three sisters shared a vast room that was like a female factory. Face powder hung in the air, and Sophie's older sisters sat in their slips at dressing tables applying layers of blood-red lipstick. One day they rouged my face. They looked at the results, sighed, and told me not to worry; I had a 'good personality'. Every evening Citadel cadets arrived to carry Sophie's sisters off into the night like prizes they had won. One night Sophie and I hid behind a sofa while her sister said goodnight to her date. Sophie got so excited she wet the floor.

Sophie taught me how to dance. I loved the shag, the fast music. Learning how to move my body was almost as exciting as climbing walls or chasing boys. (Other girls weren't interested in running and climbing.) One favorite game was to hide under the veranda of Pete's or Henry's house until they came home. Lying in the dirt, listening to their conversation when they didn't know we were there, was excruciating. But the best part was being discovered and chased, over the roofs, through the alleys, up and down Charleston's cobblestone streets. One day when the boys caught us they kissed Sophie. It was then I realized it mattered to Sophie whom she danced with or was chased by. More significant, neither Pete nor Henry kissed me. It filled me with anxiety. I was involved in a game in which I couldn't win.

One night when I was sleeping over at Sophie's she took my hand and placed it on her breast. She instructed me to suck her nipples. I would have followed Sophie into fire. When she moved down in the bed and put her mouth between my legs, I learned a pleasure I'd never dreamed possible. But when she instructed me to do the same, I cheated. I used my thumb instead.

Overnight Sophie was into dresses while I remained in blue jeans. During our last confusing days of play together, I tried desperately to follow her, not to lose her. On the way to her house, I would stop my bicycle just outside our big iron gate, lean over my handlebars with my head hidden in the bicycle basket, and slash a streak of color on my lips. My blue-jean pockets bulged with the accessories of my two lives, lipsticks and jack-knives. I was prepared for anything.

But nothing could prepare me for Sophie's rejection. I tagged behind her and her new friends, girls her own age. When she applied for Kanuga Camp's Senior Division, I lied about my age; frantically I followed her up into the mountains, to spend the worst three weeks of my life, stuffing my latex aquamarine bathing suit with falsies – which promptly showed when it got wet. Evenings I sat alone under the trees and watched couples disappear into the woods. One morning the Junior Division walked by on their way to the lake, among them the girls I'd grown up with, my best friends until Sophie had appeared. I would have given anything to be with them.

How many months, years, later was it that I tried to re-create that night at Sophie's? A friend was sleeping over and I rolled on top of her, rubbing up and down. But nothing happened. It wasn't shameful, it just wasn't fun. We gave it up and went to torment my older sister instead. Susie had her bedroom door locked but we could hear Frank Sinatra singing 'Night and Day'. 'Oh, Frankie,' we screamed, rattling the doorknob, laughing hysterically.

My mother is very good about not throwing out my trunks of childhood memorabilia that clutter her attic. Recently I came across a tarnished identification bracelet. They were the rage when I was growing up. Boys gave them to their girls, with their names on either side. On mine 'Nancy' was engraved on one side and on the other, two names, 'Pete' and 'Henry'. I had bought it for myself that terrible summer when I was ten.

The day I began to menstruate it was raining. A paralyzing Saturday, smothered in heat and the indecision of whether the rain would cancel my riding lesson. The odor of the magnolia tree outside my bedroom window held me down, reminding me all the while that if I didn't get up and move my bicycle, which was parked under the tree, the seat would soak up so much water I'd have to stand up and pedal all the way to school on Monday. Another niggling worry was the discomfort in my lower stomach. Once before I'd talked my mother out of the need to have my appendix removed; it would have meant missing basketball season. Now the entire summer was threatened. When I saw the little brown spots on my pants, I breathed a sigh of relief. So that's all it was. The rain stopped. I could go riding. The summer was mine.

My friends and I knew all about those blue and white Kotex boxes in our mothers' bathrooms. We knew they were our future. When we'd moved from the big pink house, my friend Joanne and I had gagged with laughter when a moving man held up a loose Tampax from a bathroom cupboard and asked, 'Shall I pack these candles?' Many's the time I'd stuffed a Kotex into my pants and walked about, enjoying what would one day be mine. We were very knowing girls, who knew absolutely nothing.

There was no one but mother to instruct me how to put on a Kotex. My sister was away at boarding school. If my horse wasn't waiting, I might have lain in bed and bled to death rather than go to her for such intimate help. She had been busy all morning with a workman, who was installing a siren outside her bedroom window; Charleston was in alarm over a burglar whom the newspapers had named Amorous – a name that accurately reflected Charleston's condescending assurance that even burglars knew their place. Amorous got into bed with female victims, but never dared go further. My mother was having the On-Off switch installed within easy reach of her pillow when I came in. I mumbled something and she followed me back to my room. I still remember the unmentionable discomfort between us of that moment.

She got me a pink elastic belt and showed me how to hook the ends through the metal hooks. I sucked in my stomach away from her fingers and rushed her through her patient explanation. 'All right, all right, I understand, I can do it.' I couldn't wait to get out of the house. Beginning menstruation meant two things to me: relief that it wasn't appendicitis, and deep embarrassment at having to go through the initiation rites with my mother. I didn't tell her about my stomach ache, and she didn't cancel my riding lesson. I was used to telling my mother as little as possible and getting my way. Years later I was to accuse her of indifference. Mothers cannot win.

Driving me to a friend's house the next day, she caught me off guard with a new voice: 'Well, how does it feel to be a woman?' I hated the friendliness those strained words offered. I leaned far out the car window, my pigtails flying behind. My answer was appropriately lost in the wind. They were the last words my mother was to utter on the subject.

I didn't mind menstruation. I'd expected it, but probably not so soon. It was ironic that I was the first of my group to begin; many of my friends were into bras while I was quite flat and hairless. I don't think I brought up the subject until one of the other girls mentioned she'd begun. 'Oh, that,' I said. 'I began ages ago.' But I didn't want to talk to my mother, ever, about 'those kinds of things'. And I couldn't care less about being a woman. I was eleven.

I am still working on her question about how it feels to be a woman. But I never have understood the secrecy about menstruation.

*　　　*　　　*

Women live in an isolation that belies the picture we show the world. We kaffee-klatch and gossip, turning our lives inside out for one another, exposing our feelings with a compulsion we ourselves don't understand, telling each other things we hide from our lovers. The world nods, agreeing not to notice even our early experiments in homosexuality. 'That's how girls are.'

Close, loving, tender, and intimate as we may be, we would rather have these ties with men; we will betray one another when a man offers them to us. Men are disappointing; they do not have our need for intense relationships. They cannot convince us that they love us. The leitmotif of our lives is that we will fail with men and bind ourselves to other women. The bond is not one of loving friends. It is the bond of mutual jailors, keepers of the unmentionable secret – which is our sexuality.

'Those women who boast most fulsomely of their love for their own sex (apart from lesbians, who must invent their own ideal of love),' says Germaine Greer in *The Female Eunuch*, 'usually have curious relations with it, intimate to the most extraordinary degree but disloyal, unreliable and tension-ridden, however close and longstanding they may be . . . Of the love of fellows they know nothing. They cannot love each other in this easy, innocent, spontaneous way because they cannot love themselves.'[1]

When we were little we knew mother had a secret. As close as we felt to her, as much as she knew about us and said we must tell each other all, we knew she was hiding something. She denied there was 'more' to her life than what we saw and imitated, but we know better. We bided our time. We gladly forfeited the things boys did – though we envied their mobility, speed, and daring; hadn't mother too given up these things? Didn't she acquiesce in daddy's being the one who left the house to work, who went out at night alone, and handled the money? There was clearly some wonderful reward up ahead in being a woman like mommy. It had a lot to do with what went on between her and daddy when they were alone. They aroused emotions in each other, tensions, angers, joys that touched chords in our own bodies; deep resonances that made us fear and envy and anticipate mother's secret. It was only a matter of time, of waiting, before all would be revealed to us.

And we were used to waiting.

Have you ever known something was going on, yet everyone denied it? Part of you really doesn't want to know, so you ignore it. Then suddenly you find out what it is, and realize you knew it all along – and wish you'd never found out. That is women and sexuality.

When we are still little, we get our most important lesson about our body from the person who holds, feeds, and disciplines us. Mother may spank our brother when she catches him playing doctor games. He may feel guilty, but he gets his attitudes about his body, his sex, from other boys and men. 'No,' says mother when we touch our vagina. 'No,' she says again when we chase boys, 'wait till you're older.' 'Don't bother daddy,' she says when we discover how much we like the feel of his lap. We obey. Later we may masturbate and lust after men, but what do we feel? Long before the lectures, the book left on our bedside table, the film at school, we have learned about our sexuality from mother's denials, avoidance, and her relationship to her own body.

'There may be a critical period for learning the art of mothering,' says anthropologist Lionel Tiger. 'If you don't learn it then, you are not likely to pick it up. For example, Benjamin Spock thought that girls learned to be mothers between three and six, when they played with dolls and watched mommy make chocolate-chip cookies. They put away all this information for a while and then at twenty, or when they marry, they retrieve the cookie utensils.' Then he added an associated but different idea: 'There is also reason,' Dr Tiger said, 'to believe we learn our sex roles very early.'

Not a world-shattering statement until we examine the distinction made between the mothering role and the sexual one. (The fact that they are both being learned at the same time compounds the confusion). We love the first part, admitting easily and with grateful affection that we got our terrific skills in housekeeping from mother. We remember watching her in the kitchen, how good she was at taking care of people. We love her for it. More important, we *want* to love her. The slightest twinge of anger or dislike fills us with gnawing unease. It is for this reason we don't like to think the same mother who taught us to be good mothers also taught us to be lousy sex partners. We never 'see' her as the model from whom we learned our fear of our bodies as naturally as we learned to prize clean hair; we do not connect our anxiety when he tries to touch us 'there' with the same anxiety she felt when we, as babies, did it ourselves. We go home to her to visit, filled with good intentions of expressing our love and gratitude, needing to reinforce our bond with her, but all too often there is tension in the air, and when we kiss her goodbye, we are guilty.

Why? What goes wrong? Even women who say, 'I just don't get along with mother,' do not cite sexual tensions as a problem between them. We cannot face the fact that our sexual anxieties today are inherited from mother.

It is a pediatric commonplace that children have a self-protective way of learning about sex. We take in only as much information as we can handle at any one time. 'I thought I'd told my daughters very well how babies got in and out,' says a mother of two girls, seven and nine, 'until we were watching a Dick Van Dyke show. A little girl said that the way babies were born is the mommy and daddy wish upon a star and then go into the garden and if they see a blue cabbage, it's a boy, and if it's a pink one, it's a baby girl. So I said to my oldest girl, "We know better than that, right?" And she said, "Of course, everybody knows that it's a pink rose, not a cabbage."'

This story reassures mothers. On one level it says their little girls don't want to know about sex anyway. Mother is right, therefore, to postpone the talk about sex and menstruation another year or two. It also reinforces the feeling that mother can control what happens to her daughter: my little girl will only know what I tell her.

'It's a common kind of wishful thinking mothers have about

their daughters,' says Dr Schaefer, 'a prime example of the unreality of symbiotic thought patterns. They don't know where they leave off and their daughter begins. If you see your daughter as your extension, you cannot imagine that she has thoughts and feelings different from yours. A mother assumes, "If I'm embarrassed and uncomfortable about sex, my child is too."' It is another self-fulfilling prophecy.

Women who have outstripped their own mothers' limited lives, who act in a sexually liberated way and consider themselves open-minded, are bewildered when their daughters haven't 'heard' their brave new message. 'It's as though I hadn't told her a thing,' a mother of a sixteen-year-old says. 'Why didn't she use a diaphragm? It's as though she's been listening not to me but to my own guilt-ridden mother.' There is a clue here to the conservative backlash so often found in children of women who proclaim themselves sexually liberated: the daughter does not so much take in her mother's brisk new chatter about freedom as she is conforming to the deep, often unconscious feelings about sex mother learned as a little girl herself. It takes more than a generation to change the lessons we learn from our mothers.

'Personally, I think the more a girl is intimate with her mother, the more natural will be the daughter's feelings about her body,' says Dr Fredland, who feels that her own attitudes have changed enough so that she can communicate a message different from the one she got from her mother. 'My four-year-old daughter loves to look at her vagina. Sometimes when I'm getting out of the shower, she'll come and lie down on my bathroom rug and just stare up at me and say, 'I like to see what your vagina looks like and what your rectum looks like,' and I say, 'OK, have a good look.' When my daughter was younger, she liked me to hold her up to the mirror and look and locate which places were for what. This kind of ease about the body *can* be set up through a real intimacy with the mother.'

The idea of my lying on my mother's bathroom rug, smiling up at her vagina, is too awful to imagine; more to the point, it was too awful for my mother, and probably yours too. It sounds like a utopian way to raise a child, Dr Fredland's ease and naturalness with her little girl. But Dr Fredland is an M.D. and psychiatrist; she has been analyzed and has thought more about this issue, both professionally and personally, than any other mother I've interviewed. She would be the first to dissuade you from imitating her *unless you believe in your bones you are as accepting of your sexuality as you tell your daughter you are.*

Nothing confuses us more about sex than the double message. If a naturalness hasn't been there since birth, sex cannot be communicated 'naturally.' After six or ten years of silence, if mother plucks up all her courage, takes a deep breath, and suddenly announces like the J. Arthur Rank man banging a gong that Sex Is the Most Natural Thing in the World – she fills us with contradictions. 'The mother has read all the books,' says educator Jessie Potter, 'and knows what she is supposed to say. But the girl has lived in that house all her life and knows that sex is not a happy part of her parents' life.'

Mrs Potter goes on: 'My experience in school and in talking to hundreds of parents tells me that some rare and special people – parents or teachers – have been raised to have a comfortable feeling about sex. Most have not. So while they think they are merely telling children the facts, their own discomfort is what the child learns.'

'Except for telling us that if we masturbated we wouldn't be interested in men,' says a twenty-two-year-old woman, 'my only other memory of sex education was how rigid and prissy the teacher was.'

Mother doesn't have to be perfect, just consistent. If she is herself, then we can feel secure enough either to identify with her, go to the right of her or to the left. She is giving us a known position to start from. She has held out the model of her honesty to us. She has freed us. We can accept her timidity or embarrassment about sex because that is how we have always perceived her. But mother's double message makes us grow anxious about our perceptions of reality.

'Never do anything you don't feel good about,' advises Dr

Fredland. 'If a mother is uncomfortable, she should find someone who feels easy about sexual subjects to talk to her daughter.' That too is a frank avowal of mother's feelings – that we must get the facts from a stranger rather than from her. It may distance us a bit; it may hurt. But telling us one thing while she in her gut feels something else hurts more. In fact, many women readily acknowledge that the best thing their mothers did was not to try to talk to them at all about sex.

'My mother never said anything was good or bad,' a thirty-year-old woman says. 'This is usually thought to be unhealthy, but I often think it somehow worked for me. I had no preconceptions. I found out about sex from other girls. I didn't masturbate until my late twenties – or have an orgasm until my second marriage – but at the same time I always had a nice feeling about sex. I always felt free to ask for what I wanted – even though I usually learned it later than other people. I think the real lesson about sex was one my mother never could put into words, but I got it anyway: she and my father always had a nice, warm relationship.'

It is a commonplace among psychiatrists and educators that children – even when we're grown – don't want to think our daddies and mommies 'do it'. But the lesson that transcends all the words and books is summed up in this woman's last statement: 'Because my parents really liked each other and we kids knew it, I got the idea that whatever went on between men and women was OK.'

When we despair of getting the truth from mother, we turn to other little girls. They promise the kind of intimacy we still need but cannot afford with mother. Sleeping over at one another's house, our whispers confirm what we suspect: mother never experienced what we are going through. That is why she never told us, not because she didn't love us. If she ever did feel as we do, it was long ago, long before she was a mother, in some other, overly moralistic, prediluvian time. We must protect ourselves – and her prudery – by keeping what we know from her. In choosing to act without her approval – in secret from her – we not only lose her help in discovering our 'forbidden' sexuality, we also assume responsibility for her. Sex frightens mother. We protect her with our own silence. And yet, love her as we may, there is a feeling of betrayal: if she loved us, why didn't she say there was more to being a woman than being a mother?

We try to set up with other girls the best of what we had with mother, a warm pool of closeness wherein we can tell and share 'everything'. By revealing our deepest secrets, we hope to bind our best friend to us forever, but mother's invisible hand pursues us. 'My sister and I were as close as two girls could be,' a woman says. 'We talked about everything – except intimate things. I guess that was mother's influence.'

Long after we have left mother's house, even after her death, she remains embodied in the feminine 'moral' system she taught us; it was the special territory we shared with her, from which our father and brothers were excluded. To get rid of the prudery we took over from her, to free ourselves of the fear that she inculcated into us as a form of protection takes more than mouthing a slogan or reading a new book. Good or bad, her anxieties are our maternal inheritance, our solidarity with her. To kill her unceasing vigilance, her sexual distrust, is to kill the part of her that lives on in us as the maternal conscience. That is why it is so hard to do, even when our minds say *yes, yes*. It means to go it alone.

Even when we were little girls, we had already begun to project this feminine superego onto our friends. It is why we cannot trust other girls. We will fondle one another in a tryst of gentleness, aching to think up new secrets to share – but we hold one back. 'Have you ever touched yourself down there?' we venture, already afraid of having gone too far. 'No!' she exclaims, confirming our fears. 'Have you?' 'Oh, no!' we agree, denying everything for fear she will not love us. The acme of our desire is to be – to *make* ourselves – just like every other girl.

We will never be as comfortable thinking of ourselves as sexual as we will when thinking of ourselves as mothers; the word sex never rings as true as love. Silence is preferable to any name given our genitals, and much as we may enjoy him touching us 'down there,' we will never believe he likes it. The role-playing we learned with our dolls has come full circle and we are only twelve. We may have wondered why there was no daddy for our dolls when we were three, but by the time we learn where babies come from, we are more comfortable without men. Didn't mommy give up sex for us?

Our need for acceptance by women is already stronger than any sexual need we will have of men. Jailed or jailer, it is one and the same in women's prison. Our sexuality will always seem to be in defiance of other women. Marriage, rather than a go-ahead to sex without guilt, soon becomes a stroll down memory lane, mom and dad all over again. By the time we become mothers, it is second nature to protect our daughters by denying our own sexuality. We edge out our husband, just as mother did dad, when we were three and baby dolls and cookie-making were what love was all about. At best, sex is an anxious business. Now that we're married, the center of life shifts from the troublesome vagina, out there to home, church, family. Life is pleasant. Why do we feel there is a void at its heart?

That so many women give up on men after pursuing them all our lives, cannot just be that men fail us. Perhaps we are as bloody minded as they. We say they fuck us and leave us. But once we've gotten them to father our children, don't we lose interest in the penis that has served what we see as its prime function?

'If we can repress and police a young girl enough about her genitals,' says Jessie Potter, 'she'll never find them. Even if she does, she is going to have had so many negative messages, she will have been anesthetized from knees to belly button. After we've taught her that part of her body is so awful you can't even call it by name, that it smells bad and she'd better not even look at it, then we tell her she must save it for the man she loves. Women must be pardoned for being less than enthusiastic about such a gift.'

A little boy comes to grips with his sex very early, literally every time he urinates. When he is excited, his erection appears 'naturally'. At camp, the fire is extinguished by a group pee. Seeing who can shoot his sperm the farthest is like long-distance peeing: a test of mastery and control, a confirmation of OK maleness.

But females are so cunningly made it is as if mother had a hand in the design of the vagina. We do not see ourselves when we urinate. We cannot control the stream. The only time we are allowed to touch ourselves is when it is unavoidable: when we wipe ourselves clean. Toilet training is mother's first big hurdle in raising us. Her role as a 'good mother' is at stake, and she will judge herself by how early she can report success to her friends and neighbors. When we fail her, it is, 'How can you do this to me?' – a refrain we will hear all our lives. Even when we shit in our pants it is her disgrace.

'One thing mothers tend to do,' says pioneer sex educator Dr Mary S. Calderone, 'is to get between their child's body and the child's self. They insert themselves in there because they apparently feel they own the child's body. They demand from it, first: feces, at a given time and in a given way: 'I want you to do it this way. I want you to give me a beautiful bowel movement. You're a good girl if you give it to me here in this pot.' Then they begin to demand urine in the same way. Next, they get between the child and its desire to suck its thumb. Eventually they get between the child and her desire to touch and enjoy her genitals. We interpose ourselves: we forget that we don't own that child's body. *She* owns her body and our efforts should be limited to helping *her* socialize her own control of it. Early, rigid training lays the groundwork for later feeling that sexuality is wrong, enjoyment of the body is wrong, masturbation is wrong, intercourse is wrong!'

After such denigration of the vagina, is it surprising that so many little girls look at their brothers enviously? He has something in that area we do not. 'My little girl called me in the other night,' a mother tells me. 'She said she couldn't sleep. "I keep thinking about penises," she said. "I want one. Oh, I want to be a girl but I'd just like to have a penis so I can hold it in my hand and make it go this way or that."' Then the mother added. 'My daughter is the kind of child who likes to be in control of things.'

Who doesn't want control of her own body? To a little girl who has had trouble pleasing her strict mother during toilet training, how useful the penis must appear! 'The boy seems to have the answer to getting mommy's praise,' says Dr Robertiello. 'He has a handle, something he can control, as familiar, simple and easy to understand as a kitchen faucet – you just turn it on or off. And it is clean. It stands away from his body, so the little boy doesn't have to wipe himself off after he pees. Of course a little girl would like a handle like that, to control, to be clean, to please mother. But to extrapolate from this simple desire and declare that therefore the girl would rather be a boy is to leap into mythology.'

Toilet training focuses our whole relationship with mother onto the vastly important area between our legs. Because we are like her, mother transfers feelings about her own genitals onto us, much more than onto our brother. Remembering her own dificulties and humiliations, her defense is to instill into her daughter the notion of fastidiousness. Is it surprising that the little girl wonders, at some deep level, What is so shameful about her that such iron control must guard against? A ground of anxiety has been laid, and we are only two.

I grew up without a father or brother, but by the time I was four I was already trying to pee standing up, to control that all-important function. You might ask where I got that idea – there was no male in the house to see, let alone envy. Does that mean I never saw the neighbor's little boy peeing confidently behind a tree? Penis envy is born, not from the specific desire to be male, but to solve the problem of control, of mother's anxiety and shame, and our own.

In 1943, psychiatrist Clara Thompson wrote 'Women and Penis Envy' – a paper that significantly changed the course of psychoanalytic thinking. Dr Thompson's findings were that penis envy is primarily symbolic – a rationalization for women's feelings of inadequacy in a patriarchal society.

'. . . Cultural factors,' she wrote, 'can explain the tendency of women to feel inferior about their sex and their consequent tendency to envy men . . . The attitude called Penis Envy is similar to the attitude of any underprivileged group toward those in power.'[2]

In a male-dominated society, the penis is seen as the symbol of the more privileged sex. In a matriarchal culture the symbol of power might be the breast or pregnant abdomen. A Boer child raised in an African tribe would wish her skin were black. In our own lives, we may envy our friend Louise's curly hair, *but we do not want to be Louise*. Similarly, we may envy the penis – the obvious 'extra' boys have – without wanting to be men ourselves. Penis envy is merely what the words say, before Freud overweighted the phrase: it is *anatomical* envy, not *gender* envy.

'Unfortunately,' says Dr Schaefer, 'the phrase still holds anxiety for many women. Despite all our denials, we are afraid it might be true, bringing with it all the horrid notions of 'the castrating woman' – even though today only the most rigid of Freudians still take the idea literally. We know now that women's feelings of being 'less' are due to society in general, and mother in particular, not putting the same value on a girl's sex as they do her brother's. The constellation of self-depreciation called penis envy is not biologically imbued but is a learned piece of social behavior.'

While I believe Clara Thompson is right to think penis envy in part due to the male's greater cultural status, in my gut I feel the problem begins earlier and closer to home – with the little girl's perception that her anatomy causes problems with mother that little boys do not have. In the end, however, it does not matter. Both ideas work together to produce low self-esteem in women.

In context, penis envy can be seen as part of the little girl's exploration of the idea of herself and reality. 'It's not so much a problem of envy,' says Dr Sanger, 'as of perfectionism. The little girl wants a penis, but she also wants a vagina, she wants to smoke a pipe like daddy and wants a tail like Black Beauty in the movies.'

When a little girl looks at her parents, she doesn't have mother's breasts or other easily visible signs of adult sexuality. Mother's promise that we will grow into these things is difficult to imagine. For the boy, the promise is less abstract. He looks at his father and thinks, 'Well, at least I have a start. Even if mine is smaller, it will grow, just as I am growing.' Says Dr Sanger: 'It's like being given the key to the car, and told actual possession will come in twenty years. At least you have the key, a tangible promise to grow on.'

On the other hand, the little girl has only her mother's promise that a penis is not more enviable than a vagina, that when she grows up, she will be glad to have a vagina. This assurance is one of the most important things a mother can give her girl; but it must be based on the girl's perception that her mother is telling her what she really feels. The little girl wants to believe mother, and so if penis envy is no problem to mother, it is soon forgotten by the daughter.

'When my daughter was two and one half,' says Dr Fredland, 'she became interested in penises. She would say she wanted to stand up to make wee-wee like the boys – which is universal. I told her penises are very nice, but that she had a beautiful vagina. "Do I? OK, let me see it," she would say. So I would hold her up in front of the mirror. That satisfied her but the next thing she wanted was a baby. At three and one half she recognized she couldn't, so she said I should have the baby and I should give it to her. At first, she said she would nurse the baby from the breast, but then she said she'd feed it from the bottle. "Why are you going to feed it from the bottle instead of nursing it at your breast?" I said. She looked at me very angrily and scornfully and said, "You know perfectly well that I don't have any breasts." She was very hurt. The next thing she wanted, of course, were breasts. One phase succeeded another.'

Today, Dr Fredland's daughter wants hair on her vagina. Tomorrow, who knows? A little girl should keep wanting things until she's tried enough to know what she does want. After penises, breasts, hair on her vagina, with luck she'll shift her attention outward; she'll go on to envy people who have self-esteem and courage, who are aviators or philosophers. If her childhood training has not left her feeling vulnerable from within, and if her problems of controlling her body are resolved, she will have just that much more energy to face what reality offers.

In the end, mother must and does win the battle of the chamber pot. Our loss is that all too often we have come to think that the source of our pleasure and our waste are one and the same. Mother's confusing instructions have set up a kind of Lady Macbeth phobia: we will never be able to wash away the taint (to the joy of makers of vaginal sprays and the blue chemicals we flush through our toilet bowls).

I'd hate to tell you how old I was before I learned that the Tampax I'd been inserting for years didn't enter the same passage through which I urinated. I'd always wondered why the Tampax didn't block the urine – *but not enough to ask.*

There is in fact a name for this kind of thinking, and it describes women like me who long resisted trying to locate our holes and to undertstand their functions. It is called 'the cloaca concept.' Like the word 'symbiosis,' it resonated within me with multilevel meanings the first time I heard it. It was an emotional summing up of years of untalked-about experience, an explanation of the cultural put-down of the 'cloacal' vagina, compared to the cleaner, more estimable penis.

The cloaca is the one opening in the body of simple, lower animals such as earthworms. It serves both excretory and sexual functions. Many little girls have this unthought-out idea – a 'feeling' – that they urinate and defecate out of the one place, and that babies are perhaps born out of it too. Later, this confusion spreads to include the notion that sex itself is connected with this one opening – which leads us to think our sexual organs are dirty, not-to-be-mentioned, in the same way that we learned during toilet training to feel no great pride in the function of the anus. 'Many mothers are terribly confused about their anatomy,' says Dr Robertiello. 'By the time she's given birth, a woman will usually have learned the difference between her urethra, vagina and anus, but there is a split between intellectual grasp and emotional belief. During toilet training she may pass on to her daughter the confusion that these three areas are all lumped together in one idea, "down there," or "your bottom".'

'When I was little,' says a thirty-five-year-old woman who was valedictorian of her graduating class, 'some girl said that babies come out of where you wee-wee. I just rejected that out of hand, because any fool can see if you look at the navel that it's a drawstring. When the time came you just opened up the drawstring, took out the baby, and pulled the drawstring back. I really didn't learn about sex until my sophomore year at college. But I've never liked a man to touch me down there, never.'

Men too have problems with bad body images: they grow up under the shadow of the Marlboro Man. Eventually, though, they find more important things to worry about. It is their lot in life to be judged by their accomplishments. They may worry that they are too tall or thin, but even the ugliest man can find women, if he's successful enough. But our culture's heavy emphasis on the need for beauty in women, all by itself, does not explain why even the loveliest women are unable to believe they are beautiful. It's almost a joke: compliment a woman on her face or legs and she will sigh and say, 'But if only my breasts were bigger.' Nothing is ever perfect, something always needs changing.

We don't understand it ourselves. We show our best friend a photo of the two of us taken last summer; she is lean and beautiful in her bikini. 'What a terrible picture!' she cries, and tears it up. 'I'm going on a diet!' Nothing we say can persuade her that she is already svelte and slim. Women's magazines know there is one never-fail cover story: Elizabeth Taylor Does Not Believe She Is Beautiful! Impossible as that idea seems to be, we buy the magazine because we know it's true; after all, Elizabeth Taylor is a woman, isn't she?

We all have something to hide. Why else would society build us stalls and cubicles with locks to undress and urinate in, when men are left to get on with it in large, communal, open locker rooms? And in these locker rooms, men shower together whether they are fat or skinny or bowlegged; they wrestle and snap towels, their bodies touch or not, they stand in front of adjoining urinals, holding their penises in their hands while they urinate and talk about sex. They may lie, but on the whole they are easy with each other, unselfconscious. Why are women different about this?

'I don't think I've ever met a woman whose mother said anything positive to her about her genitals,' reports Dr Fredland. 'On the contrary, they were all warned against promiscuity at the least, and threatened at the worst if they masturbated or got too interested in boys. Most women can't touch themselves and can't imagine anyone else getting any pleasure touching them there. It's what an analyst friend of mine wryly calls "lack of vaginal self-respect".'

By the time the high school teacher rolls down the anatomical charts in the classroom and runs the sex education film, we are beyond seeing the separation of the urethra and vagina; an invisible veil of embarrassment glazes our vision, as real as the sheet we will later clutch in front of our bodies when we visit the gynecologist. By then, we are so trained in myopia that we can't 'see' the plaster cast on the desk. I ask Vera Plaskon, who is twenty-eight and teaches sex education to teen-agers at New York's Roosevelt Hospital, if this idea gibed with her experience. 'Have I run into it?' she laughs. 'I went through it myself! That couldn't be me! I thought. Those plaster casts are so inhuman-looking. Women know they have arms and legs, hands, a tongue . . . but they have disassociated themselves from their genitals, particularly their internal organs. Don't look, don't touch. Everything down there is dirty. In our work here at Roosevelt, we try to give young girls information. But more important, a feeling that their body is a good body. By six or eight, we have such poor body images.'

'Women's ignorance about their bodies is learned behavior,'

says gynecologist Marcia Storch. 'Little girls are taught to be frightened and insecure where their bodies are concerned. At the opposite end of the pole we have The Great Sex Queen Person, who is held up to be very, very special. Since you cannot attain that position, you are ashamed of the body you are given. So young girls get it from both directions, forced to aspire to something they know they will never be.'

Why are we never satisfied? Why the incredible importance taken on by our fat thighs and small breasts, why can we think only of our faults and so rarely take pleasure in what is fine or beautiful about us? Why the displacement of attention from our *selves* to our bodies — as if that is all we are?

Because these nagging worries are displacements indeed!

We never get over our worries about our waists and weight because they are not the real, unmentionable, and unthinkable root of our concern. Complaining about our skin, our calves, distracts our attention from that other area mother would never mention, that had no name, that made her face distort with disgust if it got dirty. We say it is our breasts, our thighs, that are ugly; we fear it is our vagina.

When we do give our sexuality expression, we do it blindly. We close our eyes when we masturbate. We get drunk so that the next morning we can feign ignorance and not take responsibility for our pleasure. 'I don't remember a thing I did.' When a loving man kisses us between our legs, we have a fantasy of a stranger we need never see again rather than the man who is actually doing it. We fear that he won't be expert enough to find our secret clitoris, and pray that if he does, he will fight his boredom and dislike long enough to get us past our own learned repugnance. Was there ever any man more adored than he who finally gets through to us that he knows our secret and loves it?

The fashion and cosmetic industries didn't create women's dissatisfaction with our bodies. Commerce merely preys upon an already learned insecurity, putting a dollar sign in front of the hope that someday we may find something that makes us smell, taste, and feel good about ourselves. Those who would encourage women to reject 'meaningless' preoccupation with beauty and get on with the real business of being equal – without first explaining the very significant fear underlying this preoccupation – are merely offering women another piece of uncertain ground. Self-acceptance cannot be built on blind denial. Why do we spend too much money on clothes, too many hours over facials? Because we can't believe anyone would want us as we are. Convince a woman that her vagina is beautiful, and you have the makings of an 'equal' person. I believe this with all my heart.

Our attitude toward menstruation is a vivid example of the power of emotion over intellect. My mother wanted to give me the information she had. I needed that information. I am certain she tried, but our crossed emotions got in the way. As I think back to that crucial moment in our lives, I feel we were enacting a universal mother-daughter drama. She could not give me the facts in a way I could hear; because listening was hard for me, she became even more inhibited herself. For most of us the results are the same: grown women of twenty-five or forty-five, we are not easy about a function which more than any other sums up what we've subliminally been taught to feel about that part of our bodies: it is not nice.

In my entire research on the mother-daughter relationship, I have found no aspect more ruled by contradiction, loss of memory, confusion, and denial than menstruation. There is no behavior about which we express such cool certainty, but over which we have less control.

To be fair to mothers in general, and my own in particular: 'Often there's no way you can tell a child about something in advance,' says Dr Sanger. 'People often talk about everything but what really is important. The same is true of listening. There is a general anxiety about facing something new. The case of the student who can't open a book until the night before the exam is similar to the inability to listen to your mother's description of menstruation before it begins.'

Long before we are eleven or twelve we have been aware that

mother bleeds once a month – something that is difficult not to learn in any household. (If by some extraordinary arrangement, mother has kept us from knowing it, that speaks perhaps loudest of all.) By the time we reach puberty, we already know how mother feels about *anything* connected with sex. If she likes her own body, takes care of it, is proud of it, we too may feel pride in becoming a woman. If she enjoys men, if she doesn't become someone we don't recognize when she's around them – then, when she takes us to lunch and tells us that we are beginning 'the most beautiful part of a woman's life,' we may believe her.

'I get such mixed emotions about her growing up, going to high school,' says a mother of a premenstrual twelve-year-old. 'I'm proud of her, but I know that she's going to be leaving me. It's very ambivalent, these feelings when your daughter begins to menstruate and goes into a new, grown-up phase of life. I see my own life changing.

Gynecologist Marcia Storch tells me of an eleven-year-old who had just begun menstruating but refused to wear Kotex, or anything. Then she saw the mother, an intelligent, politically active woman; the deeper implications of the problem came out. The mother was upset that her 'baby' had started menstruating. 'The basic message the mother was sending the girl was anxiety,' says Dr Storch. 'So the daughter was trying to hide what had provoked her mother's fears. The story is not uncommon. A lot of girls pretend they haven't really begun because of the negative emotion it arouses in their mothers.'

Says psychiatrist Dr Lilly Engler: 'Many mothers don't want to face their daughter's menstruation because it means the girl is now sexual. If there's another woman in the house, it makes her the 'older' woman. I've known mothers who really want to prepare a daughter and even think they *have* done it . . . but have not. We don't like to admit this, but it often has to do with jealousy.'

On the other side of the oedipal door, 'menstruation reminds a young girl that her mother is sexual in a way she cannot deny,' says Dr Schaefer. 'A girl of fourteen came to see me. She could not understand her own reluctance to discuss menstruation with her mother. She said she "hated" it, that suddenly her mother was "connected with the whole business." She was worried, guilty that she no longer felt as close to her mother.'

Until we begin to menstruate, we have some distance from mother. We identify with her, but we are not like her. It is a kind of freedom. The gulf allows us to ignore the facts of her life we don't yet want to face. We ask questions, open doors, but when we bump into facts we aren't ready for, we close the door, forget what we just saw or heard, and go back to our childish games. But once we begin to menstruate, we can't look away. Her life is ours. Having to understand what the periodic cycle means to mother makes us unable to avoid any longer recognizing that mom is not merely the kindly, 'pure,' and totally unsexual being we had always assumed, but is as irrationally taken by the same erotic desires as we. She feels our emotions and knows the same excitements as we do within our own bodies. It is disturbing. Obscure oedipal conflicts are stirred up. She is not only our mother, she is a woman too. And a rival.

Two years ago I interviewed an eleven-year-old girl. She was very much looking forward to menstruation. 'It's funny,' she said, 'how the older girls who've started don't like to talk about it, but my friends and I, we've decided to throw a party for the first one of us who begins. I hope it's me!' Times have changed, I thought. Six months later, I saw her again. 'Did you get that party?' I asked. 'Oh, that.' She shrugged off the subject, not embarrassed, just uninterested. When I interviewed the girl's mother she said, 'The day she began, I suggested that we all go out to dinner to celebrate, but my daughter said, "Oh, no, please don't tell daddy!" '

The excitement of becoming 'one of the girls' quickly disappears. Becoming a woman isn't a rite of passage into a new and exciting world; it's more of the same, more waiting to be asked before you can go anywhere, do anything, more dependence on others. More tension with mother too; she watches us with a new anxiety. Being a woman means being 'less'. The little girl who used to strut about with one of her mother's Kotex between her legs feels no excitement now when she puts it on to do its real job. Whatever feelings of achievement and sexual identity menstruation brings with it are soon diminished by old, rearoused memories of feeling unclean in 'that place'.

The truth is that menstruation poses for every woman a Janus-faced problem. It points us inexorably forward into womanhood. At the same time it turns us back, regressing us in its own unheeding manner to that earlier time when we were unable to control our bodies. Suddenly we are back in touch with emotions we haven't felt in years, the primitive shame that went with wetting our bed, bad odors, soiling our clothes. The humiliation of involuntary or untimely excretion has been so pounded into us by years of zealous toilet training that to avoid it we have learned absolute control, iron control, control so rigid that neither our bladder nor sphincter dare to let go even while we are asleep. Abruptly, we are back in the middle of all that.

The enemy steals upon us in the night. We wake with the sick feeling that there is no way to hide the evidence. So humiliating is the return of these old emotions that we hide from them, repress them, determined not to think about menstruation in any but the most commonsense manner. Is it any wonder that, later, the repression has worked only too well, and we forget to discuss this 'dirty' side of menstruation with our daughters? Of course not – we are still ashamed ourselves.

Every woman remembers her first day: 'I was wearing my sister's pajamas, and when I saw the blood...' 'My mother had given me a book, it was blue and beige...' 'We were on our way to Europe, on the *Queen Elizabeth!* I thought the blood was from being seasick...' 'My mother made me stay home from school and go to bed, which puzzled me...' These details are stenciled on our brains, like a screen behind which we can hide everything else associated with menstruation. 'The book had a cow and her calf on the cover,' a woman says twenty-five years later, but when you ask her what her mother told her, she says, 'She told me nothing.' When you ask the mother, she says, 'I told her everything.' Rashomon.

'And what do you feel today about menstruation?' I ask the same woman. 'What is there to feel?' she smiles. Nothing.

'My mother slapped my face when I showed her my bloody clothes,' is how a twice-divorced woman, who is a lawyer and a grandmother, remembers her first menstruation. Her voice is still indignant. I share this anger until, months later, someone tells me it is a customary Jewish rite for the mother to slap the daughter's face at this time. The lawyer had wanted me to share her resentment rather than understand the custom. Did this woman's mother indeed use the ritual slap as an excuse for her own anger at being faced with a sexual situation she felt unable to handle? Or is her anger the emotion she needs to displace onto her mother to express the disappointment she has found in her own sexuality? Throughout our interview, anger is her dominant emotion about her sex, about her mother, about men, about her own daughter, and what it is to be a woman.

In contrast, here is a story another woman tells me: 'I was so happy when I began. I was eleven. Up till then I had felt like an oddball. I was two years ahead of myself at school. Everyone else was thirteen. They'd all begun long before. I knew these intimate things made my mother uncomfortable, so I went to my closest friends. It was thrilling. For the first time in my life, I was like every other girl.'

How we remember the onset of menstruation is largely determined by how we feel about our sexuality today. If we are easy about sex in our grown lives, we will remember any embarrassment, shame, or fear attending that first time with a rueful smile, maybe a laugh. If sex is a problem now, *that* was one of the first signs of trauma. It was clear to me in this interview that this woman likes her sexuality. She wants to like her mother. That her mother was shy, and did not prepare her, is not so important as that her mother was consistent. By not lying to her daughter, not pretending a false confidence, she freed the girl to turn to people who could help. That's how mother was. How we get through menstruation, loss of virginity, marriage, childbirth . . . it is all of a piece.

There may be mothers who feel they have failed in preparing their daughters for menstruation. I have rarely met one. At the very least they say, 'I didn't have to tell her. She knows more than I do. They pick it up from their friends.' But I could count on one hand the women who feel they themselves were prepared – not with equipment, but with an intelligent, accepting and emotional understanding of their bodies. I agree with gynecologist Marcia Storch that a girl's peers are probably her best teachers in sex and menstruation; most mothers are still too emotionally indoctrinated in their own generation's inhibited attitudes to avoid giving the girl a double message. But the fact remains: whether we get the information in school or from our friends, we are still stuck with the sexual attitudes of the woman who riised us. 'The parents do the primary and longer-lasting sexual education of the child,' says Dr Mary Calderone, 'whether they know it or not: good or bad, positive or negative, inevitably *they do it*.'

Dr Fredland makes an important point: 'There is a kind of regression that goes on in the mother-daughter relationship. The mother tends either to repeat what her parents have done or to undo it – to do exactly the opposite – which is sometimes just as bad. Usually, of course, it is an uncertain oscillation between the two. For instance, if a woman had a very inhibited mother herself, who told her nothing about menstruation, she may be determined to prepare her daughter better. But what does she do? She leaves a book on the girl's bedside table. *This is so much more than her mother did for her,* that she feels she has told her daughter "all about it".'

Menstruation is the elimination of a waste product. We all go through it. Why then should it not be something we share, a common experience that ties women together? 'If men menstruated, they would probably find a way to brag about it,' writes a male reviewer of a recent book on menstruation.

'Most like they [men] would regard it as spontaneous ejaculation, an excess of vital spirits. Their cup runneth over, their sexuality supererogates. They would see themselves as "spending" blood in a plenitude of conspicuous waste. Blood, after all, is generally considered a good. "Blood sports" used to be the true test of manhood and at the successful conclusion of a boy's first hunt, he used to be "blooded". All that is turned around when it is the woman who bleeds. Bleeding is interpreted as a sign of infirmity, inferiority, uncleanliness, and irrationality.'[3]

'One of the first things I found out in working with women and health,' says Paula Weideger, author of *Menstruation and Menopause*, 'is that absolutely every woman, no matter what she looks like, thinks something about her is ugly. In my view, that is closely related to thinking there is something *centrally* wrong with you – and that thing is menstruation.'

'My daughter has become so modest, I haven't seen her undressed in over a year now,' says a mother of a thirteen-year-old. 'She's always worrying about herself, always bathing, always washing her hair. Suddenly all she wants to do is diet. She has a beautiful little figure, but she's never satisfied with it.' Everything seems to happen at once in puberty. How can anything feel right? Of course, we want our privacy. Then, simultaneous with pubic hair, the lift of a breast, the curve of a thigh, comes menstruation. We cannot face the real source of our discomfort. Instead, we begin our life pattern of dieting and unhappiness about our bodies, but we cannot diet away our vagina nor wash it clean. We cannot face the idea that dissatisfaction with our bodies begins with what we have been taught to feel about our genitals.

We pretend disinterest in a function that begins on an hour and day of its own choosing, that may make us irritable, that can cause pain, public embarrassment, that makes us reject our men sexually or feel rejected by them. Again and again I warn my husband about my evil temper prior to my period; again and again I am aware of how true it is – after the fact, after my period has begun, after the quarrel. When I was seventeen, my best friend – like many other brides – planned her wedding around her menstrual cycle. Inexorably, it began as she was, literally, stepping into her wedding dress. We bridesmaids stood about her in horror.

Medical research shows that the brain affects our menstrual cycle; it may even control it. We also know that what goes on hormonally at the time of menstruation feeds back into the brain. But no doctor can tell you exactly how or why. The amount of control menstruation has over our lives is indeed so profound emotionally and physically that we can only deal with it in silence and denial. We douse ourselves with perfume – *against what smell?* We make a fetish of clean, clean, clean underwear – *against what soiling?* After telling me the story of her first day – a memory still alive with anger, pride, accomplishment, whatever – every woman I interviewed, including women doctors, then says, 'What's there to discuss? It's like fingernails, hair – they grow. It's just a fact of life. What's there to feel?' Different as our individual stories may be about the onset of menstruation, we're all agreed without words that there is nothing more to talk about – which means it doesn't have to be talked about at all. 'A whole book about menstruation?' women said to Paula Weideger when she began her research. 'How do you find enough to say about that?'

Dismissed: a function that has been the subject of myth, speculation, mystery, and taboo since the world began, a function that is unique in every woman's life and that ends one day just as it began: unannounced. We prefer superstition to knowledge. Says Jessie Potter: 'My experience has been that seventy-five percent of women in this country (and that's a modest estimate), couldn't give an explanation of menstrual periods to a sixth grader. They don't know how it happens, have little or no idea of what does go on in their bodies.'

'Not many other people thought menstruation worth a course on its own,' says Paula Weideger about her experience teaching women's health. 'The attitude was you just give women the nuts and bolts stuff about the egg and the uterus and that's it.' Her book, published in 1976, was the *first* on menstruation ever brought out by a major publishing house with intent to reach a large popular audience. Nevertheless, when she began to publicize her book, TV talk shows invariably focused the discussion less on menstruation than on menopause. They said it was because their audiences were 'health oriented.' What does that say? That they found menstruation unhealthy?

'One media woman who interviewed me,' continues Ms Weideger, 'said she knew all she needed about menstruation. "Therefore," she told me, "your book is useless to me." But as we continued to talk, she kept coming back to one subject. "Maybe you can tell me why I sometimes feel so ashamed when I go to buy tampons?" I explained to her the primitive notions of shame, feeling dirty, et cetera, that are so often attached to menstruation in our society. "Oh, no," she said. "I don't feel like that at all. But why am I ashamed to buy tampons?"'

A woman recently told me of an event she still finds almost unbearable to speak about, though it happened twelve years ago. She had been in love with a handsome man, who at last asked her out. In time they went to bed, but to her horror when she woke up before him in the morning, she discovered her period had started. 'I knew just what I had to do,' she said with only half a smile. 'I got up like a thief, put on my clothes and sneaked out of his apartment. I would never go out with him again, even though he phoned and phoned to ask.' Her humiliation was so great she could not face the man even though she was in love with him. (Or because she was in love with him?)

To pr$pare for writing this chapter, I play back a taped interview with Dr Sanger; I hear myself break up with laughter when he says, 'It's a shame more women can't see the beauty of their menstrual cycles. How can a woman not want to learn what's going on in her body? The beauty of the ovaries, the fantastic performance of the Fallopian tube . . .' On the tape, my voice interrupts, changing the subject. Do you too find his comments nervously funny? What does that say about us as women?

We are so embarrassed about menstruation that we cannot abide to hear it spoken about even if in a complimentary manner. We believe the words must be merely empty flattery, and only fools are taken in by flattery.

Men have always been willing to play the clown. A little boy will fart in class. It is thought to be embarrassing perhaps, but essentially funny. It is no laughing matter when a little girl farts. It is dreadful.

When men go through a humiliating experience, they may get mad, curse, or fight. Then they have a drink, make a joke about the whole thing, and laugh it off. 'You know those terrible roast programs they have on TV, where all the men make fun of the star?' a woman says to me. 'Well, last week they had a woman as guest of honor. When they began knocking her for being ugly, about her shape and her funny hair, I got terribly uncomfortable.' When a woman is insulted, made fun of, if she gets drunk or stains her clothes, we look away. It is so painful, it hurts. Low self-esteem, rooted in notions that there is something wrong with our body, makes us more the prey to feelings of humiliation than men. There is no space for light-hearted kidding.

Humiliation is perhaps the most persistent of all emotions. In time we forget feelings of passion, the faces of people we've loved. We laugh at old angers and rages, time heals the memory of even physical pain. But old humiliations stay with us for life. They wake us out of the deepest sleep and flush our face with shame and anger even when we are alone. 'Patients with problems of humiliation,' says Dr Robertiello, 'are the most difficult to treat.' Humiliation is so powerful it can make us wish for our own annihilation: our very ego shrinks and wills itself for the moment no longer to exist. 'I felt as if I wanted the ground to open up and swallow me.' The strongest feeling of humiliation, according to all the psychotherapists I have consulted, are those associated with soiling ourselves in public, with loss of body control. In the end this is perhaps the most difficult barrier to accepting menstruation: we have no control over this new body function. What is worse, nobody has warned us about this aspect of it.

Perhaps, too overcome by the excitement of the awaited event, we don't feel shame the first day we bleed. Eventually it surfaces. In all the talk about beauty and being a woman, why has nobody warned us, for instance, about the smell? And if nobody has mentioned it, it must be the most terrible smell of all. The surprise of it, the silence in which we experience it, our isolation in feeling we alone are fouling the air of everyone near us – all double the shame.

What I myself liked about the pill was that you always knew when you would menstruate, the flow was less and so were the cramps. Psychologist Karen Page finds a direct relationship between heaviness of flow and high menstrual tension. In her studies,[4] the women who were less anxious and moody during menstruation, who tended to ignore the old taboos against sex, swimming, etc., tended to bleed less. Dr Page traces anxiety about menstruation to cultural taboos: the menstruating woman is unclean. Psychoanalytic authorities tend to give more importance to early childhood experiences – overly rigid toilet training, and consequent shame over loss of body control. My own feeling is that it is a question of emphasis – both factors undoubtedly enter. The important fact is that no matter what the reason, the humiliation is there.

'But,' you say, '*I* feel no shame about menstruation!'

'Emotions as painful to handle as humiliation about a body function,' says Dr Robertiello, 'tend to be repressed. We "forget" them.'

Psychiatrists say that when we are little, we think everyone else shits ice cream. Only we make a foul mess. If no one, especially mother, mentions the embarrassment that goes with loss of body control in menstruation, it must be that other women don't bleed like us: they merely bedew themselves with the attar of roses. We are the only ones whose dark, often clotted blood flows from the heart of mystery. What have we to do with those beautiful women, gowned by Givenchy, stepping out of the limousine in the Modess Because advertisements?

And yet with infernal cleverness, the Modess Because ads go right to the root of our unease. Giant market research companies know that during her period a woman feels unattractive and nervous about what she is wearing, so they associate their product with the most beautiful – and most beautifully dressed – women they can find. They are saying to us that what they sell is the antidote to our feelings of wounded narcissism; but perhaps they will forgive me if, while I salute their diagnosis, I do not buy their cure.

The best protection against feelings of humiliation associated with menstruation is to have a mother who believed in positive narcissistic training in our earliest years, who rewarded us with love and praise for learning control of our body functions. Rather than feeling disgusted and shamed when we didn't perform for her, we would have emerged with a sense of mastery and self-achievement. A mother like this would probably have been trained in the same way by her mother, since the most difficult ideas to change late in life are those of low self-esteem. If she didn't feel as good about her body and ours as she said she did, we would have gotten the old double message: 'Don't feel as I do, but as I say.'

Menstruation – the great fact of life which mother and daughter share – becomes the dirty secret that pushes us apart. 'In my practice,' says Dr Robertiello, 'I've known people with delusions. They can never form relationships because to be with them, the friend or lover has to believe the delusion too. The sheer lack of reality causes too much strain, and the relationship breaks up.' Mother says menstruation is beautiful but the daughter knows in mother's life that is a lie.

Menstruation is beginning younger and younger. We may like the idea of sexual liberation – 'I wish things had been this free when I was a kid!' – but we don't like to think that gynecologists are now seeing nine-year-olds. 'There isn't a decent book available, no good information for girls in the eight to twelve bracket,' says gynecologist Marcia Storch.

'The first reason mothers give me for not wanting their daughters to use tampons,' says Jessie Potter, 'is that it will break the hymen. But what it really is, is an inability to encourage the girl to bend over, look for the vagina, put something in it, take something out, touch herself. Even physicians, who should know better, still imply it's better to wait until you are more grown up to use them. We still want to deny a girl access to her genitals, to put distance between her and her body. We could teach women who are reluctant to have sex during menstruation that they can put a diaphragm up there to hold back the blood, but we don't – as simple a piece of information as that is.'

Kids will tell you that things are different now, that 'menstruation isn't a big deal like it used to be.' When Paula Weideger was talking to twelve- and fourteen-year-olds, she did find them less embarrassed than her own generation, 'but they would gleefully tell me how they could get a male teacher to let them off homework by hinting they had cramps. They *use* menstruation.' When Ms. Weideger asked if they ever mentioned menstruation to boys, 'Oh, no!' was the universal chorus.

One of the most self-proclaimed liberated women I have interviewed, a well-known writer of twenty-seven, laughingly talks about a man whose summer house she visits. 'I don't want to fuck him,' she says, 'so each time I go out there I say I can't because I'm having my period. He must think it's the longest one in history.' If you use menstruation effectively enough as a barrier – against sex, work, or anything else – pretty soon you will believe it too.

Contrary to the fable this writer foisted off on her summer host, there is evidence that for many women sex relieves cramps. Sex, especially before and during menstruation, keeps the muscles limber – the opposite of cramped. How much more pleasurable than a bottle of Midol and a heating pad. You would think every gynecologist in the country would suggest at least we try it. But sex therapists tell me that many gynecologists are too shy to discuss sex with their patients. I myself have found that sex when I am bleeding, when my body is at its most 'unattractive', is often the best. It makes me believe myself loved as can no mere verbal protestations of 'I love you'.

Men offer one of our great opportunities to dissolve the maternal inheritance of negative feelings about our body. How they feel about menstruation is therefore significant. 'Men get their attitudes about menstruation from women,' says Dr Robertiello when I ask his opinion on this subject. 'That it is something secret, not to be discussed, to be avoided as much as possible. Women can be insane about not wanting men to know they are menstruating. The analytic explanation is that they make the man into the parent who is going to judge them as being "dirty children". Even without menstruation women see the man's organ as being cleaner than their own. For instance, a menstruating woman may try to conceal the evidence of her "waste". She will wrap her sanitary napkin in layers of paper, and carry it outside to his garbage can rather than leave it in his nice clean wastebasket. It is also why most women don't want to have sex with men at this time. In a woman's eyes, since he doesn't share this dirtiness with her, he will look down upon her with tremendous contempt. The woman projects onto a man this demandingly "clean" parent, unconsciously left over from the toilet-training period, who is going to see her as dirty, disgusting, not acceptable.'

When I went home and thought about this, I felt that as far as he went, Dr Robertiello sounded right. But I felt there must be something more. I called him. 'Couldn't men's difficulty about menstruation,' I asked, 'be due not only to their picking up on the woman's embarrassment, but to some emotion of their own they bring to the subject?'

What I like best about Richard Robertiello is that he is always willing to rethink any idea, no matter how long he has held it, nor how grounded it may be in conventional psychoanalytic theory. He heard me out and then said, 'You know, I remember as a boy thinking how mysterious menstruation seemed to me. And what you don't understand tends to frighten you. Today, even though I have an MD's knowledge of the physical facts, and a psychoanalyst's knowledge of the psychology of menstruation, I still find it mysterious.'

He went on: 'Yes, there must be an anxiety in men about menstruation that women sense. What creates men's anxiety is not only that it is a mystery connected with female anatomy. It is also a reminder of another feminine mystery – allied, but not the same. It is the power to reproduce. Men don't have this power, so it makes them edgy. And finally, women's mysterious powers rearouse another unconscious anxiety in men: at one time, a woman was all-powerful in every man's life . . . when he was a baby. Her sex once gave her power over him, and now that he's grown up, do you think those humiliations are all forgotten? Not in the unconscious, they're not. Also, if her sex gave her power over him then, might it not happen again? Men's safest bet was never to give women a chance to have power again. And they went right to the heart of any person's strongest feelings of identity – the power of total sexual acceptance and freedom.'

As recently as our great-grandmother's day, women's power was thought to rest in her voracious sexuality. Certain male surgeons in the mid-nineteenth century won immense prestige for inventing instruments and operations that would remove women's clitorises, the source of their 'dark sexual appetites'. The same woman who was deified as the creator of character and the custodian of familial and even national morality was feared as the potential ruination of every strong man. These surgical excisions were performed for the sake of the power balance. A male fear and injustice, yes – but it is women who keep guard over women, mother who cuts us off, not only from our clitoris but from our vagina. What women feel they must protect and deny through fear, women can learn to release.

Menstruation has never kept me from anything, from that first horseback ride to sex today. But as I began to write this chapter, my period began (a week early) and I had my first and worst cramps in years. Every beginning I wrote seemed superficial. Something was missing, nothing I wrote resonated with the deep, inner conviction – *That's right, that's how it is!* I had to get up from my typewriter twice, almost shaken by anxiety, to walk across Central Park in the April sunshine to resume a conversation with Dr Robertiello.

When he had stressed the emotions of shame and humiliation buried beneath women's matter-of-fact attitudes toward menstruation, I had shrugged him off. I had decided his opinions were overly colored by experience with women who came to him for help. I had identified myself more strongly with Dr Schaefer and the majority of women who say they have no particular feelings about menstruation: it happens, that's all. But in the face of some unexplainable resistance, I now realised I had no easy reply to Dr Robertiello's question during our last talk: 'OK, then, Nancy, you tell me why you are having such a difficult time writing what you say is just a straightforward chapter on one of the simple facts of life?'

It is troublesome to have cramps, humiliating to stain your clothes, to be caught somewhere bleeding and unprepared. But I would rather bleed than not. I remember how disturbed I was when I was on the pill and would miss a period entirely. Doctors told me not to worry, that it was 'normal.' But I did worry. I wanted it, blood and all. I wanted that reminder. When I read of primitive tribes who were in religious awe that women could bleed once a month and not die, something in me resonates to their emotions. 'No, I don't feel any strong personal emotions about menstruation,' says Dr Schaefer. 'But I am glad I still do.' She is in her early fifties. Although she more than any woman I know realizes the falsity in the myth that sex ends with the end of menstruation, I am sure she will feel 'something' when she reaches menopause.

Menstruation alone does not explain women's problems with humiliation – no more than my difficulty with this chapter has to do only with unconscious anxieties. Our feelings about menstruation are the image of what it is to be a woman in this culture. While menstruation and the fear of revealing evidence of loss of body control bear possibilities of humiliation for women of which men are not aware, it is humiliating too to be that sex whose voice and presence carry less significance. It is humiliating to speak the same words as a man and have his heard, and not yours. It is humiliating to feel invisible when God gave you a body as solid as his. It is humiliating that women are accorded little dignity unless they are married. We twist these humiliations around, of course, and say it is glorious to have a man fight our battles for us, put us on a pedestal, take care of us. It is, if you enjoy being dependent on someone else.

There are other emotions as secretive as the shame that surrounds menstruation. They are the feelings that remind us of life, that we can give life, and that we are still alive, young – sexually capable of reproducing ourselves. It is difficult to tell an eleven-year-old daughter about these inchoate and complex stirrings of sexuality, life, and death which are hers to live with. How do you describe the awe that has always surrounded reproduction, the mystery and emotion that such a gift (the power to reproduce) and such a curse (to bleed once a month) must arouse in those who do not share them?

How do you not?

CHAPTER FIVE

Competition

Although I didn't realize it at the time, my mother was getting prettier. My sister was a beauty. My adolescence was the time of our greatest estrangement.

I have a photo of the three of us when I was twelve: my mother, my sister Susie, and I, on a big chintz sofa, each on a separate cushion, leaning away from one another with big spaces in between. I grew up fired with a sense of family spirit, which I loved and needed, with aunts and uncles and cousins under the omnipotent umbrella of my grandfather. 'All for one and one for all,' he would say at summer reunions, and no one took it more seriously than I. I would have gone to war for any one of them, and believed they would do the same for me. But within our own little nucleus, the three of us didn't touch much.

Now, when I ask her why, my mother sighs and says she supposes it was because that was how she was raised. I remember shrinking from her Elizabeth Arden night-cream kiss, mumbling from under the blanket that yes, I had brushed my teeth. I had not. I had wet the toothbrush in case she felt it, feeling that would get even with her. For what? The further we all get from childhood, the more physically affectionate we try to be with one another. But we are still shy after all these years.

I was a late bloomer, like my mother. But my mother bloomed so late, or had such a penetrating early frost, that she believed it even less than I would in my turn. When she was a freckled sixteen and sitting shyly on her unfortunate hands, her younger sister was already a famous beauty. That is still the relationship between them. Grandmothers both, in their eyes my aunt is still the sleek-haired belle of the ball, immaculately handsome on a horse. My mother's successes do not count. They will argue at 2:00 a.m. over whether one of my aunt's many beaux ever asked my mother out. My mother could never make up a flattering story about herself. I doubt that she so much as heard the nice things men told her once she had grown into the fine-looking woman who smiles at me in family photos. But she always gives in to my aunt, much I'm sure as she gave in to the old self-image after my father died. He – that one splendidly handsome man – may have picked her out from all the rest, but his death just a few years later must have felt like some punishment for having dared to believe for a moment that her father was wrong: who could possibly want her? She still blushes at a compliment.

I think she was at her prettiest in her early thirties. I was twelve and at my nadir. Her hair had gone a delicate auburn red and she wore it brushed back from her face in soft curls. Seated beside her and Susie, who inherited a raven version of her beautiful hair, I look like an adopted person. But I had already defended myself against my looks. They were unimportant. There was a distance between me and the mirror commensurate with the growing distance between me and my mother and sister. My success with my made-up persona was proof: I didn't need them. My titles at school, my awards and achievements, so bolstered my image of myself that until writing this book I genuinely believed that I grew up feeling sorry for my sister. What chance had she alongside The Great Achiever and Most Popular Girl in the World? I even worked up some guilt about outshining her. Pure survival instinct? My dazzling smile would divert the most critical observer from comparing me to the cute, petite girls with whom I grew up. I switched the contest: don't look at my lank hair, my 5'10", don't notice that my right eye wanders bizarrely (though the eye doctor said it was useless to keep me in glasses); watch me tap dance, watch me win the game, let me make you happy! When I describe myself in those days my mother laughs. 'Oh, Nancy, you were such a darling little girl.' But I wasn't little any more.

I think my sister, Susie, was born beautiful, a fact that affected my mother and me deeply, though in different ways. I don't think it mattered so much until Susie's adolescence. She turned so lush one ached to look at her. Pictures of Susie then remind me of the young Elizabeth Taylor in *A Place in the Sun*. One has to almost look away from so much beauty. It scared my mother to death. Whatever had gone on between them before came to a head and has never stopped. Their constant friction determined me to get away from this house of women, to be free of women's petty competitions, to live on a bigger scale. I left home eventually but I've never gotten away from feeling how wonderful to be so beautiful your mother can't take her eyes off you, even if only to nag.

I remember an amazing lack of any feeling about my only sibling, with whom I shared a room for years, whose clothes were identical to mine until I was ten. Except for feelings of irritation when she tried to cuddle me when I was four, bursts of anger that erupted into fist fights which I started and won at ten, and after that, indifference, a calculated unawareness that has resulted in a terrible and sad absence of my sister in my life.

My husband says his sister was the only child his father ever paid any attention to: 'You have done to Susie what I did to my sister,' he says. 'You made her invisible.' Me, jealous of Susie, who never won a single trophy or had as many friends as I? I must have been insanely jealous.

I only allowed myself to face it twice. Both times happened in that twelfth year, when my usual defenses couldn't take the emotional cross currents of adolescence. When I did slash out is wasn't very glorious, no well-chosen words or contest on the tennis courts. I did it like a thief in the night. Nobody ever guessed it was I who poured the red nail polish down the front of Susie's new white eyelet evening dress the day of her first yacht club dance. When I stole her summer savings and threw her wallet down the sewer, mother blamed Susie for being so careless. I watched my sister accept the criticism with her mother's own resignation, and I felt some relief from the angry emotions that had hold of me.

When Susie went away to boarding school, I made jokes about how glad I was to be rid of her. It was our first separation. Conflicting urges, angers, and envies were coming at me from every direction; I had nothing left over to handle my terrible feelings of loss at her going. It was the summer I was plagued by what I called 'my thoughts'.

I read every book in the house as a talisman against thinking. I was afraid that if my brain were left idle for even one minute, these 'thoughts' would take over. Perhaps I feared they already had. Was my sister's going away the fulfillment of my own murderous wishes against her? I wrote in my first and only diary: 'Susie, come home, please come home!!!!!! I'm sorry, I'm sorry!!!!!!'

When I outgrew the Nancy Drew books for perfect attendance at Sunday school, and the Girl Scout badges for such merits as selling the most rat poison door to door, I graduated to prizes at the community theater. I won a plastic wake-up radio for the I Speak for Democracy contest. I was captain of the athletic association, president of the student government, and had the lead in the class play, all in the same year. In fact, I wrote the class play. It might have been embarrassing, but no one else wanted these prizes. Scoring home runs and getting straight As weren't high on the list of priorities among my friends. (The South takes all prizes for raising noncompetitive women.) In the few cases where anyone did give me a run for the money, I had an unbeatable incentive: my grandfather's applause. It was he for whom I ran.

I can't remember ever hearing my grandfather say to my mother, 'Well done, Jane.' I can't remember my mother ever saying to my sister, 'Well done, Susie.' And I never gave my mother the chance to say it to me. She was the last to hear of my achievements, and when she did, it was not from me but from her friends. Did she really notice so little that I was leaving her out? Was she so hurt that she pretended not to care? My classmates who won second prize or even no prize at all asked their families to attend the award ceremonies. I, who won first prize, always, did so to the applause of no kin at all. Was I spiting her? I know I was spiting myself. Nothing would have made me happier than to have her there; nothing would induce me to invite her. It is a game I later played with men: 'Leave!' I would cry, and when they did, 'How could you hurt me so?' I'd implore.

If I deprived her of the chance to praise me, she never criticized me. Criticism was the vehicle by which she could articulate her relationship to my sister. No matter what it was, Susie could never get it right – in my mother's eyes. It continues that way to this day. Difficult as it is to think of my mother as competitive with anyone, how else could she have felt about her beautiful, ripe fourteen-year-old daughter? My mother was coming into her own mature, full bloom but perhaps that only made her more sensitive to the fact that Susie was simultaneously experiencing the same sexual flush. A year later, my mother remarried. Today, only the geography has changed: the argument begins as soon as they enter the same room. But they are often in the same room. They have never been closer.

How often the dinner table becomes the family battle-ground. When I met Bill he had no table you could sit around in his vast bachelor apartment. The dinner table was where his father waged war; it was the one time the family was together. In Charleston, dinner was served at 2:00. I have this picture of our midday meals: Susie on my right, mother on my left, and me feeling that our cook, Ruth, had set this beautiful table for me alone.

No one else seemed to care about the golden squash, the crisp chicken, the big silver pitcher of iced tea. While I proceeded to eat my way from one end of the table to the other, Susie and mother would begin: 'Susie, that lipstick is too dark . . . Must you pluck your eyebrows? . . . Why did you buy high-heeled, open-toe shoes when I told you to get loafers? . . . Those pointy bras make you look a, like a – ' But my mother couldn't say the word. At this point one of them would leave the table in tears, while the other shuddered in despair at the sound of the slammed bedroom door. Meanwhile, I pondered my problem of whose house to play at that afternoon. I would finish both their desserts and be gone before Ruth had cleared the table. Am I exaggerating? Did it only happen once a week? Does it matter?.

I was lucky to have escaped those devastating battles. 'I never had to worry about Nancy,' my mother has always said. 'She could always take care of herself.' It became true. Only my husband has been allowed to see the extent of my needs. But the competitive drive that made me so self-sufficient was fired by more than jealousy of my sister. If my mother wasn't going to acknowledge me, her father would. If she couldn't succeed in his eyes, I would. It's my best explanation for all those years of trophies and presidencies, for my ability to 'reach' my grandfather as my mother never could. I not only won what she had wanted all her life – his praise – I learned with the canniness of the young that this great towering man loved to be loved, to be touched. He couldn't allow himself to reach out first to those he loved most, but he couldn't resist an overture of affection.

I greeted his visits with embraces, took the kisses I had won and sat at his feet like one of his Dalmatians, while my sister stood shyly in the background and my mother waited for his criticism. But I was no more aware of competing with my mother than of being jealous of my sister. Two generations of women in my family have struggled for my grandfather's praise. Perhaps I became his favorite because he sensed I needed it most. The price I paid was that I had to beat my mother and my sister. I am still guilty for that.

In the stereotyping of the sexes, men are granted all the competitive drives, women none. The idea of competitive women evokes disturbing images – the darker, dykey side of femininity, or cartoons of 'ladies' in high heels, flailing at each other ineffectively with their handbags. An important step has been left out of our socialization: mother raises us to win people's love. She gives us no training in the emotions of rivalry that would lose it for us. With no practical experience in the rules that make competition safe, we fear its ferocity. Never having been taught to win, we do not know how to lose. Women are not raised to compete like gentlemen.

The young girl does not begin by thinking of it as competition at all. The adolescent merely wants what mother has. And she has so much! Food from her plate has always tasted better. Putting on her clothes has always been more thrilling than our own. Hasn't she said a thousand times, as she's scolded, bathed, clothed, and taught us, that she does it all because she loves us? Well, then, why doesn't she just step aside and give us daddy, and let us succeed her as the woman of the house? It has nothing to do with wanting to hurt her. Our biology is our logic. Competition only enters when mother resists.

Freud defined the Oedipus complex as the sexual feelings of the four-, five-, or six-year-old child, directed toward the parent of the opposite sex, accompanied by competitive urges against the parent of the same sex. But contemporary psychoanalytic theory believes the contest between mother and daughter isn't only for daddy. It is the girl's struggle for recognition, for the limelight, for her place in the world, with or without daddy's presence.

Alas, the entire literature and folklore of the oedipal conflict is written from the child's point of view. Nobody tells mother what she should feel. Nobody gives her sanction for what she *is* feeling. All she knows is she is supposed to have only nice, storybook, motherly emotions. There is no place here for jealousy of a young girl, resentment at finding your place as the only woman who matters undercut, anger that the person who always obeyed you, *and whom you love,* now demands to do things her way, and makes you feel old.

Mother recognizes these feelings with anger and shame: they are a rearousal of her old, buried, oedipal competitive wishes against her own mother. She is not evil; how can she admit to feeling these evil things? 'It is not easy for a mother to admit competition with her daughter,' says Dr Helene Deutsch. 'She has these sincere motherly wishes for the girl. They cover her own competitive urges.' Out of this conflict, rationalizations are born. After all, mother is a grown woman – it is undignified, unrealistic, to feel this way about her little girl. Mother wants to make things nice. Her denial makes them worse. Our desires are so bad, she won't even name them.

We've been afraid of this all along! To the savage untamed id, competition knows no bounds or civilized rules. From the Freudian point of view, the oedipal struggle is experienced as a kind of death wish. We never solved it at five. In adolescence the ego is still threatened by these dread impulses. The rivalry goes underground, becomes intense and deadly.

We have no lived-out experience that competition can be anything but this frightening, murderous urge the unconscious says it is. We never fully expressed our rivalry with mother, she never acknowledged that we had these feelings with a smile and a kiss that told us they are not so bad after all. And yet, self-respect demands we continue to try to win our place, fulfill our needs, posit our identity. Sex itself is not ours but seems to be something that must be won from somebody else.

Once upon a time our emerging sexuality almost made us lose the most important person in our lives. We gave in to her then, denying our desires; had we not, her anger could have meant abandonment at an age when we could not live without her. We go through life denying we are competitive, while feeling other women's gains somehow bar us from life's feast.

'Competitive? *Me?* I'm not competitive!' we hotly deny as if we've been accused of murder – even as we blindly race against the only people who count: other women. The exercise is to win the prize, but perhaps more urgently, to test once again the limits of the contradictory reality which hems us in: can you beat out the other woman and still have her love?

'I adored my father,' says a twenty-year-old woman, 'but more than anything I think I've always wanted my mother's approval. I'm still very much aware of my need to have women like or admire me. I'll spend more time getting dressed for lunch with a group of women than I do for a date. When I go to a party alone, I love it when men turn to look. But when there are just women in the room, I hate coming late. When they turn to look, I feel they are making a judgment against me. This makes no sense, but that's what I feel.' Little girls or grown-up women, our greatest source of love as well as our toughest competition are one and the same. How can we not be confused?

Mother denies any rivalry on her side, and acts instead on the emotions that surround and protect her from competition. It is irritation, motherly concern, and exasperation she feels at our adolescent behavior. We are her 'little girl', not her rival. When we grow up and another woman gets a dazzling new job, we aren't as comfortable around her. We say she 'irritates' us. She is our best friend; we didn't want the job anyway. What is irritating is that her promotion threatens to make us conscious of our competition with her.

In a similar manner, to avoid acknowledgment of competition, we declare it no contest and put ourselves down before anyone else can pass judgment. When our husband talks too long to another woman, we say, 'I know I'm not as interesting as she . . .' Feelings of inferiority are a classic defense. We feel diminished by her, frightened, we could kill her. Or him. But we do not feel competitive. Do you understand? *We are not competitive!*

Even women psychoanalysts, who smile ruefully and say that feelings of competition between mother and daughter may be denied but are universal, are unaware of any discontinuity in their thinking when later – often in the same interview – they tell me that they have never felt any competition with their daughters. 'My daughter is a very beautiful little girl,' one such woman analyst says to me. 'She is twelve, and just developing. I don't know what will happen when she starts looking better in a bathing suit than I do.' She laughs. 'For instance, I work one night a week in a clinic, and my husband told me that she said to him, "You know, Daddy, when mother is away, there are a lot of things I can do for you, just like she does."' I ask if her daughter's beauty and open flirtations with her father make the mother feel competitive with the girl. 'Oh, I don't think so . . . they are both much nicer people than I am.' Competition first, a charming denial second. I recognize these disarming techniques. They were my own for a long time.

When we were infants, it was appropriate that we should get the feeling of narcissistic enhancement so essential to growth from mother. Now we are young women ourselves and want it from a man. How father responds to his daughter's adolescence can determine which way we go: toward men and our own identity, or back to mother and the symbiotic tie. If father can make us feel we are the most glorious young girl in the world, we will gain confidence to move forward. Says a young woman: 'My father was a very warm, loving person. I think that is where I get my terrific interest in sex, my good feelings about my body. Not that I ever saw him being demonstrative with my mother, but he was with me, when I was young. He made me feel wonderful. I would love to have known my mother before she became a mother. I think motherhood did her in sexually. She must have been more sexual before we kids were born, because *he* is so physical. My whole feeling that sex is forbidden comes from my mother.'

There is much a father has to offer a daughter at adolescence. But what a tightrope he must walk! He must give attention to the needs of both wife and daughter, while being careful not to set one jealously against the other. 'My husband is crazy about our daughter,' says psychologist Liz

Hauser, 'but initially he didn't realize what he was setting up. For instance, if she and I were having a quarrel, he would come in and give her a little sign: don't worry about what mommy is saying, I'll fix it up. That wasn't good, he realized. The child doesn't know where her loyalties should be.' It arouses mother's jealousy, but may also instill in the child the doomed desire to win out over her mother permanently.

Very often, father's reaction to his daughter's adolescence is determined by his wife. If the mother has laid claim to the girl, if they have this tight thing between them, a father is going to be wary of responding to his daughter's blooming sexuality. The mother who has tried to avoid competition with her daughter by playing down sex with her husband isn't going to want the girl to have him either. She may not want him, but still has a certain ego involvement: she doesn't want any other woman to have him, not even her daughter.

Many mothers try to keep their daughter and husband apart by denigrating the father. Says Dr Robertiello, 'It's their way of competing with the girl while keeping both the daughter and father for themselves. Divide and conquer.' 'You know your father can never handle that kind of problem,' says mother. 'Why didn't you come to me in the first place?' Mother remains the friend of both sides, always firmly in the middle.

It is a destructive situation, leaving room for all sorts of oedipal fantasies to enter. If mother doesn't want him, if she doesn't understand him, maybe the girl can win him after all. But even if mother is a bitch, the girl can't afford to lose her primary alliance. Father may be the spice of life, but mother is the bread and butter. The relationship to mother was formed earlier, and runs deeper, than anything the daughter has with her father.

Here is a poignant story from a thirty-five-year-old woman and mother of three daughters whose own marriage ended recently. When I heard it I couldn't help wondering how many fathers are like hers: 'It wasn't until I got married myself and geographically far away from my parents that I began to see their relationship realistically. I had always thought of my father as a tyrant who had to be lied to and manipulated. My mother and I had always been very close. She was very much the martyr in the marriage. But when I began to examine my own marriage recently, I began to see that my father had a pretty raw deal, which made me feel different toward him. A year ago I gathered up all my courage and telephoned home, and after I talked with my mother I asked to speak to daddy; when he got on the phone I said, heart in mouth – I don't know what I was afraid of – "I wanted to tell you that I love you." There was this silence and then my mother came on anxiously exclaiming, "What did you say to your father?" I told her, "I told him that I love him, which is something I've never said, and I thought he might like to know." She said, "He's sitting over there sobbing." She called me back in several days and said, "Your father and I've been talking" – which is not something they frequently do – 'and he told me that all these years he thought you hated him.'''

For mother and daughter the problem becomes not so much winning the man as sorting out their own relationship; controlling their jealousy, denying anger, finding other words for their guilt. Years after he is gone, divorced, or even dead, the struggle between the two women remains: how to maintain the truce, the pact, the symbiosis?

'Once a year my mother and I take a vacation together,' a fifty-five-year-old woman tells me. Her mother is eighty; they are both widows. 'What infuriates me is that whenever anyone approaches us, man or woman, my mother just takes them over. Just as she did when I was a girl.' I don't ask why she continues to vacation with her mother. In symbiosis, you would rather stay with your partner – competition, defeat and all – than break the tie.

'If the mother doesn't have a good relationship with the father,' says Helene Deutsch, 'she will be jealous of the girl. This arouses competitive feelings in the mother which inhibit the daughter.' On the other hand, if father is absent, preoccupied when at home, if he tries to sidestep the competitive issue between mother and us by ignoring our needs for recognition, we will take in mother's negative sexual message, wait passively for men, not believing in them if and when they do come along, and remain dependent on women for our deepest emotional needs.

Many women can only fall in love with married men. They say they want the man to leave his wife — just as they wanted father to leave mother for them. But when the man is ready to divorce his wife, the woman loses interest. She didn't really want her father to leave her mother, it was just a wish. If mother and father should get divorced, and the daughter goes to live with daddy, she is guilty. She didn't want the wish to come true. *'Some oedipal wishes are very ardent but are not meant to be fulfilled,'* says Dr Deutsch.

Father has his own oedipal feelings to contend with. When we were five, he may or may not have felt nervous about our sexual overtures. 'Little girls can be terribly seductive,' says Dr Esman. 'At least, fathers can experience it as such.' But when we are thirteen, there is no way he can dismiss our advances as the games of a little girl. Nor do we want him to. We press up against him as daddy, the one person who loves us so well we can try behavior with him we wouldn't dare with boys our age. We expect him to run the show, to be able to know the difference between actions that say, 'Treat me as a woman,' and our continuing need to be loved as a daughter. We expect the world of him since he's daddy. Therefore, we are terribly hurt if he is threatened, if he precipitously withdraws and says, 'Get off my lap, you're a big girl now.' We are thrown back onto mother. The healthy sexual thrust of adolescence toward men has been dammed up or even reversed; the major movement of our lives remains focused on women.

'It is not so much that he is sexually aroused by the girl,' says Dr Sanger. 'It is the idea that something uncontrollable may happen that bothers a father. I think it is essential that a girl feels her father finds her attractive. Unfortunately, too many fathers – and mothers – can't put into words what they feel. It would be nice to grow up feeling that your body was loved by your parents, who knew how to kiss it, hold it and verbally let you know you are lovely.'

In tracing the line of the adolescent girl's psychosexual development, sociologist Jessie Bernard warned me against putting too much weight on any one variable, including mother. 'It oversimplifies the problem,' she said. 'Things are coming at the daughter from all sides,' I agree; mother is not the only determining factor in the girl's life. But whatever else happens to us in relationships to father, peers, teachers – the tie to mother is the one constant, a kind of lens through which all that follows is seen.

Games are paradigms for life, in which children can learn about losing and winning on a scale they can take in. How often do you see a mother and daughter pitted against each other in deadly earnest on the tennis court or in a game of cards? Today, a young girl may learn competition in Little League baseball. Her mother never did. Losing anything to another woman is not 'just a game' to mom. It rearouses deeper feelings of loss and anger that were never resolved with her own mother. The girl gets the message that open competition is OK merely in marginal matters like baseball. In matters with mother or other women, to compete and to win means risking the loss of a prime connection.

'The problem is not so much that the daughter pushes the mother aside to get to her father,' says Helene Deutsch, 'but that the daughter sticks to the mother. That is the explanation of the anxiety. The daughter is troubled because she is *dependent* on mother even while she wants to be *free* of mother.'

Father is not the only man who arouses oedipal competitions. 'There was a man, my father's best friend,' says a woman of thirty-five. 'We called him Uncle Steve. Years later I was to find out that my mother was very attracted to him. But to her dying day my mother patted herself on the back for never having had the slightest affair with this man. I was fourteen when this incident happened. We were out on the terrace. I was lying alongside Uncle Steve on a redwood chaise. He was a very affectionate man. The whole family was there . . . my brother, father, my sister and mother. Out of a clear sky my mother said, "Helen, you're a bit too old for that now." I remember going scarlet. I instinctively knew there was something between my mother and him. She was jealous. I was utterly embarrassed, but nothing further was said.'

Later in our interview, this woman tells me that when she and her husband were living together before they were married, she always dreaded that her mother would telephone while he was there. 'I was afraid she would know he was in my apartment, in my bed. I just didn't want her to.' How could her mother know? Because her mother lived on in her head. Love for the man she was to marry was pushed aside by fear of her competitive, No saying mother.

The dictionary gives this ecological definition of competition: 'The struggle among organisms, both of the same and of different species, for food, space, and other factors of existence.'¹ What two organisms share as close physical and psychological space as mother and daughter? What better force to make each seek her own place than the sexual drive? We could even accept losing to mother, if she would just acknowledge what is going on between us. The hard but necessary lesson to the loser in the oedipal competition is that she just can't continue to hang out around her rival's house forever. She has to grow up and get out if she is ever to find her own man. But mother dismisses our efforts at sexuality as silly, brushes off our independence as foolhardy, and denies our growing ability to want and feel what she does. She says it is for our own good, but we are not so sure.

The family that was once felt to be lovingly close now seems claustrophobic and boring. We want to get out, to get away. We are often drawn to people and activities mother doesn't like. With her grudging permission, or behind her back, we do them anyway. *An identity is being formed –*

but we feel it is in the teeth of her opposition. Guilt piles upon anger, we twist and double back on her. How can you hate your own mother? It is a Laocoon struggle, endlessly unresolved.

The oedipal situation is less complicated for boys. They need the same early symbiotic tie to mother that girls do, but there is another figure in the house against whom they can afford to express self-assertive notions of competition because in no way does it threaten what they have with mother. This figure, of course, is dad. A second, related reason boys don't find adolescence as painful or unsettling is that they don't go through the love-object shift that girls do. The boy's primary, straightline involvement is always with women. First his mother, then girl friends, later his wife, etc. Girls must make this extremely complicated shift to the male sex – away from mother to father.

Almost from the beginning, long before they are reidy to begin the work of cutting the symbiotic tie to mom, little boys are learning how to separate, establishing themselves in their own identities through competition – first against the male parent, later against other little boys. At four or five, they begin to vie with dad, often at his urging. They wrestle and race with him, beating him at Monopoly or Ping-Pong. By the time he is an adolescent, the boy will have become accustomed to all sorts of structured situations in which competition is allowable, encouraged, and even fun because it is protected from the dark and murderous underside of the competitive urge by the rules of the game: the limits are clearly defined.

Psychoanalyst Dr Reuben Fine, who is also a chess master, writes of this struggle dominated by powerful Kings and Queens – perhaps the most nakedly oedipal game of all – that the enduring fascination it holds is that while the King is captured, he is never destroyed.[2] In the same way, boys learn through the strict rules and structures of sports that if you beat the other guy in baseball, it will not kill him, and he will not hate you forever. Besides, there will be another game tomorrow, and maybe he will win then. Through these social situations that men share, the latent hostility in competitiveness that is in us all is brought into the open and given expression as play. The lesson is taught to the boy without words: feeling competitive, acting competitively, *winning* is not betrayal. *It's natural.* And as long as it is kept within rules, it can even lead to deeper friendships. Counselors at boys' summer camps have long known that if you take two little boys who dislike each other, put them in a ring with strict rules and heavily padded gloves, they will more often than not emerge after even the toughest fight as the best of friends.

Fathers are so unthreatened by their son's competition that at the beginning they can allow the boy to win. They want him to 'stand up for himself', 'to fight his own battles', 'be his own man' – to separate. The son who stays tied to his mother is no tribute to his father. Eventually the younger man may honestly beat his father. The older man may not like it. But he is so at home with feelings of competition that he can even let his son see he is momentarily annoyed at being beaten. This only gives the boy greater feelings of independence and pride. Griping at each other's prowess at the game, father and son advance in their relationship. They may grow closer, they may not; but the airing of competitive feelings has given the son experience in handling these emotions in a highly charged situation.

Women watch men walking off tennis courts, leaving football stadiums in tight, amiable groups of two and four, and we feel the lack of something they have. I used to think it was an open sharing of feelings. I now know that men's camaraderie is not about honest communication. What they do have is a learned communal release of pressure, a way of letting off steam, hostility, competition; it allows them to be easier with one another. Men learn to play to win, to stretch their competitive limits and be proud of it. Some men overdo it, but all men learn the vital lesson: 'A young boy,' says Dr Robertiello, 'can't get through adolescence without learning how to take defeat.' He has lost, but it has not destroyed him. Therefore he feels he can win in his own turn, without destroying his opponent. Men do not feel their happiness or sexual success comes at the expense of crippling someone else.

'It's very healthy to let your body act out, thrash out, your competitive feelings,' says Dr Robertiello. 'I often tell women they would look better if they could just let it out, verbally and physically. If they don't, they acquire that strained, tight mask, they become anxious-looking people.' Tact calls for us to contain our feelings, but if it is too rigid, there is often a psychosomatic price to pay.

'The development of adolescent girls is probably the most complicated process in human growth,' says Dr Esman (himself the father of three daughters). 'They have to cope with the complexities of their reactivated oedipal conflict over desires for their father, the resulting rivalries with their mother, and the hostility it engenders in both women. At the same time, they must learn to accept themselves as women. In a society like ours, which values the male more than the female, this can be a very tough, even reluctant acceptance.'

It is a dilemma; we are between worlds. We have not yet arrived at the safe harbor of discovering we can love men, and that they will love us back – and that in this new, exciting (but still frightening) kind of sexual love, we will find feelings of warmth, intensity, arousal, and power that in their different way are as rewarding as what we had with mother. We look to boys for the confirmation of the burgeoning sexuality mother doesn't like, and the reinforcement which daddy would not give us. But the acceptance we get from boys never holds the deep reassurance we had with mother. Boys are so strange. Often, we ask too much: who can live up to the glamour of being the forbidden, unattainable object – once he is attained? Men have drives and needs of their own. From their side of the sexual fence, they resent our demands or feel insufficient to meet them. They hurt us and depart.

Unlike the promise mother makes, their love is conditional. They have been raised to see us as appendages, symbols of their success, sex objects. They want us for something we don't wholly believe in.

We went looking for love, but somehow sex came with the package. Sex *is* exciting, but it's scary and dangerous too. The whole business becomes problematic, tinged with anxiety. Wouldn't it be wiser to retreat? If we go back, become 'good' again, mother's girl, mother would stop being angry. These endless arguments about whether she doesn't like this boy or that would end. We would have her love forever. There would be no competition.

Instead of asserting our individuality, our needs and desires, we become more like mother; join in her protest that sex isn't important to us after all. Pretty soon, the sexual drive is tamed, symbiosis wins. We grow up, we marry and have children, but never really left home.

On a realistic level, mother is not afraid we are going to steal daddy away from her. But there is a difference between a six-year-old who can fit into a man's lap, and a thirteen-year-old who fits perfectly into your clothes, who vies for the only man in the house and elicits from male visitors the kind of smiles you haven't seen in years – all the while, making plans of her own for a future you will never see again. Perhaps mother has come to terms with her fantasies of motherhood – but nobody ever mentioned treating her daughter as another woman. Certainly her own mother never treated her as one. Another wife, another mother, yes. But another *woman*? Never.

If we are our mother's claim to immortality, we are also a reminder of her years. How can we be going out with boys? Mother was just fourteen herself. 'Adolescence is classically the time when mothers begin to live their own lives through their daughters,' says Dr Schaefer. 'It can happen with bewildering suddenness. With my adolescent daughter, I can practically name the day when she began to change, last September.'

Mother helps us come to a healthy resolution more by example than by lecture. At best, she is comfortable in her own role of a woman – *however she defines it.* She may have a career, or be a traditional wife and mother, but a daughter needs the day-by-day perception that mother has chosen her role, and is not constantly embittered or bored by being consigned to what she feels is an inferior place. 'It is also very important,' says Dr Esman, 'for the girl to sense that her mother has a reasonably satisfying sexual life, so she can see that the relationship between a man and a woman is rewarding. She sees something exciting up ahead toward which to grow.'

A daughter's adolescence brings into high relief whatever problems or conflicts sex may still hold for mother. How can you explain the difference between romantic and sexual love if neither is present in your own life? Can you talk about the promise of womanhood, a career, motherhood – and not want a bit of that promise again if you yourself feel stifled?

Some women have always felt overwhelmed by their more glamorous friends, that other women were more sexual. Now their daughter too is more beautiful, and younger. They withdraw from the competition by letting themselves go, becoming even more of a mom. Other mothers become so sexual that the daughter doesn't dare compete: 'My mother flirts with men outrageously,' says a fifteen-year-old. 'She is what's called a cock-teaser. She tells my father all about it when different men proposition her at the country club. I think dad likes it, it boosts his ego. But I think her behavior is ridiculous.' This young girl is twenty pounds overweight; she admits, 'I can't beat my mother at her own game. I've given up trying to compete with her.'

Says psychoanalyst Betty Thompson: 'People tend to keep on being whoever they are. Becoming a mother doesn't change that. So a woman who is more concerned with her own feelings than anyone else's can be unreasonably competitive with her daughter. I've known mothers who forget they are twenty years older than the girl the minute their daughter starts bringing boys home. They compete as if the man were their own age. It's habit. Any time a man comes in the room, they have to feel attractive.'

'I've been wondering if I should get Penny a bra,' a mother who is thirty-four says to me. Her daughter is thirteen. 'No, she hasn't asked for one, but I've noticed that people are beginning to look.' What kind of people – men, women? What kind of look? I don't ask. But what is this pretty young mother feeling? Fran is a good mother who sees her work as caring for children and husband. Feelings of envy, competition, would be out of the question. At the dinner table that night, the daughter scolds the father: 'Daddy, do you know how many calories there are in that dessert?' It is her mother's voice. She starts to take the dessert away from him, playing the stern mother (wife), but her father draws the line. 'Sit down, Penny,' he says. He is smiling. Fran watches from across the table. It is difficult to read the expression on her face. Where does she fit into this? The challenge comes on all levels, from the girl she loves, but also from everyone and everything that would take the girl or her husband away from her. Psychiatrists say we should air these feelings, maybe joke about them. But Fran's mother didn't joke with her about feelings of jealousy, competition. So Fran too is silent. The husband says privately to me, 'My wife and daughter argue about everything and anything. I don't think they even know what it's about. I find it kind of amusing because I know it's about me. It's nice to have two women fighting over you, though they'd deny it to the death.' Meanwhile, Fran sighs and confides to me, 'I must find some exercises for Penny, she's getting round-shouldered.'

I remember being round-shouldered, not because I needed a bra, but because I didn't. I hated the nasty pink one my mother finally bought me after kindly pointing out that I didn't need one. Seeing my humiliation, she'd tried to cover it up by telling me how lucky I was: I wouldn't have strap marks on my shoulders when I was her age. *I wanted* strap marks! The battle of the bra is an adolescent classic.

Why should something as trivial as a bra bring such storms into the mother-daughter relationship? Perhaps it is answered by this fifteen-year-old: 'Before I even kissed a guy, I had a bad reputation. I don't know where it came from. I think it's because I had breasts before anyone else did.'

Mother knows what breasts mean in our culture. If she likes hers, if she allows us the peculiarly female rite of passage of the first bra when we want it, and not when she does, we too may grow to like our breasts. If not, our round shoulders try to hide the inadmissable truth: at one time in our lives, our breasts were the focal point of anxiety about the new sexuality we wanted to be proud of, but which mother feared and shamed us into hiding. The perfect symbol of this unresolved conflict is the fifteen-year-old of the liberated '70s who goes braless under her tight T-shirt, and stands with her arms crossed, hiding her chest. 'The classic mistake mothers make with adolescent girls,' says Dr Fredland, 'is that they won't let them become women.'

Skills and abilities that once gave us recognition and self-esteem now also betray us. 'Up to the age of puberty,' says Jessie Bernard, 'the young girl does all right, but now she traditionally begins to fall behind in school.' We used to raise our hand enthusiastically for teacher's attention, to speak out loudly and clearly when we knew the answer. Now we hide our intelligence and bite our tongue. We want to attract boys, we want to be 'feminine,' and lo and behold, the way you do this is the same way mother taught us to keep her love: submission and passivity. For every sociological study I see that shows this is changing – that girls now stay on the honor roll right through high school – there is another study indicating that while boys tend to prefer high prestige occupations the more they get into adolescence, the reverse is true for teen-age girls.[3]

'Because adolescent boys are anxious of their ability to perform,' says Dr Sanger, 'an assertive girl will scare them off.' Often the little, simpering itsy-bitsy girl will be most popular because she is less threatening. In her book *Letters Home*, Sylvia Plath's mother recounts an incident that speaks poignantly to any woman who knows what it is to be torn between being bright and being popular at school: 'By the time [Sylvia] was a senior in high school, she had learned to hide behind a façade of light-hearted wit when in a mixed group and, after a triple date, was exultant as she reported to me, "Rod asked me what grades I got. I said airily. 'All A's, of course.' 'Yeah,' he replied, grinning, as he led me out to the dance floor. 'You *look* like a greasy grind!" Oh, Mummy, they didn't believe me; they didn't believe me!"'⁴

Girls are raised for partnerships, boys to perform. If we are now beginning to raise our girls to achieve, that doesn't mean we aren't still raising them for partnerships. We instill in them what psychiatrists call a 'hidden agenda.' We say, Go to college, succeed, be self-sufficient, but we also give them this message: if you don't succeed as a wife and mother, you have failed. The message need not be spoken. A mother's own life is experienced by a daughter as a standard of achievement. No one tells us that it is difficult, painful, maybe even impossible for many women to be a success in a career and a good mother as well. Nor does anyone prepare us for the fact that to be a success you must be competitive, and that most men in our culture still feel the competitive women to be a threat.

'We will not make men's mistakes,' say feminists. 'We will not be competitive with our sisters.' This is hailed as an advance. It is childish to think denying something will make it go away. 'Be sexual, fulfill yourself,' women today are encouraged. Why do so many of us still hold back? On some level we know we are being encouraged to reach this goal using only a child's make-believe tools. A world in which you are told competition can be eliminated does not exist. I am not holding out as an ideal for women the lunatic degree of passion men bring to their drive to 'win' at any price. That doesn't mean competition doesn't have a rightful, necessary place in women's lives.

'I grew up in Georgia,' says a twenty-eight-year-old woman, 'and in the South, women are supposed to have some kind of magical power. But it's really manipulation, the women hanging in together to run the men. A good example is in my family, where my mother was Big Betty and I was Little Betty. Being just like your mother, even sharing her name, says you have this power to manipulate men just like she does. You and she are a team, so there can't be any competition between you. You both want the same thing. If women ever stuck up for their individual rights, they'd lose their solidarity; the men could pit one against the other and do what they want. The hitch is of course that southern women are terrifically competitive over men, looks, who has the prettiest children. Smothering that competitiveness, denying it, eats up all the energy that women might use to win themselves a real position of power, if only over their own lives.'

The speaker, who teaches high school, continues: 'There are dozens of girls in my class who are loath to compete. They blush if they get high marks. Last week, a class of seniors staged a debate and the girls automatically elected boys to lead both debate teams . . . even though several of the girls were smarter and better debaters. I was horrified. By the third day of the debate things were in a shambles. Some of the girls got up their nerve and put the best people – themselves – in charge. But they didn't feel good doing it. They were afraid the boys would think them aggressive. I think they minded even more that the other girls would be angry because these smart girls had shown themselves to be superior.

'It reminded me of when I was young – Little Betty. It was understood that part of the magic of being half of Little Betty-Big Betty, was that we had fixed places. I would never beat out, never outgrow Big Betty. We were always close – still are. But it gets rougher every time I go home. I'm successful on my own now, and it's hard to maintain the childhood tie. How can I? It's based on the assumption that she is bigger than me. But I don't want to give it up. There's a strength there. Big Betty and Little Betty – it sounds awful, but it's home.'

Billie Jean King and Bella Abzug may be the wave of the future but they are still marginal figures in a world where young women are not taught how to express competitive feelings within approved structures, nor given rules with which safely to express rivalry. The girl who strikes out with the bases loaded at the picnic is still thought to be adorable. She may have lost the game but has succeeded in something more important: reinforced the sexual status quo. By rising above merely masculine notions of winning and losing, she gives living evidence to the rule that women are noncompetitive, and all the more loveable for it.

'What makes women afraid to compete with other women,' says Dr Robertiello, 'is a fear that if they show they want to beat out the other person, but don't totally succeed, the unconscious talion law will exact revenge. To the unconscious, competition is to the death. People are afraid to compete because they are afraid of the powerful, unseparated mother. She would kill *them*.'

'How can a mother help her daughter to separate?' reflects Dr Deutsch. 'You cannot make a rule, personality enters into it. A mother who has already separated from *her* mother is more like to be able to help her daughter do the same. It also helps if the mother has a life of her own, other things she does and is interested in besides taking care of the daughter. But then that too can create a problem for the girl. Maybe the mother has more talents than she. Then the girl has to handle not only the oedipal jealousy but the thought that the mother is more gifted than she. It arouses feelings of competition, analogous to the sons of famous or successful fathers. But it is better for the child if the mother has something else. Yet, often when the mothers do work, children wish their mothers were like other mothers, always at home. It is ironic.'

Should mother try to do better by her daughter than her own mother did by her – give the girl a greater measure of self-confidence – is it any wonder she may occasionally feel an irrational anger at her own efforts? Nobody ever did it for her! 'I didn't want my daughter to grow up as I did,' a mother tells me. 'My mother was an anxious woman and tried to hold on to me all my life. I try to separate my own subjective fears from what may be realistically dangerous for my daughter. For instance, I have a terrific fear of deep water. I didn't want her to have it, so I made sure the first times she went into the water she was with people who *enjoyed* swimming, who felt safe in the water, and not with me. When she was nine she wanted to take the public bus to school. I used to send her on private buses. At first I thought: Oh, dear, the idea of going all that way on a public bus in the middle of the city. Then I thought: it's me who is nervous about it. She wants to try it. The bus picked her up right in front of our house. It was safe and made her feel terrific. Her world had grown. On the other hand, when I am certain that the danger is real and not involved with my own personal fears, then I insist she do it my way. I don't want to deprive my daughter of an experience that enlarges her, that gives her a growing sense of mastery over herself and the outside world just because I'm anxious.'

How does this woman's fourteen-year-old daughter describe the relationship? 'I used to be closer to my mother. It changed when I started going out with boys. I don't know why she thinks the parties I go to are so wild. She's practically waiting at the door when I get home, and she asks a lot of questions. Who was there, what did you do, what was this person like? She asks the same questions before I go. I get the idea she's kind of anxious. I sometimes think she's jealous of my friends.'

When a mother tries to make up in her daughter's life for the mistakes experienced in her own, it often works fine until adolescence. When sex enters, mother cannot intellectualize away the feelings of competition and anger if they were never resolved with her own mother. The ugly thought that she doesn't really want her daughter to outstrip her makes her feel guilty. While she pushes for the girl's success, she brakes for her safety. There are always three generations of women's voices in a house.

The daughter tries to act out her mother's double message: 'Be sexual and popular as I would have liked to have been,' but also, 'Don't, because that is bad.' The girl often resolves the conflict by putting both halves of her mother's message into action serially: first she stops, then she goes. The classic story that psychiatrists tell is of the mother who repeatedly warns her fourteen-year-old daughter not to get pregnant; but the very strength of her injunction signals the girl of the intensity of forbidden delight by which pregnancy is achieved. First the girl acts on the spoken *Don't* part of her mother's ambivalent words. Then, in a rebellious moment, she acts on the unspoken *Do*. She becomes pregnant.

Adolescence is a tempestuous time, filled with rivalries, crushes, rages, disappointments, and unreal, giddy exultations of new relationships. It is the time for up-till-then undemonstrated problems to come to a head. An ego structure that was adequate to handle the conflicts and tasks until the time of puberty 'is no longer adequate to handle this tidal wave of increased sexual drive that takes place now,' says Dr Fredland. 'It's like a house built on stilts; it's fine until a wave comes along that is too strong for the stilts. Then the house comes down. Angers and anxieties that could be suppressed earlier can no longer be held back. You suddenly have all these new feelings to cope with – hormonal and psychological – but with the old apparatus.'

At adolescence we go through what psychoanalysts call 'the pregenital tug.' With every step forward, away from mother, we want to run back for reassurance. 'One minute my daughter wants to choose and do everything by herself,' a mother tells me, 'and the next minute she's having a temper tantrum and acting like a baby, wanting to crawl into my lap.' I would hate to tell you how many of the mothers I interview have read their daughters' diaries. 'I was so worried about her,' they excuse their behavior. 'She has become so withdrawn, I just had to find out.'

We know our privacy is being violated; it undermines our half-hearted efforts to break away. 'No, you can't stay out till midnight,' mother says. 'No, you can't go out with that girl, that boy.' Her answers seem to come ironclad in the same wisdom and certainty with which she has always run our lives, but our anger has new weight. She is proud when a teacher says we think for ourselves; when we try to assert our independence at home and lock our bedroom door, she doesn't like it. Says pediatrician Virginia E. Pomeranz: 'When we find out that our parents' values are irrational, untrue or phony, that's when we turn.'

We talk of adolescent rebellion. Applied to women, the word is a farce. 'My mother and I have become like total strangers,' a fourteen-year-old says. 'She doesn't like this guy I'm going out with. We get into terrible fights. I'll slam my door, turn the record player on full blast, and just sit in there fuming. Or when she tells me to be home at a certain time, and I can see that the time is coming near – I have a watch on – I'll just stay where I am, two more hours maybe, and then I'll go home and she'll be hysterical. I'll tell her I'd completely lost track of time.'

We slam doors, stay out late, go out and get pregnant, or rush into early marriage – but it is stasis. We have done nothing for ourselves, only something in reaction to her. Rebellion implies a break. Dr Sanger defines it as self-differentiation and self-definition. 'It is a way of saying, "The family is great, I love the family, but I have to do it on my own, leave me alone." With some people you have to rebel in order to get them to listen.'

When we rebel against mother, it has no teeth in it. No more than when we later tell our husbands we are leaving. We pack our suitcase as he sets out for the office, but when he comes home at the end of the day, we are there. Says Dr Sanger: 'A girl can't say, "I've got this fight with my mother and I know I'm right. I'm going to go out and make something of myself." Instead, it all dwindles down to this endless arguing and reconciliations. "Hey, break it up!" I say to women. "What on earth do you keep hoping for from your mother? The few crumbs you're going to get from her at the end of this argument aren't worth it. Find a way to argue and not to look for crumbs."'

In adolescence we want rules, if only to assert ourselves by breaking them. The girl who complains about her mother's strictness is disturbed by her friend whose mother doesn't lay down any rules at all. 'This friend of mine tries to pretend she had the best deal,' a thirteen-year-old says. 'She's always going on about don't I wish my mother was like hers, but I don't think she's really happy. She's like a lost soul.'

'I hated only having the backs of cars, dark hallways,' one mother says. To give her daughter the privacy she missed, this mother goes out when her girl has a date. 'I don't want her to think I'm playing the heavy chaperone, spying on her.' Privately, the girl tells me that when she has a date, she always spends the night at a girl friend's house. 'They are a big family, there's always someone at home.' The daughter wants her mother around in case she needs the control, in case she wants to tell the guy, 'We can't do that, my mother's home.' The irony is that the mother never asked if the girl wanted her there. She didn't consider that her daughter's needs might be different from hers. *She made the assumption that the daughter wanted what she wanted.*

The girl who is ready to break the rules will. The girl who is not can use them to buttress her lonely position in a society where everyone seems to be 'doing it'. 'I love you, Johnny, but I've been raised so strictly.' It is not she who is putting him off. It is her stern mother. A situation that helps both her ego and Johnny's.

'There is a cliché which I tell mothers of girls of this age,' says Dr Esman. 'You have to resign yourself to the fact that between the time your daughter is twelve and fifteen, whatever you do will be wrong. It is my effort to give them a sense of humor about the situation to help them – the mothers – survive.' A mother who finds she must play the square for her daughter's own good, even while her daughter protests, needs a certain appreciation of irony.

'Kids today,' says Dr Sanger, 'often find themselves in the difficult position of having to set their own rules because mothers mistakenly believe the new freedoms should be applied to young as well as older women. A girl of thirteen needs enough rules to feel she can regulate her growing sexual experience. She needs to be protected from taunts of, "What kind of girl are you if you don't put out on the first date?" Well, why should she? She just doesn't know enough about human beings to be able to posit sufficiently strong answers to such questions. Not that much has changed. The needs are still there, the kids want rules. The years between seven and eight, and thirteen and fourteen are very valuable years, scholastically, socially, athletically. Things you learn in those years last the whole of your life. To have those years loaded down by excessive sexual worries hampers the consolidation of those skills.'

We may bitch at mother's rules but we will accept them if something at the back of our minds tells us they are sensible, consistent, and in accord with reality. But if we perceive her decisions as arbitrary and/or phony, we will resent her and them: they come out of that inauthentic gray area we cannot define but don't like. We fight to win ground for ourselves but she shifts the argument from the content of our request to the tone of our voice: we are rude and unladylike. We want to be popular and have our own friends, separate from her; she says certain girls aren't good enough and are just taking advantage of us. She feels left out of our decisions, rejected, and becomes punitive about the high cost of the telephone calls we make. We want a string bikini, but the argument becomes one about the clutter in our room. Years later when we fly home to visit, her first words at the airport are, 'Oh, darling, what a short skirt!'

What is confusing is that part of mother does worry about

our well-being. Half of us knows that is so. When this is genuinely the case, the criticism is not so unceasing; sometimes there is none at all, just pleasure in seeing us again. But if time after time, the first words we are met with make us feel like naughty little girls, the pattern is clear: more than our welfare or beauty, mother wants to put us in our place.

In adolescence the sexual drive is an explosion of energy that tries to break through, once and for all, the sticky, little-girl ties that bind us to mother. Sex is an expression of our own individual needs and desires. 'I am a woman who likes this, does that, and goes for the other kind of man.' It says who you are – and takes no account of mother at all.

If mother's fear of sexual self-assertion has made us reluctant to assert our own, our growth will stop. To deny that we are in sexual competition with her, we will say we are not sexual at all. The girl comes up to the threshold, but the full woman never does emerge. The processes of separation and individuation slow or cease; we merge with mother instead and become what Mio Fredland calls one of the 'latency girls'.

These are the women whose lives express a certain safe, nonsexual quality. It is as if they are living still in that period – between eight and ten – that is characterized by palships with other girls and not too great interest in boys. 'There are millions of women,' says Dr Fredland, 'who are very successful at jobs and careers, even as wives and mothers, but who never really got into adolescence. They were well organized, get along fine with other women, not too competitive on a "female" level. Psychosexually they are still back in their latency years. They are easy to identify. They have a different "feel", a kind of Girl Scout quality.'

Many mothers do not see this kind of behavior as arrested development but as a process that has produced exactly the kind of daughter they want. A 'nice girl', pal to girls and boys alike, who will dutifully get good grades at school and never be seen by mother as any kind of sexual competitor. She won't be heavily involved with men until it is time to marry, and then she will choose an equally 'nice' boy who himself will carry none of the anxiety provoking overtones that mother distrusts. 'In this way,' says Dr Fredland, 'the mother avoids feeling competitive or threatened. The daughter never makes her feel she herself may have missed out on the possible erotic richness of life. Very often, these mothers themselves are latency girls who never became women. They are the wreckers of daughters.'

We all know women of thirty and forty who are still referred to in their family as 'the baby', or 'the kid'. It is not uncommon to run into daughters who phone their mothers two and three times a day, or whose mothers call them. 'It's one thing to think along the lines of the extended family,' continues Dr Fredland, 'where there seemed to be space enough under one roof for everyone. But I'm talking about the "little girl" who never grows up. She leaves home physically, but never psychologically. *From the very beginning, the mother has to encourage the daughter to be her own person, not just let her go but encourage her!*'

Unless we learn the rewards of being our own women now, we will ever need to merge with a man as we did with mother, rather than expand his life and our own by joining in a union of two separate individuals. It may look like sex, but it will be symbiosis. Never mind that it is taking place with a man; it is modeled on what we had with mother during latency.

True sex, continuing sexual excitement, can exist only between two separate people, each aware of herself/himself as individual entities and therefore of the alien magnetism of the other. It is then we feel the lightning bolt of sex, that electric charge that connects two bodies: we orgasmically 'have' one another – and separate again. There is no passion in symbiosis.

Can it be exciting when – as the saying goes – the right hand caresses the left? Symbiotic partners may struggle for orgasmic sexuality but are defeated before they begin by this presexual need to belong and blend into someone, to be so close that his head (as mother's once was) will be inside ours telling us how we feel, who we are, what we like and don't like – giving us an identity we never established on our own. We love the people in our families; we feel sexual desire for strangers.

'Do you remember the lookalike clothes that mothers and daughters used to wear?' says psychologist Liz Hauser. 'I can remember thinking when I was a little girl how wonderful that would be. When my daughter Liza was little, she loved to look at them in Altman's catalogs. Before I understood the problem of separation, I thought those clothes would be wonderful for her and me too. It's a terribly symbiotic way of relating. It's thought to be cute in our society, but it tells both mother and daughter that they get extra applause for being tied together as tightly as possible. If they are on their own – separated – they are somehow diminished. Today, Liza has three pairs of jeans that fit her like skin; the old unseparated me would have tried to make her wear what I wanted her to wear. If she doesn't want to give them up, that's fine with me. Mothers who want their daughters to dress for them should realize this is what we accuse men of doing when we say they are chauvinistic and want their women to look pretty because it reflects on them.'

When we were little, we loved to romp in mother's oversize dresses. When we are thirteen, her clothes fit us. We are older. So is mother. We approach one another's wardrobe with the desire to 'take on' something the other possesses. 'Hey, you stole my favorite blouse!' says mother when we walk into the room. She would give her life for us. Seeing us in her clothes makes her proud of the daughter she has produced. But what have we 'stolen' from her in the process?

The rare mother who can believe that there is enough sexuality to go around, that her daughter's doesn't threaten her own, says, 'You look better in it than I do.' We heave a great sigh of relief. We love her more. The wish to outstrip her, to take away her crown, has been experienced safely, symbolically. Mother recognizes our sexuality, concedes we may even be a more beautiful (if only because a younger) woman – but does not hate us for it! She still loves us!

What if mother wears our clothes too well? We hear her boast to her friends she could take even a smaller size than we. At a time when we have little but youth to give us an edge in the race with her, if she can 'get away with' wearing the same clothes we do, she has won. The victory may seem pleasant to her, a small triumph over her years. To us it can be shattering. We have not had so many victories as women to be able to afford this defeat.

Little wonder that young girls adopt clothing so outlandish that mother would never want to put it on. 'Mother doesn't like it,' says Dr Schaefer, 'when the daughter ignores her ideas of good taste and is totally guided by her peer group's standards of what to wear, what is in, what is out, and ugly. It is a competition for control. A lot of it has to do with how much of an independent person the mother feels herself to be. If your children are your reason for living, then you need your children to be a certain way to satisfy you. If I have a life where I get other satisfactions and am not dependent on the satisfaction I get from being Katie's mother, I can tolerate the difference growing between us.'

The reason so many women do not let go of their daughters is that they have little else in their lives, nothing of their own. Or else they have been so frustrated in their relationships with their own mothers that they try to make up for it in symbiosis with their daughters. 'Many girls,' says Dr Fredland, 'have mothers who are trying to fill up the empty hole inside left by their own absent, cold or distant mother. Usually the mothers aren't aware of it because if they were they would have to let the girl go. It recalls the pain of loss of their own mother. These mothers insist their daughters tell them everything about their lives, their friends; the girl has no private corner for her thoughts or activities.'

'My mother tells me the same thing over and over,' says a

thirteen-year-old. 'It's always in this whiny tone that drives me nuts: "Call me when you get there. Call me when you get there . . ." Then when I complain about one of her rules I don't think is fair, she says *I'm* whining.' Because we cannot afford to hate mother, *we become like her*. We take on her whiny tone, her anxiety, her 'nice girl' rules and fear of sex. We are only thirteen.

'I know from my own personal experience,' says Dr Deutsch, 'that sometimes a woman will say, "There is a certain expression I get which I hate." When she stops to think about it, very often it is an expression her mother wore, which she disliked. It is true of me. We don't want to be like our mother, to be reminded of her in ourselves, because in the first oedipal competition, she was the victor.'

Before you know it, we are thirty-three and whining at our own husbands and daughters. Rather than become angry with mother – which would force the issue of separation – we take on her voice and those expressions we liked least. Married or not, 'we' are still not sure sex is nice. We blame our husbands for not making sex more enjoyable, for not making us feel like 'a real woman'. Our husbands wonder what became of the sexual woman they married. They cannot compete with our first ally. Who is also our first censor.

Women of forty or fifty with grown daughters of their own tell me that they are not able to see men except as husbands, fathers, and brothers. Divorced women who want a sexual life react to men in the old childhood ways, hemmed in by adolescent rules. 'I tried to fantasize about sex with this man,' a forty-eight-year-old divorcée tells me, 'but it only got as far as the motel. I couldn't imagine myself going through that door with him, and taking off my clothes. And that was only a fantasy!' This woman is 'disgusted' with herself for her inhibitions, but she remains a little girl, angry at her mother's rules, and protected by them too – inappropriately.

Our pre-oedipal alliance with mother sets up patterns we can never understand. Without her encouragement to leave and find a larger world, something always holds us back. Our intellect and ambition want to try for a better job, but an older voice says, 'Don't take chances.' Without mother's acknowledgement of our sexuality, the move toward men always seems tinged with a sense of betrayal. We go out with boys, we grow to want them sexually, but feel an inhibition: our deepest emotions remain with her. Eventually we may choose men who are diametrically opposed to the kind 'we' approve of – sexually exciting men, whom mother cannot control. We may even marry one of them, but the battle is not over. 'Not tonight, Tom,' the woman says, knowing that even as she rejects him, she is rejecting her own pleasure. She knows she likes sex. What is holding her back? It is puzzling because it is not her body which is saying no. It is the old recorded message in her head which continues to tell 'us' what 'we' feel.

We develop migraines and ulcers. We would rather live with the pain of suppressed rage than lose the illusion of a love that is eating up any real love we may feel for her. We go home to visit, but are relieved when it's over. We know there is love between us, but can't touch it.

'Women have these endless fights with their mothers,' says Dr Sanger, 'and then they feel guilty. The mothers feel guilty too. There's a tremendous reconciliation until the next big fight. It's endless and it gets nowhere. It looks as though something is happening or going to happen, to change, but nothing happens, nothing changes. It's a series of fights and reconciliations and guilt . . . no progression.'

We want both to separate from mother and not to separate. As long as we stay attached to her, we remain her little girl – *safe* – but immature. What keeps us attached? 'Guilt!' says Dr Schaefer. 'Mother feels the only way to continue to be needed is to keep us dependent. She cries at our birthdays. "How big you've grown!" The girl wants to break away but that is mixed up with "breaking mother's heart", and she's guilty about that. The idea has been instilled never to leave mother, never to go out on your own. Who will love you like mother?

We are frightened at the idea of separating. And so even if we are unsuccessful at it – as most women are – we are still guilty for having wanted to.'

Guilt eats up our lives, but we don't want to be cured. To be free of guilt would mean to be free of mother herself. When I ask Dr Fredland why mother's prohibitions against masturbation stay with us long after we outgrow so many of her other *don'ts,* she speaks of the unconscious fantasies that so often accompany masturbation. 'It isn't just the act that's forbidden – the fantasies are forbidden too. There are fantasies that are oedipally tinged, so there's the incest taboo but also the terrific fear of oedipal competition.' Masturbatory fantasies in which, in some half understood manner, we set ourselves up as rivals to mother are so threatening that we give up the pleasure of masturbation when we are four or five, or younger. Eventually, we may give up sex too. All we are really guilty of – is wanting to be women ourselves.

In the end, however, I wonder if *guilt* is not a euphemism for something else – for the dread we feel must be the consequence of an ambivalent action. The fear is that if we do this wrong thing, the other person will become so angry she will go away. Guilt is merely the first step, which we name with tears and regret, but the *consequence* is so awful that even in our own minds we cannot speak it: loss. It is too embarrassing to admit to childhood emotions like that.

When I first began to ponder these ideas, I went to see a woman psychoanalyst whose work I've admired for years. She spoke of her two daughters, now in their late twenties and thirties: 'Where did I go wrong?' she cried out to me. 'They say now they had so many battles with me as children, of which I wasn't aware. And yet I nursed them all! I enjoyed it. I *did* take care of them, and loved reading to them. I was always there when they left for school and always there when they got home. I didn't go to work until the youngest was six and I was forty-five, but their memory of me was that I was always away. Something was wrong with me . . . to have thought I was *present*, available to them, and for them to have felt I was not there at all.'

This conversation took place early in my research. I had not yet realized that to end any discussion of 'Where did I go wrong?' with vague explanations of 'guilt' is not enough. The next question must be, 'And what dreadful event does your guilt make you fear will happen?' Loss is unspeakable.

I came to this after talking to Jessie Bernard. 'Guilt is the biggest thing for mothers,' she said. 'Guilt is built into the role. You don't have all that much power and yet you assume the responsibility if anything goes wrong. When I talk to people about the future of motherhood, they aren't interested. Mothers are the most put-down people you can imagine. What young women want is babies, someone to hold and cuddle. They don't want sons and daughters like themselves, who are going to grow up, shake their fists at them, the way they did at their parents.'

Angry sons and daughters, furious over the restraints and frustrations of family life, threaten mother they will leave her forever. A baby in your arms cannot.

A mother who did not give her baby a bottle of the right temperature, who wasn't home when her daughter got the flu, may feel guilty – but it is in proportion to the 'wrong' act she has committed. It is not a fear of unimaginable consequences, that terrible malaise that hangs in the air like thunder. That is left for mothers who have children old enough to utter the dread sentence mother has been afraid of all along: 'That's the last straw. I hate you. I'm never going to see you again.'

Daughters fear they will anger their mothers so much that mother will desert them. Mothers fear they will anger their daughters so much that daughters will desert them. Both women call it guilt. Every woman speaks of it. It is not guilt. It is terror. The terror of losing each other. It makes them cling even harder, tightens the claustrophobia between them even more. In the end, the ironic truth is that if you have the courage to let each other go, you may be friends for life.

I've been thinking about these problems for three years and still they elude me. Last night I dreamed about them, this morning as I lay in bed I understood them, but by the time I get to my desk, I find I am chasing shadows in my head. It takes all my force of concentration to get over the resistance to knowing what I *do* know – and even while I write this, I can hear my husband in the next room, typing away toward the finish of his novel. 'Look what chapter you're writing!' my friend Richard Robertiello says. 'You're afraid that if you do this book well, if you succeed, your mother and Bill will be jealous, they'll hate you. The fact is, it doesn't matter to them.'

Why do I think my success and/or failure are so murderously important to everybody else?

Competitive urges will always be frightening because they stand for our desire to be sexual and separate. They are associated with feelings of being left, reprisals, etc. *They were never aired and found to be simply childish fears!* And so, at thirty-five, we still feel as we did at fifteen: that competition with other women must be denied because of our need to be loved and accepted by them too. We are left in anxious stasis: the only way to kill competition, it seems, is to kill in ourselves the desire for life.

I have always thought my emotional highs and lows were with men. It was men who peopled my days and nights. Today I know it is not that I don't need women, it is that I need them too much and my need of them precedes my need of men. I have long despaired of ever finding with women what I want, and I fear the retribution I would wreak on them for not giving me the love I need. I would have told you before I researched this book that, yes, of course I love my mother but that we are two different people living in different ways in different cities. I know today that I am tied to my mother more deeply than I dreamed, to the point where I have always avoided competition, not just with her but with every other woman.

– *Which does not say I am not competitive*. I am; so strongly that I cannot admit it.

'It is much easier to get a woman to accept that a man is treating her badly,' says Dr Robertiello, 'than to make her see that her best woman friend is doing her in. Another woman will steal her man, talk behind her back, but women refuse to give one another up.' The story of a thirty-year-old woman's best friend making off with her husband is a cliché, but from mother after mother I hear about the same thing among twelve- and fourteen-year-olds: 'I tell my daughter, if that girl is after your boy friend, she's no friend of yours. But my daughter won't give her up.'

A fourteen-year-old girl tells me a story that she says has nothing to do with competition. 'It's about how girls hurt each other,' she says with resignation. 'They are not honest with one another.' It will be a self-fulfilling prophesy in her life.

The events on which she bases her conclusion began one afternoon when her girl friend lost her virginity. 'Then that night, the boy turned around and had sex with her best friend!' My interviewee became the confidante of the injured girl – and the boy too. In fact, she and the boy 'happened' to become very close. 'He needed someone to lean on.' She quickly explained to me that she was not a sexual competitor with either of the other two girls because she was still a virgin. She and the boy 'only kissed and touched'.

I asked if the friend minded her seeing this boy to whom she had given her virginity, and who had then deserted her. 'I don't know how my friend feels. She's not a very honest person, so I don't know her real feelings. I don't feel guilty, though. He didn't leave her for me. If she were nicer to him, and if she were a good enough person, he'd want to be involved with her again. I didn't tell the other girls, though. They wouldn't understand why I was seeing him. There's nobody that I really trust at all, except him. He has something that I never have found among my girl friends. I know he would never betray me to anybody. No matter what I do, or what I tell him, he will always like me. Boys don't turn on you the way girls do.'

That interview was a year ago. Today the girl is fifteen and there is a different boy. She looks to him too for those things she cannot find with women – like trust. Given her unresolved and denied contest with women, what are her chances with men? In some mysterious way, they will always seem to fail her. And if she gives up on men, and falls back on the company of women – relieved to be rid of the competitive struggle – how long before she finds she is irritated and angry at women once more, hurt by them and hurting them herself? Getting rid of men doesn't rid our lives of competition. Men may be the sexual prize, but long before they came along, the struggle with women was going on for life itself.

When we were little, we had to live by mother's rules. It was her house, her man. Now there are enough men to go around, and the rules are up to us. If we lose one job to another woman, there is another good one around the corner. Fear of competition is nurtured by notions of living in a psychic economy of scarcity. Grown-up life is an economy of abundance.

CHAPTER SIX

The Other Girls

When I was nine I went to a private summer camp, a beautiful plantation home on an island, hung with Spanish moss. I had my first case of homesickness, impetigo, and rejection by a best friend. Her name was Topsy and she came from Atlanta. We slept together, we ate together, we jumped hand-in-hand off the diving board on the big oak pier together, and we made a pact to do everything together, especially to be best friends, forever. One day a mother arrived and left her little girl at the big house. She was put into our room. Topsy and I eyed her during lunch, conspicuously leaving her out with our giggles, as we left out everyone from our secret world. By supper time I was the one on the outside. They whispered when they looked at me, sharing secrets you would think they'd shared for years. Their friendship was born on the strength of my exclusion. That night I lay in my bed and sang 'Onward, Christian Soldiers' to myself to keep from crying. My head ached, trying to know what I had done.

One afternoon when I was eleven, Mary Stonewall and I were playing at Betty Anne's house. Betty Anne was my best friend. We paid her brother a quarter to let us see one of his dirty comic books. The three of us retreated under Betty Anne's canopied bed to read it. *What was this?* 'Oh, no!' we cried, straining for a better look. Our heads bumped. 'Let me see!' we cried, but it was too terrible to look at, too thrilling to bear. The space under the bed was suffocating. We rolled away from one another in hot-faced shame and an excitement we did not know how to share. Laughing hysterically we ran from the bedroom, bumping headlong into three workmen who were painting the backstairs landing. Men! They might as well have been brandishing ten-foot penises as paintbrushes. The three of us flew in all directions, screaming. Ten minutes later we convened on the veranda, damped down by thick sandwiches of chopped olive and Hellman's mayonnaise on Pepperidge Farm bread.

What to do next? It was a hard act to follow. Boredom worked on us like an itch. 'How do you spell brassiere?' I asked, and Mary giggled. She had been Betty Anne's best friend before I even knew Betty Anne, who now tightened and blushed. She was the first in our group to wear one and she had secretly told me how much she hated it. Mary took up my chant, 'Brassiere, brassiere,' and the funny word that one minute earlier had left flat-chested Mary Stonewall and me out of its portentous, exciting meaning, now became the ugly thing no one wanted part of. Betty Anne squeezed her shoulders together to hide her breasts and tears. At last the afternoon had a name: leave out Betty Anne. Within minutes the front door slammed, and two little girls had left one little girl behind.

Every Friday night when we were thirteen we went to Madame Larka's dance class at the South Carolina Hall on Meeting Street. At a resounding chord on Madame Larka's piano, we girls would rise and stand in front of our chairs, waiting on our side of the room as the boys approached to make their selection, one by one, until there were none – but the unpicked girls. If I danced it was usually with Gordy Benson. My Aunt Kate couldn't understand why I didn't like Gordy; wasn't he taller then I? I told her that Gordy Benson smelled of Cream of Wheat.

Certain girls were always asked to dance and they were my best friends. I have always preferred good-looking friends; until I grew into my own looks, not being picked for the dance didn't hurt so much as being grouped with the losers. What had I in common with them but this unfair rejection by men? My feelings about myself as every bit equal to any other girl were jangled by this new role in which winning had nothing to do with ability, initiative, daring, and action. I got through dancing class with an optimism that each time it would be different.

After dancing class there was always a party at someone's house to which we would race in a fleet of cars borrowed from worried parents. South Carolina adolescents can drive at fourteen and we girls, still half-bludgeoned by Madame Larka's lesson in passivity, would half run, half saunter in slow motion to reach our favorite boy's car before our opponents. It was a deadly sort of ballet we did down those graceful swooping stairs of the South Carolina Hall, pacing each other out of the corners of our eyes while we pretended animated interest in anything but what was really going on. Did the boys know how totally our lives were focused on them, how we could have gladly betrayed one another for their favors? I doubt it. Their ignorance, their uninterest – *maddening!* While we died in closed rooms to the sound of recorded music, they roamed the streets, played football, lived quite easily without us.

Their cars were our one chance to get close to them. As they 'gave us a ride' for a few blocks, we girls would giggle and invent endless airy chat to camouflage our deadly intent to get close to an arm, a leg, a pair of trousers that went with a particular song or passage on the violin. 'Touch mc,' we would pray, 'just let him touch me.' Meanwhile we would smile at our best friend, who had outmaneuvered us and was sitting next to him. No malice was ever exchanged, the desperate strategies for position and counterposition mutually ignored. But when we were planning the last party of the season, I blackballed Patty Hanson. I can't remember how I did it, but I made sure she wasn't invited – a girl as much a part of our group as I. Nobody stood up for her. Had they, I would have lied a thousand lies rather than admit I simply couldn't bear the possibility that once again, because of something I couldn't control, Patty would get to sit beside the boy who filled my dreams. The night of the party, Patty sat home and never knew why.

I grew up with Helen. I learned to smoke in her kitchen, we studied together for exams all through high school, and when the right Sunday came along, we put on our first garter belts and stockings and walked into St Philip's Church together. When I had finished my own dinner at home, I would often go to Helen's to help them finish theirs. It had gone on for so long that her mother never bothered to ask, 'Nancy, would you like to join us?' A place would be set for me and the maid would make her rounds again. More than the food, I liked having a man at the table, being part of a family with all the roles accounted for.

Once a month in history or math class I would get terrible menstrual cramps. The school infirmary offered nothing more than a heating pad. Home was too far away to go for the shot of gin that eased the pain like nothing else, so I would usually go to Helen's house across the street. Once, when her mother wasn't home, I climbed in the kitchen window to help myself to the gin. It never crossed my mind that Helen's mother would object to my entering her house this way. She loved me like a daughter, a love I took gladly. And once repaid badly.

It was a Sunday night and we were leaving the church parish house after a party. We girls were standing in the vestibule, putting on our coats, when someone saw something outside through the distorting stained-glass window; she announced it to be Helen and Tommy Boldon, kissing.

Helen and Tommy hadn't even had a first date. Judgment was passed instantly. The next day Helen was snubbed in the halls at school, given 'the treatment'. Not too coincidentally, Helen was the most voluptuous girl in our crowd; the older boys were already paying attention to her. No one was sure if the crime had been committed, but our gnawing envy told us it must have been. Ostracizing Helen released us from jealousy. Her exclusion fed into the group a cohesive strength we hadn't felt in some time.

'Why?' Helen's mother asked me, when I could no longer avoid going to see her. 'What did Helen do, Nancy? She is so unhappy. You are her best friend.' How could I tell her the truth? The truth was a lie. Helen had done nothing. I could not answer Helen's mother because the things women do to one another, in cruel anger and even crueler silence, do not bear talking about. It is the work of bitches.

Instead, I told my best friend's mother I would make things right. I did, but I know Helen never forgot. Neither have I. I blush that I might still be capable of that kind of cruelty, that I could feel deprived by my friends' successes, and not adult enough to live in my own accomplishments.

After mother and before we are ready for men, there are the other girls. At five and six, they appeared in our lives like life rafts, bright welcoming alliances to carry us away into a new identity. We could never have left mother on our own. Father had failed us. Little boys weren't interested in our overtures – but little girls! They are our great chance to separate. They have all the safety and familiarity of home: they are female and needy, just like us. All of us are eager to find something more than mother, to embrace life, but the prospect is frightening. We rush into one another's arms the first day at school. Those arms close round us as tightly as the pair we just left at home. We don't struggle. We went looking for freedom, but found something too good to resist: tightness and closeness. We think we've left home. We have only changed partners. Symbiosis with a new face.

What human relationship contains as much ambiguity and ambivalence as women with women? We have so much to offer one another, but our history is one of mutual inhibition. The bond that ties us to other women parallels what we had with mother. She too began in our life as a loving friend. She became a no-sayer and a rival. Her very success in helping us grow through the difficult early stages of development brought us to the threshold of sex. Dad was the first man we saw. Mother was in the way. All her goodness and patience did not help. Within the family, there is only one prize. She had him. We wanted him. In one way, our desire was as natural as a river finding the shortest way to the sea; in another, guilt was the inevitable result. The irony is, the better mother she was, the greater the guilt. It is one of the inexorable, situational tragedies of human nature.

'What happens next,' says Dr Robertiello, 'varies within different family constellations. Generally, the girl develops a negative oedipus complex. Her feelings of guilt, and the attendant fear of losing mother, make the girl deny the wish for her father. She bonds herself to mother and female sex. With most girls, this drive leads to the tight, intense friendships which are such a famous feature of the latency period.'

The fear of competing against mother and the guilt at wanting to beat her out anyway spreads to the entire female sex. We like the little boy who sits next to us in class and want to win him away from Sally. But to go after him might incur Sally's anger, so we defend against wanting him at all. Instead of being jealous of Sally, we telephone her to come spend the night. In these misdirected circumstances, is there any wonder there is often overt homosexual behavior?

Clinically, this is called reaction formation. It is a way of denying an unconscious impulse; the act comes masked as its opposite. Men who are afraid they are ninety-five-pound weaklings in their soul go in for muscle building and parade on the beach as Mr Universe. Censors read and see more pornographic works than anyone else. They say that because they hate it so, they must see everything dirty in order to know what to ban. The reaction formation against wanting to be filthy is to be compulsively clean. Instead of expressing our anger and competition toward women, we join with them and express love.

Now we are fourteen and fifteen. The boys who five years ago wouldn't give us the time of day want us. Our own bodies are stirred by mysterious desires and passions. The most natural thing in the world would be to respond. It is not so much sex we want, but to feel something that cannot be denied as easily as when we were six years old. We want recognition of whatever degree of sensuality we possess and whose expressions we feel is life itself. But what we have with other women is already more important than anything we might have with boys.

Three little girls cannot play together. When we were seven we had one best friend. 'If you have more than two, you have trouble,' says a mother. 'When my daughter used to ask for more than one girl to come play, I always said no. I couldn't stand the fights. At that age, they have terrific jealousies, whisperings, and secrets. "She's *my* friend." They just cannot share someone with another girl. My daughter is fourteen now and travels in huge groups, gangs of girls. But they still say vicious things about one another.'

In an interview with this mother's daughter, she speaks of love and hostility in the same breath. 'My best friend is always trying to get the boy I like,' she says. 'It's not just a malicious thing pointed at me, but a general idea she has. She always says she can get any boy to be interested in her. She's not unique, though. Girls just do mean things to each other. For instance, whenever a girl talks behind your back, the person she confides in will immediately turn around and tell you the mean things she said about you.'

Boys do not develop girls' reaction formation, our denial of competition with mother. *Unlike us, they do not compete with mother.* This means the boy can still hang on to her as the nurturing figure, while expressing his competitive feelings against the dominant male. He suffers of course from sexual taboos placed on his feelings for the mother, but he is not in the position of the little girl: in competing with mother, we are in the impossible position of one who wants to bite the hand that feeds her.

'Girls can be merciless,' says Dr Sanger, 'organizing vendettas against other girls, suddenly turning on each other.

A girl needs all the help her family can give her. The tears I have lived through with my own daughter and the young girls who come to see me . . . what they go through is terrible. Boys do it, but it doesn't have that personal, poignant cruelty. Boys have defeats to deal with too, but they don't have this sense of violation, betrayal: "This morning, I thought she was my friend, and this afternoon I found out what she was doing to me.'"

With no outlets for feelings of envy, competition, or jealousy, our emotions become compressed, escaping like steam through cracks in our nice-girl veneer. Before we know it, we have dealt the stab in the back, said the unkind word. We don't want to be bitches. Where did we learn it? Even as she separated us from our own body, mother smiled and said she loved us. Blending love and anger, smiles and deceit, she taught us that our only rejoinder was to love her back no matter what she denied us – daddy, independence, sexuality – or we could suffer even worse loss.

'Of course you learned to play mother's game,' says Dr Robertiello. 'You still needed at least the illusion of perfect love with her. You didn't have anything to replace it with.'

One of the characteristics of childhood is singleness of mind. The baby likes this, is overjoyed by that, hates the third thing. As we grow older, as we take in more of the crosscurrents of life, conflict comes to sit in the heart. The intense friendships with other girls may be an experiment in replacing the closeness we once had with mother, but we are no longer innocent dwellers in Eden. Our competitive feelings have not magically gone away. They have merely found safer targets, been transferred onto these girls who, like mother, are both friends and rivals at the same time. All that love and affection between little girls masks the turbulence within – which is why we hurt each other so often. Our love for our friend to whom we talk for two hours on the phone every night and swear eternal devotion is not unmixed. It is not the same we felt toward daddy or Johnny, the little boy next door. It is born of détente, on mutual avoidance of anger. 'But underneath, you are just plain mad at women,' says Dr Robertiello. 'When you see a chance to get more love from someone else by turning on your friend, all that old anger is there to justify what you're doing.' The anger left over from the unresolved oedipal situation just breaks through. Mother won daddy's love by excluding us. Now we're doing it to our best friend.

'I think adolescent girls' rules are almost biologically determined,' continues Dr Sanger. 'They are there to be relied on when you can't think of any other way to protect yourself.' Dr Sanger was referring specifically to rules on conduct, the need for curfews, times to be home when things are getting out of hand with a boy. But aren't the rules for dress, for instance, when we are twelve, also biologically determined? They camouflage us against a sexuality we are not supposed to feel. 'When we're going somewhere after school,' says a twelve-year-old, 'we call each other up and say, "Everybody wear football shirts," or "Everybody wear shirts with the alligators." All seventh graders do nutty things, my teacher says, like we'll all wear different colored socks. My teacher is in love with a man who teaches at our school. His name is Ken, and we wrote all over the door one day, "Ken my love".' We ache with love at twelve. It doesn't hurt so much if everyone is wearing different-colored socks on each foot.

When our world was small, one friend was all we needed. In this narrow focus, she came to stand for life itself, and our demands on her became ironclad. We live on the edge of bliss with our best friend, just as we once did with mother; just as we did with mother, if she falters or grows disinterested, we despair. We want more life but we want absolute security too. We are not above leaving our best friend if more love should beckon elsewhere, but we could not bear it if she left us.

Adolescence faces us with more complex problems. Boys are everywhere, moving with mobility and freedom, tempting and frightening. We are caught in too many gusts of emotion; the world, alluring, dangerous, huge and glittering is upon us. We need greater numbers to hold our own. The single, one-to-one relationship we used to prize with one best friend is too narrow. We want to be free to join in the swim of life. We need more varied relationships, larger groups of girls to help us handle the experiences rushing in from all sides. Our gang of girls becomes a microcosm of the universe, big and complex, shifting, changing, but nevertheless understandable and ordered. The group is power and fun but it is based on control. Its laws are arbitrary, cruel, capricious, dictatorial. That doesn't matter. It offers the great recompense: the law of symbiosis. No one will be alone.

People together, people in crowds, feel emotions, have a heightened sense of life and daring (for good and bad) that individuals rarely achieve. In the end, the group does not merely substitute for mother, it takes us over totally. It supplies us with love, friendship, protection, strength, precisely defined outlets for emotion, a source of approval and a promise against the loneliness of being thirteen. The group may be a prison with a code of iron, but as a member, we have the biggest identity in town.

Our adolescent ties with the other girls could provide the balance and self-confidence we need now so desperately. We know there are more pitfalls for us in sex than there are for men. Boys are stronger. They don't have to worry about their reputations. Only we can become pregnant. If anything goes wrong, it is always the girl's fault. Within our friendships with women, a larger and freer framework than the stultifying one at home, we might explore ourselves with people who are subject to our own anxieties, curiosity, and joys. We want confirmation that it is all right to go, to separate, to seek our identity on our own and with men. We ask one another for encouragement, for community and a boost up out of childhood. We want the other girls to tell us that is OK, that they too feel what we feel. What we get instead are The Rules.

The Rules institutionalize the anger in our reaction formation. I've never met a woman of any age who could tell me when they were drawn up. It seems at fourteen they were always there. There were certain things no 'nice girl' ever did. No woman I interview can list them, but The Rules run our lives at thirty-five as they did at fifteen. They make us push men away, edit our opinions, dress like everyone else. More than anything, The Rules make us choose: which do we want – sexuality or the love of other women?

The group's job is to find outlets for those pressures society does not yet want to see in us. Slumber parties, romantic gossip, covert and overt sexual relationships with other girls substitute for sex with boys. *The group must keep the woman a girl for a few more years.* An increasingly difficult job when you consider that on the average, girls today are ready to bear children a full six years earlier than a century ago.[1] If you agree that early motherhood is often disastrous, it can be said that the group performs a valuable function here. The price, however, is that many women never really outgrow The Rules.

We never make rules of our own that we believe in more wholeheartedly than we do those of our fourteenth year. 'When I began to go out with men again after my divorce,' says a forty-five-year-old woman, 'I would sit in the car and wonder at the end of the evening, should I let him kiss me, say good-night with a handshake, or go to bed with him? It was like being a kid with all those rules all over again.'

Like some ten commandments of the flesh, The Rules are a list of Thou Shalt Nots: no kissing, no touching, no sexual expression, except to the degree the group allows. 'The rules are made so none of the girls can outdistance any of the others sexually,' says Dr Schaefer. 'It is a truce, an attempt to contain the violence of the competition of all against all for the small amounts of male attention we are allowed. Instead of sex being something that women eagerly join together to get more of, we join together to protect ourselves against it . . . and to make sure that someone isn't getting more than any other girl of that dreadfully dangerous but even more dreadfully exciting stuff.' Those who break The Rules, walk around like pariahs – living examples of the punishment for making us jealous, bringing our competitiveness to consciousness. 'I was fourteen when I started going out with boys,' a woman tells me. 'The rules were unspoken. But there was a pair of twins at school. Everyone speculated about whether they went all the way. We thought one did not, so we were friends with her. Nobody spoke to the other one.' To be excluded from her love was one of the worst punishments mother could dole out. Exclusion is the sentence girls mete out to rule breakers now.

In contrast, boys don't hate the other guy who has sex. They may envy him, but they identify with his success. For a young boy, another's triumph is not a diminishment but a goal, something he can go after. 'When I was sixteen or seventeen,' says Dr Robertiello, 'listening to some other guy talking about what happened in bed with his girl the night before, I admired him. It didn't matter if he was lying, because we wanted to hear those stories. Men are tremendously reinforced by sexual talk. This kind of first-hand data helps get us over our insecurities. Whereas women are silent. So when they get to their first man, or tenth man, they are just as insecure about their performance and sexuality as when they were born. Talks with the other guys gave us a handle on how to act, what boys were supposed to do. Maybe it wasn't the best advice on how to be with a girl but at least when you were sixteen and crawled into bed with a girl for the first time, you remembered what the guys said. That sex is OK. That what is bad is *not* to be sexual. For girls, it's like going into the water without a swimming lesson. No, it's like being told that if you go in the water, you'll drown.'

When the mysterious tides turn in the group and one girl is suddenly left out, she cannot retaliate. She is alone, while those on the inside are bonded even tighter by the fact of her exclusion. The process is merciless and kindest little girls, the nicest grown women, understand it: the girl who is out at the moment must wait, bottle up her anger and pain. In *Pentimento,* Lillian Hellman describes a young woman: 'Anna-Marie was an intelligent girl, flirtatious, good-mannered with that kind of outward early-learned passive quality that in women so often hides anger.'² No trace of it can be allowed to show.

'I'm president of the class,' says a fourteen-year-old. 'But this other girl, who's vice-president, is always running the meetings, which is my job. I never say anything, even though it gets on my nerves. She's one of my best friends. I never show anger because if I'm angry, and I tell my other friends, it always gets back to her. You just can't afford to be angry with your friends. A few of the girls will show their anger, but they aren't popular.' Once more, we are acting out a parallel to the lesson mother began to teach us almost from the day we were born: nice little girls don't get angry.

And yet, anger is one of the dynamics of life. It lingers and rankles; years later it may explode, safely disguised as defense of our own adolescent daughter. 'I could kill those little girls,' a mother says. 'Yesterday, my daughter was *un*invited to a party by this girl Laura, one of her friends! I remember how that can hurt. I tell you I'm furious with those little bitches!'

What does her daughter feel at being excluded? Exactly what her mother felt when *she* was thirteen, and suffered these same hurts. 'I hope Laura changes her mind and invites me again,' she says. 'When she first invited me, my mother changed my dentist appointment so I could go. The next day, I found Laura had taken me off the list. Then a few days later, she said, "Oh, by the way, you're invited to the party." But I found out yesterday I wasn't invited again. Am I angry? Oh, no, I really don't care.'

I really don't care. Is there any reader who believes these four familiar, sad words? Is there any woman who does not recognize herself in this passive reaction?

We pool our (mis)information and aspirations, changing any opinion that is too personal or individual, until everything we say or think boils down to the group attitude. Wanting more, we settle for the lowest common denominator. 'I had to really work to get into the In group,' says a mother of thirty-four. 'All the girls in that group married by the time they were twenty-one, and began popping babies like crazy. They thought I was strange to want to travel, to have a career. I live three thousand miles away now, but I still keep up with them. Whenever my husband and I go to Paris or Rome, I send them a picture postcard. I'm that wild glamorous person to them, and I'm delighted to have them think that. I have a feeling that for most girls who were superpopular as adolescents, life ever after is downhill. I think my keeping up with those girls is a way of verifying that I have succeeded.'

We may never see the girls again whom we knew at fourteen. We never forget their standard of success. If the group's goal was marriage and two babies by twenty-two, even if we succeed in our own self-chosen goals, something is missing at the heart of our achievement. Alternative success never seems so sweet as when it is seen in the group's eyes.

Mother raised us on the principal of *two*. 'It's the *two* of us against the world. Mother may scold but no one loves you more.' It is her defense against the anxiety of our future separation. If she had raised us to feel we could have her love and that of others too, we would embrace our new friends, two, three, and four of them. Abundance would be exciting instead of laced with duplicity and the watering down of the bond. We have been raised as if we were shut-ins, but when we go to school, we are tall enough to see out the windows. Mother's silence about that exciting world out there, her evasions and lack of encouragement for us to go out and explore, makes us evasive and silent too. Our new friend is part of that 'out there' that mother distrusts. We rush home, clutching the idea of her to ourselves like secret treasure. 'Leaving my daughter at camp that first day was devastating,' says a mother. 'I felt I was leaving a part of myself, that I might never see her again. When summer was over, when she came home, she was very secretive. She didn't even want to tell me her new friends' names.'

Says Dr Fredland: 'Children go away to camp for a month, to school for a day, and they come home changed . . . *if* parents can accept these changes and not move in with the old arguments.'

How mother reacts to our new alliances determines not just the wholeheartedness with which we form them but what we come to expect from these new friendships. If mother is afraid for us, controlling, prying, telling us who we can or cannot see, we will try to control our friend, unable to expect more from her than we get at home. If mother is jealous, we will be jealous too – fearful of other people taking our friend away. 'My mother resented one of my friends,' says Dr Liz Hauser. '"Why do you spend so much time with her?" she'd say. "You're always over there, you even eat there." I was a very insecure little girl. I was always afraid something would happen to my mother, that I would lose her as well as anyone else I got close to. Sure enough, as a mother myself, I used to interfere with my daughter Liza's friends too. Just like my mother, I was constantly overprotecting. Often I thought that the other girl was taking advantage of Liza. But I was wrong. In effect, what I was saying was: You can only trust, be honest and open with mommy. Making Liza dependent on me, just as my mother had made me dependent on her. When Liza was born they weren't teaching about symbiosis and separation in my psychology courses at Columbia. Liza was six when I began to try to undo what I had done. It was late but I tried to encourage her to enlarge her world, see more friends, to spend the night out. I want her to get close to a lot of people so that the world seems a welcoming place. Not some place that's only safe if I'm there.'

If mother had said, 'I love you but I want you to love other people too, to have relationships with them as rich as you can make them, and to try other lives than the way I live,' our discovery of life's variety would not seem a betrayal of her. Mother never said we could have this wonderful identification with anyone but her. We are deceiving her . . . or did she deceive us? The very plenty of what is suddenly being offered is bewildering. Richness comes mixed with guilt. Why do women feel they cannot love more than one person at one time? Why does the thought – that the person we love may also love someone else – terrify us? Loving in two directions threatens us with the loss of whomever we are not facing at the moment; there seems to be a minus to every plus in life. 'Promise me that I will be your only friend, your best friend, and that you will leave everybody else out,' we say to another girl. We want the same thing of men ten years later. We cannot ask it of our husband because that would be childish, but when he turns his full attention on others, we feel deprived, hurt. Behind every new love is the fear of loss. We never learned there is enough to go around, enough success, enough friends, enough love.

We lead double lives. We learn to take off our new selves before we get home, before mother's anxiety and control start setting the old limits: 'Don't get so excited, Don't dress that way, Don't talk so loud.' We are aware of her immense influence. Before walking in the door, we tamp down the excitement of being seen by others as the secret selves we've always been, at finding intimates, confidantes, twin people just as hidden and 'misunderstood' as we. We whisper on the phone, though it's only that day's math problems we're comparing. 'She's so quiet nowadays,' a mother says. 'It's not like her. I held her diary in my hand one day, but I knew I couldn't face myself if I read it.'

I interview this woman's fourteen-year-old daughter: 'When I was thirteen,' she says, 'I was with another girl and we smoked a cigarette. Afterward I felt very guilty. I came home and told mom about it. I thought I was going to be forgiven, that I'd have a clean slate and she'd say, "That's all right, just never do it again." But she got angry and yelled at me. I was very hurt, and I think that had a lot to do with my turning away from her. It disappointed me. Up to that age, I'd just assumed if I told the truth I wouldn't be punished. It made me lose trust in her. The same thing happened when I went out with the first boy who kissed me. I didn't tell my mother because I knew she'd be worried about what else had gone on. Nothing else happened, but she'd never believe that. I can't tell her things any more because if I did, she wouldn't believe me.'

Mother 'betrays' us because the old bargain no longer works. She cannot trust us because she does not trust sex and we have suddenly become sexual. Men will deceive us, just as they deceived her. How can she hope we will fare better than she? She says that we cannot learn to drive, though our brother learned when he was a year younger than we. She says we cannot have our own key to the apartment because we are too 'irresponsible and scatter-brained'. We know that is not the real reason. Behind mother's anxiety to guard us against all sorts of dangers which we sense are not very important is the one that *is* important. It is sex, but she will not name that.

Nor can we expect more from the girls in our crowd. 'My friends and I tell each other everything,' says a fourteen-year-old, 'but we have certain understandings. Definite lines. When we go out with boys, we tell each other what we did and didn't do. But if you go past the line of "feeling" – I only mean touching breasts – you don't say anything about it. There's one girl in our crowd who's had sex. There's so much talk about her behind her back that you get paranoid about being talked about that way too if you break the rules. At a slumber party last night, one of the girls left to go to the bathroom. When she returned, she was sure we'd said something horrible about her behind her back.'

Fear of exclusion from the group is a stronger glue than love. It makes us angry even as it holds us together. We feel the group's limits throttle us back, as once we also were by mother's double check of love and control. Reinforced by the group, we dare to break mother's rules: 'One of our favorite expressions is "freaking out",' says a thirteen-year-old. 'My mother hates it. And cursing is in. Everything, especially fuck.' Similarly, when the opportunity comes along – one we are sure no one of our sisters could resist either – we betray the group and break its rules too: 'When I was fifteen and a boy put his hand on my breast,' a woman recalls, 'I thought it was terrible. No nice girl ever did that. But he'd been voted the handsomest boy at Fishburn Military Academy, so I let him.'

Knowing mother's criteria for 'nice girls' – the kind she likes us to be with – it is almost inevitable that we will be drawn to the kind of girl she doesn't like. 'When my daughter started doing more things away from home I was delighted,' a mother says. 'I have a lot going on in my own life. I don't expect her to spend so much time at home, but I don't like some of her friends. One girl I dislike is Sally. She sleeps with boys. That isn't why I dislike her, but she's a disloyal friend. Any time my daughter likes a boy, Sally goes after him. I asked her, if Sally does this, why do you still see her? "I think I'll just not confide in Sally when I like a boy," my daughter said.'

When I interview this woman's daughter she says, 'I like to go around with Sally because she's so different. You sort of feel that you're doing something out of the ordinary by being with her. She's very exhibitionistic, and all the boys talk about her. My mother hates her, absolutely hates her.'

Mother is inhibition; things and people she doesn't like have come to represent life and excitement. In fact, much of what we do with other girls is thrilling only because we know mother would disapprove. In time, when we break the group's rules, the exploit will be all the more thrilling for being forbidden. When we are grown, how often the best sex, the most exciting, will be that which mother and other women wouldn't approve. Stolen sex with the wrong kind of man, in the wrong kind of place, all the more electric because he's married or we're flying home tomorrow. What kind of grown-up sexual people are we when our greatest moments are in ratio to their disobedience to The Rules? The bottom line is that when we marry, when we have the kind of sex mother would approve, sex goes stale. Our true excitement was not purely erotic. Underneath was the greater adolescent kick of rebelling against mom and other women too.

If it were really sex we wanted, if it were our strongest drive, we would break the adolescent rules and join with men in a sexuality that reinforced us. If it was a realistic fear of sex and its consequences (such as pregnancy) that held us back, we would be more intelligent about the use of contraceptives. But it is not sex we want most, nor sex we fear. It is the loss of our place in the society of women.

A woman at a cocktail party tells me she wants to be a writer. She is twenty-five and has a responsible job. She'd had an idea for a story that grew out of a dream. 'It was about a woman on a desert island with a man and another woman,' she says. 'I was one of the women and I was terribly attracted to this man. But I never finished the story. Every time I tried to write what seemed so evocative and powerful to me, I would come up with this same dull ending: this other woman and I just walking off together.' I ask her if she thinks it has to do with competition, that the story says she would do anything rather than compete with a woman. The idea fascinates her and she calls me in a few days to say she finally finished writing the story – *by awarding the man to the other woman*. 'You know,' she says, 'I'll argue with a man. I'll even compete with him for a job. But I hate arguing with women.'

Sociologists speak of a cult of domesticity that once existed, a special 'woman's sphere'. 'It was a secure place,' says Jessie Bernard, 'in which women had warm ties with one another. It was a woman's world, and they loved it.' Sociologist Pauline Bart feels this area in which women were by right and by birth preeminent disappeared when male professionals like gynecologists began to take over. 'Women used to help each other with their own special problems,' she says. 'My great-grandmother used to have herbal recipes for sickness and burns. These were the accumulated bits of female wisdom women shared with one another and passed on to their daughters.'

Perhaps the woman's sphere of our grandmother's day belongs to a time we will see no more. That does not mean a community of women cannot be formed today which would be relevant to contemporary life. 'Men always have had their old-boys' network,' a woman tells me, 'which gives each man within it a feeling of place and identity. In this way, they don't have to see someone younger as a terrifying rival, but as someone it is a pleasure to help out. Since I've become successful in my work, I've gone out of my way to help younger women. It's a great satisfaction. It makes me feel close to women, close to life, part of something larger than my own narrow ambitions. I've always wondered why I had women friends, but felt isolated from them anyway. It was that I always felt I had to protect what I had from them. I'm beginning to feel now that there can be a continuity of "helping" among women, that I can belong to some kind of network myself.'

Jessie Bernard moves me strongly when she says, 'Women have been left sort of bereaved – psychologically high and dry. Women give emotional support to their husbands twice as much as husbands give it back. It leads to severe emotional deprivation, especially in housewives, whose mental health I regard as the Number One public health problem in this country.'

I do not think that the passing of the old 'woman's sphere' alone explains why we are such emotionally hungry people. Our problems of emotional deprivation go back too early in both our collective history as women, and in our individual biographies as daughters. The difficulty is that we have no healthy reserve of narcissism, no trust in our feelings of value built up in the first years of life and then strongly reinforced in adolescence. Perhaps our grandmothers felt this emotional deprivation less because theirs was a time when women lived through others – when independence and sexuality were not so highly prized, and therefore ties to other women were not threatened by anyone's individual success. Another woman might have a bigger house, a more successful husband or children, but these 'achievements' did not threaten. A name, a home, wealth, sexuality – all were given. No woman achieved them for herself; the competition was muted.

The woman's sphere was secure precisely because it was so small. Today a woman's world is as large as she can make it – but that means she has larger yardsticks by which to measure herself. It is from this sense of competition and potential loss that our anachronistic, adolescent fears come back to haunt us.

'You don't get dropped by your group if you have sex,' teenagers today tell me. 'We are more liberal than our mothers. What gets you into trouble with the group is when you have sex with more than one guy.' Superficially, The Rules seem to be new. Factually, if one girl gets more than anyone else, she threatens the cohesion of the group. The need for symbiotic bonding above all else remains the same. How can there be any meaningful new 'woman's sphere' if girls are still raised to feel another woman's gain somehow and mysteriously diminishes them?

How grand is our success when we know other women would love us more if we were less – less beautiful, sexual, successful? We give up our will and initiative. We say to the man, Here I am, defenseless, vulnerable, take care of me. More than sex, we have always wanted symbiosis. We think men will reward and love us forever for giving ourselves over to them. Instead, when we get pregnant, they leave us. If we marry, they get bored with our suffocating clinging and look for more adventurous partners. Hurt, we regress to the only real protection we could ever trust: other women.

The Rules pursue us to the end of life. Winston Churchill's mother outlived his father by a quarter of a century filled with numerous affairs and two marriages to men much younger than herself. On her pain-filled deathbed, she asked herself, 'Is this the punishment for living life the way I wanted and not the way others wanted me to?'

CHAPTER SEVEN

Surrogates and Models

On a day that began like any other, my dentist removed my braces. Losing those wires marked my entry into puberty more significantly than menstruation. What had my vagina ever done for me? We were not even on touching terms. It was my mouth that carried the full potential for excitement: I had recently discovered kissing when my friend Daisy's older brother – who had nothing better to do that evening – put his tongue in my mouth. Fearful that my braces would tear it to shreds, I curled my tongue protectively around the barbed wires. I knew no more about kissing than fucking, but that kiss gave my life direction. It told me how I wanted to spend it. Stripped of my braces, I was ready. If only someone would try again.

I left my dentist's ante-bellum mansion on Broad Street like a prisoner unexpectedly released for good behavior. Grinning and astonished, I moved my lips over my naked teeth and ran all the way to the Memminger Auditorium, where we were rehearsing *The Wizard of Oz*. My Aunt Kate was the Cowardly Lion and I was the Tin Woodsman. She took one look and wrapped her arms around me.

Aunt Kate was the only woman, after my nurse Anna, whose embraces I welcomed, whose breast I allowed myself to lie on. I knew her perfume and the smell of her skin and when the world threatened to be too much in those years, her voice, her presence, the mere idea of her was something to hold on to. 'You're just going through adolescence,' she said to me once, and because she had a name for it, I believed it would end. She was the way I wanted to be when I grew up.

Kate was my mother's youngest sister. She had come to

visit us after graduating from Cornell and had stayed on to live in our house. I don't remember her arrival. My memories begin with an overwhelming need for her, which she filled with a generosity and love I can never repay. She saved my life. If that sounds overly dramatic, understand that it wasn't just the pain of adolescence that she got me through. She also gave me my present life. She got me ready for my husband and my work. The idea of her life, the picture of her, how she was physically and mentally, were my motivation and goal for years when I wanted everything and didn't know what it was I wanted. Long after adolescence, things she had told me, ideas she believed in, ways I observed her to be, were my guideposts. We are very different women today, but I am her child. My whole family knew that, including my mother.

Aunt Kate was different from anyone I had ever known or seen. All my years in Charleston I had wanted nothing more than to blend, to melt into 'the group' and be like everyone else. She had a style, a self-assurance, a truly original spirit that made being 'different' a glorious prize. She didn't try to control me, didn't argue with the southern girl mold I was trying to squeeze into. Her opinions and knowledge fell about me like gifts, waiting until I was ready to open them. One by one they were incorporated into the self I was forming. Even as I stuffed falsies into my bra and made myself shorter by dancing with my knees bent under the conveniently long skirts of the New Look, I was beginning to take pride in being smart, to question whether there might be more to life than chasing boys. I wanted boys too, desperately; I wanted to be popular and to kiss in parked cars until the music station went off the air and my white panties with the lace trim were soaked through. But I wanted more than the standard conclusion of this southern dream – to wear graduation- and wedding-white on the same day. I wanted to act, to write, to travel, to be Kate.

She was my height and had my mother's beautiful auburn red hair. There was nothing in grown women's usual clothes that I coveted; they were a boring sea of shirtwaist dresses and spectator pumps. Kate wore ballet slippers. Her dirndl skirts were cinched at the waist with wide belts, and a gold Egyptian coin dangled from her wrist. Hers could never be called a peasant look; to this day I think of her as the most elegant creature I could imagine. During the day she wrote copy at the radio station and in the evenings she went to the Dock Street Theatre. She didn't just act in plays, she wrote them as well. And she painted. 'Painter or not,' my mother said with caution, 'no one in Charleston has a loft, Kate.' A grand piano, easels, old velvet couches and candles filled the loft Kate rented on the waterfront. I would go there alone and sit for hours, inhaling the turpentine like a promise.

Once Kate brought home one of her big colorful nudes and hung the canvas in the drawing room. My mother didn't notice until guests had arrived for cocktails: 'Oh, Kate, how could you!' she blushed. The red-headed nude in the painting had my mother's face. Everyone laughed and embraced my shy mother and said: 'Jane, you are funny, Jane.' Kate put her arm around my mother and it was all right.

Though I was possessive of my aunt, and distant with my mother, I liked it that they were such good friends. One night when Kate had ingeniously wrapped her bosom in a halter made of two large silken scarves, mother's voice drew the line once more: 'Kate, you can't go to the yacht club like that. People just don't dress like that down here!' My mother has never been able to stop anyone from doing anything – except my sister. When I visit her today and she says, 'Nancy, people don't dress like that here!' I know her anxiety will pass if I am not affected by it. I have often thought that behind my mother's exclamations and disclaimers at what the rest of us do, is an envy, perhaps even some pride, that we are able to carry off a style she would never dare try.

It was the summer after Kate had come to live with us that I dropped out. I stayed home, refused to see my friends, followed Kate around like a shadow. My sister was away at boarding school that year; a time that was to be a grievous experience for her too. I felt abandoned, but more to the point, I felt I was going crazy. I shrank from my mother, rejecting her touch, answering in monosyllables. I would stand at the bathroom basin with the iodine bottle in my hand, fully aware of my overdramatization but also of my fear. I read everything in the house to stave off my impending lunacy. Reading was the only way of marking time until Kate came home for two o'clock dinner. I could rest in her.

Kate didn't just tolerate me, she included me. I followed her everywhere, to her studio, to the theater, out to dinner. In vain, I sought a way of being hired at the radio station so that I could be near her when she worked. And if I wasn't jealous of her friends, it was because they accepted me too. One by one they came from Cornell to visit; some even stayed. It seemed to me they were all tall and beautiful. The men were architects, poets, and actors, people they didn't breed in Charleston. They took me with them to the beach, and when they sat around drinking chilled white wine in the evenings and reading plays together aloud, I was given a part. One night, as we were getting into a car, one of the men said to me in passing, 'You know, you remind me of Kate.' I would gladly have given him my life.

Kate drew up book lists for me. She introduced me to Willa Cather, Conrad, and Henry James. She bought me water colors, and on weekends we would sit in St Phillips graveyard with our sketchbooks on our knees. While she typed her first play on the card table in her bedroom, I wrote my first story about a girl and a horse. She did not mind my interruptions when I asked how to spell a word – interruptions I can see now must have been maddening. When she read my story, she suggested I put in a description of the girl. I did and she said it was good. When her own play was finished, I was given a small part.

It was a big success. I still remember the male lead's line to her heroine, played by Kate's roommate from Cornell: 'You move like a panther, like a tawny panther.' I wanted someone to say that to me when I grew up. I walked like a crippled person, shoulders hunched, knees bent, anything to be shorter. When Kate and I walked up Meeting Street past the Old Slave Market where I had once delivered a paper on General Wade Hampton to The Daughters of The Confederacy, Kate would slap me on the back and say, 'Stand up straight, the Goldwyn Girls are the tallest and most beautiful girls in the world.'

That time in my life when I stayed home to read to avoid my 'thoughts' and clung to Kate as to life itself ended as quickly as it began. Summer was over, school began, and once again I only came home to eat and sleep. As I was on my way out the door one day to meet a friend, Kate called after me, 'Hey, how about a chocolate sundae?' I was late, but I must have heard something in her voice that reminded me of myself: she missed me. We walked to Byer's Drug Store like we used to when I couldn't live without her. During the next years I would run into her on my way out to chase boys, to meet boys, to talk about boys, and I would avoid her eyes. I didn't need her anymore. She never said a critical word.

When I went to my first formal dance, I stood frozen to the wall the entire evening. Not one boy asked me to dance. Kate was waiting when I got home. She had seen the tiny size of the boy who had been sent to escort me. She sat on the edge of the bed stroking my hair while I cried, and told me the story of Launcelot and Guinevere. Once again the promise of her life covered me like a blanket. It wasn't just her words that said my life would become more than I could dream; it was the way she was.

How simple it was when we were three, or even nine and ten. Whatever else we wanted, we wanted 'to grow up like my mother and have children.' Says Jessie Bernard: 'Our society makes a much greater effort to masculinize boys than to feminize girls. It is not necessary for girls. The model each girl lives with is female.' But adolescence and the advent of sexuality change our ideas. Even if we want to be mothers, we don't want to get there her way. In our eyes, mother is not sexual.

For the girl who genuinely wants to re-create her mother's life, the repetition comes with a sense of peace and fulfillment. It feels *right*. Her path goes straight through girlhood, early marriage, pregnancy, with mother's smile and society's approval every step of the way. The daughter who wants something different has a harder time; the idea goes against her mother's model.

Either way, most of us repeat our mother's emotional life. We may not like the idea, but it is a fact. When we are young and energy flows in the veins like wine, we have no intention of giving up vitality, humor, adventurousness. It is unthinkable that we will ever be as anxious and conservative as mother. Then one day we hear ourselves telling our husband not to drive so fast, nagging our children to clean up their rooms, and we know we've heard that voice before. The degree to which we can forge our own emotional selves depends greatly on the help we get from other people who love us, people whose lives offer a pattern we can follow. People whose great virtue is the paradoxical one that they are not mother.

When we meet an old friend of mother's, who recounts how daring and exciting mother was before she married, it is riveting as a fairy tale. It has the power of truth in a framework of the mythic. We both want to believe and don't. 'My mother finally took the mirrors out of my bedroom because she thought I looked in them too much,' a woman of forty-five says. 'And yet my father tells me she was very vivacious before they married, that she loved dancing and laughed a great deal. Now he is the one with the sense of humor. I suppose as he became more lively, she felt someone had to keep the balance in the family. In a way, I can understand that. I used to be more lively . . . before I was married, before I had children.'

During family reunions when I was growing up, I loved my aunts to tell stories about my mother as a young woman. My mother – with different men, making conquests! I still pore over old photos of her jumping horses in dangerous steeplechases. It is thrilling to think of her taking chances. By the time I came along, she had changed.

If she could have offered herself to me as a model of daring, independence, and sexuality, would it have availed? I've known so many admirable women whose daughters reject their lives. Other women's daughters may emulate them, but the girl under their own roof will look elsewhere, *outside* the immediate family, for someone who stands for a different, roomier world, simply because mother is not in it. What I did learn from my mother was her other side: overcaution, anxiety, fear. I have tried to hide these traits behind the more daring qualities I learned from others. I know the world sees me as independent. I know myself as my mother's daughter. Mother is love and life itself, and we want to hold on to that, but a model for sexuality and independence is a bridge toward separation. Mother cannot be that for us.

Taking our mother as a model opens the door to problems of competition. Many of the women therapists I have interviewed are very much aware of why their daughters have turned to totally opposite fields of achievement. 'My daughter is a first-class musician, a superb cook,' one psychiatrist says. 'I've got a tin ear and I couldn't be less interested in cooking. She has a tough job, coming after me. I can understand why she doesn't even want to dabble in those areas where I'm so proficient.'

I do not mention the word competition to this woman's fifteen-year-old daughter. She brings it up herself but denies any competition at all between mother and herself. 'People don't understand how my mother can have her family and a full career too. Why should she be home taking care of me twenty-four hours a day? I get a lot of talk from my friends and their mothers, "She must be hard to compete with," they say. Why should I be jealous of her? She's given me the knowledge I can do what she's done, but there is no competition. I don't want her life. She is not my model. I'm a different kind of person than she is. My mother's more competitive than me. I just hate that feeling. I dropped out of the school orchestra because I didn't like fighting for chairs. I want to get ahead for my own pleasure, not because I want to knock someone down on the way up.'

This young woman recently broke with a longstanding boy friend when he objected to her plans to become a lawyer and continue a career after marriage. She says she does not want to emulate her mother's life, but she rejects a man who will play her father's role – he actively did encourage his wife to combine marriage and a career. If she finds such a man, if she succeeds in her desire to become a lawyer, her life will have paralleled her mother's. And yet she denies the repetition. It is not so much the emulation of her mother's life this young woman wants to avoid as knowledge that to set her goals as high as her mother's necessarily brings with it a kind of psychic competition. She doesn't want to 'knock down' or be 'knocked down' by her mother. In any contest, her mother starts with all the aces.

'Getting unstuck from even a "good enough" mother,' says Dr Robertiello, 'is best accomplished if you can form an alliance with someone else, someone close, like your grandmother or father. To separate, you have to ally yourself with a person you feel knows the way, who is stronger, wiser or more independent than you.' These people give us a source of power and strength outside of mother. They need not physically take care of us, but in a sense psychologically stand *in loco parentis*. They have many names in the technical vocabularies, least awkward among which are identification figures or role models. They are the dreams for us to grow on.

Childhood is marked by dependency; mother's tutelage means we are 'done to': instructed, told to do this, wear that, go there and eat our spinach. Role models open the door to the concept of choice and activity. They see us as bigger people than mother did and show us that there are self-directed people who make their own decisions, go out and do it, taking the credit or blame for their lives. Obviously, it is possible to get through childhood without identification figures, but our need for them is intense during adolescence. It is a stormy period because all the problems that weren't resolved in our first three or five years now come up again. Life gives us a second chance here, but without help, new images, hope in the form of other people, it often doesn't turn out any better than the first time around. We give in. We stay attached.

'Oh, God, yes! Alternatives to mother!' says Dr Sanger. 'Mother is so absolute. She knows how she wants her daughter to be, "Be like this, be like that, be like me!" If the girl has an aunt, an older friend, a grandmother, a teacher, a great lady like Eleanor Roosevelt who's impressive as a woman – that's terrific. Even knowing men who like women to be independent can be helpful too. It doesn't have to be direct, it can be indirect and still be useful.'

'I can't think of any woman I admire, that I want to be like,' says a fourteen-year-old whose mother is one of the most admirable women I know. 'Except this older friend of mine. She's seventeen. She's very creative. I think she's wonderful. She's got her own opinions, which doesn't mean she doesn't hear other people out. But she doesn't let them make her go against herself.' A couple of days after our interview, this girl telephones me long distance to tell me she has remembered another woman who is 'sort of a heroine of mine'. It is Katharine Hepburn.

Katharine Hepburn. She was one of my models too. Unmarried, childless, flat-chested – she is the antithesis of what mother and society want for us. And yet my mother adores her, and men too seem to sense something heroic in her. She transcends looks, style, or whatever particular circumstances the scriptwriter places her in; through force of character, by making it on her own, by never giving up and keeping her integrity intact, she wins us all. She is an image of the separate person.

Our model may be someone we meet one day or night, and never see again. She can be just a glimpse of an idea that we will fill in later, the way we imagine her and want to be ourselves. 'There was a woman who came to lecture one day when I was in the eighth grade,' says a thirty-four-year-old mother of two girls, who runs her own industrial design company. 'She showed slides, and I remember she gave a little talk on Barnard. She was an alumna, and I guess she was drumming up business, but I never got over her. She was young, pretty, so cool and intelligent and unlike all the nice mom-like moms in the little town where I grew up. I fastened on her and that college like a signal from heaven. I don't remember what she said, but that was it, the other side of the rainbow. I was going there, by God!'

We don't need an ongoing relationship with her so much as an image we can hold ever before us. She need not even be alive. The women we read about as young girls, the Nancy Drews, the Diana Riggses of television, or the more contemporary Isadora Wings, spark our imaginations and give us something to live for, to grow toward when our emotional bags are packed and we have no definite place to go, no identity to travel in. 'Very often,' says Dr Robertiello, 'we analysts tend to say someone's personality is formed by the time they are seven. But some of us are beginning to get away from that dogmatic notion. I strongly feel that somebody you run into at twelve or fourteen can change your life enormously – the people you take in and identify with at that age can have tremendous influence on the rest of your life. Think of how many lives have been changed, for instance, by a child meeting a certain teacher.

'Most analysts – I am guilty too – focus on the idea of mother being the central figure, but in the course of a psychoanalysis we often uncover other, forgotten people who turn out to be crucial in the person's development. Mother and father may have nowhere near the impact of a childhood nurse. Whatever matrix has been developed from your good and bad experiences can be greatly changed through identification figures even after childhood is over.'

Often we don't know what it is we want. We have abilities, talents, the potential to go long distances, but until somebody *sees* us, recognizes our secret selves, we will go the short distance and remain the safe, unexplored person. 'When I went to college,' recalls a twenty-five-year-old woman, 'I expected by the third day for everyone to see through my facile ways and say, "I don't know how you got here, but if you're going to stay, you're going to have to buckle down and use that brain of yours." I had the feeling up till then that I had fooled everyone at school. It wasn't until my senior year that I met this teacher who was head of the English Department. She gave me the first C I ever got in my life. I'd always got straight As without trying. I went to her and said, "Miss James, yours is the only class in this college I've worked hard for. Why did I get a C?" She smiled diabolically and said, "Because you've been doing B work, and if you tried harder you could do A work. I wanted to shake you up." I was hers. I was her slave. Somebody had seen through me at last, *had seen me*. I've never forgotten her.'

Even images of how *not* to be can be crucial to our development. Many women choose life-styles as much unlike their mother's as they can. 'I am not convinced you have to like the people who are your models,' says sociologist Cynthia Fuchs Epstein. 'Men have traditionally tried to be like their fathers – whom they may have despised. Nobody has really paid too much attention to these processes in studies, but the impact of role models can be subtle and unacknowledged.' Women may not have liked the fact that their mothers worked when they were little; they may still be angry that when they came home after school, mother was at the office or taking a postgraduate degree. Later, when these same daughters end up with interesting work and careers of their own, where do you think they got the idea?

The negative models perhaps most often objected to when we are young are overly strict or puritanical parents. One usual course is for the child outwardly to act against the harsh strictures the parents lay down, but to introject their values nevertheless. That is, we will break our parents' rules, but feel we are a rat, a bad daughter, for doing so. 'An extremely important kind of identification figure,' says Dr Betty

Thompson, 'is someone who can relieve the girl of this guilt, of her mother's introjected superego. This new figure can allow the daughter to develop a better opinion of herself. The girl can recognize there is more than one set of standards in the world that she can opt for. If someone you admire lets you feel you don't have to be all that perfect for her to like you, it's very satisfying, very relaxing. There are usually many people around for an adolescent to identify with, and they can fulfill many different functions. A healthy person will tend to pick out the best available model in her environment.' If a girl with a mother who doesn't want to let her go finds a strong role model – a teacher, for instance, or an aunt – the new figure can give her insight into why mother didn't want her to grow up. 'You might find out what your rights are as a human being,' Dr Thompson continues, 'rights which you may have been afraid to exercise until you saw the model of someone else to whom these freedoms were as matter-of-fact as air.'

Before Leah Schaefer became a psychotherapist she was a jazz singer. 'I think I got my idea for this kind of life from the movies I saw as an adolescent. I lived in the movies. I remember my adolescence as miserable. I didn't feel that boys liked me, or that my mother understood what I was feeling. We had always been close – until then. Now I felt cut off from her. But I wanted to be sexy and glamorous and wear terrific clothes and have all the boys fall down dead over me. All of which I wasn't about to have. There was no one to help me have even a part of it. So I felt terribly alone. Except for these wonderful people in the movies. After college I became a singer. When I was successful, my mother loved it. But when I was out of work she wanted no part of me. When I was doing what she would have liked to have done – to be a winner at something – she was the most helpful person in the world. When I decided to go back to graduate school and become a therapist, she loved it. Her daughter the doctor.

'I used to get angry and depressed when she disapproved of me. But now I can see that if she was unfair to me, she was unfair to herself. She treated me exactly as she treated herself. I figured out that it wasn't me, Leah, she disapproved of. What she didn't like was when she saw something in me of herself that she didn't like. You see, I was her narcissistic extension. When I wasn't a winner, she saw herself as a loser.

'From my side, I felt that if my mother didn't give me what I wanted – her approval and love – there must be something wrong with me. I was leading a very different life from hers, but I was still emotionally tied to her. As children we assume that if our omniscient, omnipotent parents don't give us what we want, there is something wrong with *us*. My mother led me to believe in her great powers from the beginning. She knew everything. She could do anything. Not even my life as a singer – just about as far from her life as I could get – convinced me that I could live in my own identity. Powerful as those images were that I had grown up on, those successful, glamorous people in the movies, magnetic as they had been in helping me get away from home, they could not contend with this even stronger pull I had to remain attached to my mother. Once I stopped demanding that she be the perfect mother, the kind of mother I wanted, we got along fine. But I was forty-two before I came around to that way of thinking.'

Until recently, the women to whom young girls turned for role models during adolescence were almost stock figures. There were so few areas in which women were, by the nature of their work, assertive and self-affirming, that school teachers and camp counselors appear with the regularity of family friends. Today, my woman editor, my woman literary agent, or any of the dozens of admirable women you and I know if only on television, are available models. Pediatrician Dr Virginia E. Pomeranz tells me that many of her women patients 'are eager for their daughters to go to both women pediatricians and women gynecologists, so that they can see a good role model, a woman who is a wife and a professional success. For the same reason,' she smiles, 'they bring their sons here too.'

As yet, the women with whom an adolescent is most likely to come into contact, to get a real feel of, remain the tried and true favorites. A gym teacher embodies the idea of aggression in the best sense, of being very connected with selfhood: if you play tennis with style and can throw a basketball well, that is a self-affirming kind of activity. Drama teachers are attractive because they direct people; in fact, anyone 'in charge' is helpful, people who put things together and furnish directions but leave room for you to bring your own talents to the role. They allow autonomy to grow because they do not do the whole job for us; they let us stand or fall on our own. It is wonderful when your heroine returns your affection and respect, but you don't want her living through you the way mother did. Ideally, she is there when you need her, but she doesn't cry Betrayal when you walk away. She has her own life, and allows you to have yours.

'I've always had my dreams,' says a seventeen-year-old freshman from a small coed college in the Midwest. 'I wanted to take a pre-med course, but I got so much hassle I dropped the idea. Then I got to know the woman who is dean of students there. I admired her liberation, her feelings that all the doors are open to women nowadays. I know now there is no way I'm going to be like most women on this campus . . . the homecoming queen type going out with a jock. What is depressing is that so many girls only come here for husbands. Maybe the guys encourage it, but if I hadn't met this woman, I don't know where I'd be. Watching her, seeing the things she has done, I know I can do the same. She's full, she's complete. She's not married, but she's perfectly happy with her life.'

If we cannot find models who will safely help us separate and become our own women, we may just give up and retreat back to where we started. A return to mother at this stage of development is a significant defeat, sapping our self-confidence and undermining our will to try again. People like this carry a feeling of resignation through life, never trying too hard for anything; they are convinced of failure before they begin. They are the eternal victims, repetitiously falling into masochistic relationships with dominating and selfish men whom they are unable to leave. Whatever significant models of self-affirmation may have come along in their formative years, just never 'took'. As they reach out toward people who represented autonomy, their need for security pulled them back to the person who never wanted them to go in the first place. They wake one day and find themselves in a spot they never intended to be, and don't know how they got there. In their lives – especially when they become mothers – they recognize an all too familiar pattern of behavior in which they feel trapped.

I am not saying that women would be better off not to marry, nor that it is a defeat to become like your mother. What matters is whether your life is your choice. If you have won independence first, so the decision to follow your mother's life comes of your own volition, and not out of a sense of passive inevitability, duty, or fear, that is a victory. It is a self-affirmative life, as valid as anyone else's.

The discussion here is about another kind of woman, one who did not want her mother's life, but finds she is repeating it anyway. Alternatives may have come along, were tried out, but always held too great an element of danger. They were exhilarating for a month or two, all right for a few years after college, but could not be counted upon for a lifetime. These young women may have geographically left home, experimented with sex, dabbled at love, work, men, but were never fully engaged in what they were doing. 'I have always thought there was a boarding school side of me, representing my conservative mother,' a young woman says, 'and a hippie side, which represents the people I lived among for the first years after I left home. But I don't feel I belong to either. When I'm on the top floor of a high building, I sometimes think I'm just going to drift away.' The usual solution for women like this is marriage. Sally Smith doesn't sound like much – largely because she has always been Mrs Smith's daughter. But Mrs John Jones – *that's* an identity.

Or is it?

In all fairness, it must be said that our view of mother makes it almost impossible for her life to aid our separation. An independent woman is one who has a totally different relationship to life, to men, to work, and to herself than we were ever willing to perceive in mother. If she has an existence independent from us, we dislike it, discredit it. *She is our mother!* She should be *there*, attached, waiting for us when we got home from school or from a fight with our friends. It is our privilege to leave her, not hers to leave us. The lament is almost universal among the daughters of successful women I've interviewed. I am guilty myself: I've said that I used to be thrilled by photos taken before I was born, of my mother as an intrepid horsewoman; but I also remember – with greater emotional intensity – my silent recriminations that she was often out for the evening, was younger than the mothers of my friends, that she didn't wear an apron and have gray hair.

We insist that mother be homey, unglamorous, 'Like everybody else's mother.' Then with the unfairness of children, once we have safely imprisoned her in the stereotype, we reject her as lacking excitement and jaunt off looking for someone else – someone who will be different, who will give us an idea on how to leave home, an arm to lean on while we try on our shaky new identities.

What makes the mother-daughter relationship so poignant is its bewildering reciprocity. What one person does, feels, inevitably affects the other. 'Even with all my professional training,' says Dr Schaefer, 'I can't help getting these feelings of rejection and abandonment about my adolescent daughter. Katie had always loved going everywhere with Thomas and me, to the theater, to friends' houses. She was wonderful company and we loved to include her. Suddenly, she didn't want to go anywhere with us. The phone rang endlessly for her, and she only had time for her friends. A friend would come to visit, they'd immediately go up to Katie's room, the door would close, and that would be that. Of course I was happy for her to be growing up, but it took terrific objectivity on my part plus Thomas's repeated assurance that she was just going through a phase, and that she hadn't rejected me; I could just feel the surge of retaliation in me, the desire to be punitive about the telephone or to set strict hours in which she could see her friends. If you have been close with your daughter, it is very, very hard when she turns to other people for what she almost exclusively used to find in you.'

An important ethical point arises. If it is mother's duty to let us go, the responsibility for our going rests with us. I agree with Mio Fredland that 'a mother should be a good loving consultant,' but among the first signs of maturity is to know the difference between what your mother should be told about your experiments in new life-styles, and what should be kept to yourself. If we tell her everything, more than she's asked to know, it is a sure sign we are not serious about our efforts to be independent. We are like adulteresses who lay their sins on the conjugal bed in a childish plea for forgiveness.

'All my friends communicate better with their mothers than I do,' says a fifteen-year-old. 'A lot of things I'd like to tell her, but she just wouldn't understand. She thinks I'm not mature and responsible enough to handle things. She just wouldn't believe the things I do and think.' In simple justice, if mother must show almost superhuman generosity by giving her teen-age girl a boost out of the house, then surely there has to be a commensurate obligation on the daughter. Says Mio Fredland; 'Mother usually doesn't expect too much back from her child. She regards what is best for her daughter as paramount in the relationship. But the girl will always be more concerned for herself than for her mother.'

So be it. But all too often the complaint, 'I wish I could talk to my mother,' really means, 'Why can't I tell her I'm smoking dope or drinking in bars and get her approval for it?' One of the harsh laws of growth is that adolescents are going to make dangerous explorations of life. It may be necessary; I think it is. One of the great crimes against young girls is parents' passion to wrap the darlings in so much crippling cotton wool that we never run a moment's risk of unhappiness. Young girls are not made to understand you can't have it both ways. We want to imitate the exciting, perhaps dangerous people we meet, but to do so with mother's full approval. This kind of protectionism leads to the feeling there are no consequences to our actions which our parents cannot fix. It is a distortion of reality, retarding maturation and prolonging symbiosis.

Just as we understand when a racing driver's wife prefers not to go out to the track to watch him in his risky occupation, by adolescence we should understand that maybe mother might prefer not to know we are having sex with a man of twenty-five – and should not be asked for her sanction. If we are not old enough to take the responsibility, we should not do it.

The wonder is not that so many of us fail, but that so many succeed – and we aren't all walk-around, wind-up children, sexual pygmies for life. When you think about it, how do we get through all that denial? The areas of conflict with mother that we've learned to avoid – our bodies, anger, masturbation, aggression, sexuality, competition – read like a program for retardation. And yet there we are: me writing this book, you raising your children, working – most women on the whole making a pretty satisfactory job of their lives. We may resonate with terror at the anonymous telephone call in the night, at the stranger in the street who whispers *fuck* into our ear, but we don't retreat. We don't go into a room and barricade ourselves against life forever. We try again.

Where do we get all that bravery?

'That's something I don't understand myself,' says sociologist Pauline Bart. 'All these theories say if you don't have good childhood experiences, you won't have a good sex life. I had the worst early experiences: double messages from my mother – which I feel are worse than no messages – consistent abuse from my father during adolescence, and then a bad early marriage. And yet – here I am!'

Why indeed is Pauline Bart one of the most vital and lively

women I have met, while others, who seem to have had better psychological starts in life, strike me as dull and timid, living under wraps? We cannot forget that our genetic inheritance is not democratic.

Among my own friends, the most interesting people had difficult parents and stormy adolescences. Basic temperament and other mysteries of the personality cannot be dismissed in trying to explain the paradox of transcendence – that so many of us *do* move against all the odds to find a larger world. And while I believe that role models make up a great part of the answer, it is fascinating to wonder why we choose some people to serve as this bridge toward growth and ignore others – who, to the outside eye, would seem to be very glamorous indeed. In my research, for instance, I have found that people like Gloria Steinem and Jane Fonda don't 'take' the imagination of most women. We may admire them, but I've never heard a woman say she wanted to be like them. They are the revolutionaries; we are still our mothers' daughters. We may intellectually admire or respect the ethos that extreme feminists project, but on the deeper, gut levels where we live, we have not yet introjected these values and made them our own: they seem anti-male, or so 'unfeminine' they make us uncomfortable. It may take another generation or two for women to begin to differentiate between a kind of generalized antipaternalistic anger directed against society as a whole, and our own individual furies. Meanwhile, the Jane Fondas and Gloria Steinems are models of assertiveness and independence that do not totally convince us. At fourteen we are shopping for a picture of sex we can accept – and hip, emotionless movie-star sex, or the feminist-separatist notion of no sex at all, is not it.

Our model of self-individuation is not always our sexual model. In a society that denigrates explicit female sexuality, we will be lucky to find any sexually defined woman at all. Little wonder that the people we look to for sexual models are often the 'bad' girls our own age. Their spirit is just too much to resist. By being 'bad' they are demonstrating what we long to achieve: separation. Even if we ourselves are not yet ready to 'go all the way,' we want to know there are people who do. They are our future.

During my interviews, I meet a woman with marked nonphysical, even asexual demeanor, but whose twenty-one-year-old daughter broadcasts just the opposite notion of sensuality. I wonder where the girl gets the freedom to see that sexuality is allowable for women, and ask for an interview. I questioned her about the first time she consciously realized some people had sexual ideas different from her mother's. 'When I was fourteen,' she says, 'there was a really beautiful girl in the small town where we spent our summers. Whatever I had that she didn't – intelligence, kind parents – they didn't seem as important as her suntan, her amazing figure, and popularity with the boys. She made an agreement with her boy friend. If he would stop smoking, she would not wear a brassiere. I've always remembered that. I never dreamed you could have such a daring agreement with a boy. I was fascinated by her, and a bit repelled too, but I have always remembered her.'

Adolescent boys have an easier time finding sexual models than we do. They may not think of their fathers as Don Juans, but at least they see them responding to women, turning to look at a pretty girl in the street, talking about sex. We may not like this, it may be done in bad taste, but it gives the boy a sense that it is OK to be sexual. But when did you last hear a mother remark to her daughter about the sexual appeal of a good-looking man? Oh, we talk about his hands, his eyes, the cut of his suit, but what about the seductive line of his hip or shoulder? How does mother react to an off-color joke? No wonder women have no background, no role models for response to blue movies. We have no sexual camaraderie.

I remember how puzzled I was the first trip to the beach when nobody talked about those fascinating bulges in men's bathing suits. I sat with my little shovel, staring at my first man in a latex Jantzen and learned women's silence.

Today men have begun to dress to be looked at. In part,

this is due to the perception that women are no longer as responsive to the undifferentiated male role as they used to be. If most women used to set their sights so modestly that 'anything in pants' was good enough, the gray-flannel suit would do. As women come to value themselves more, and thus feel they have greater latitudes of choice, men have begun to compete for the eyes of women.

Women may not yet be aroused by the nude male centerfolds in magazines. Psychologists report we are not as sexually stimulated visually as men. The implication is that this is biological, that we are born nonvoyeurs. My own feeling is that it is learned behavior. Once women are given an unprejudiced start as sexual people, we will know at last if the eye alone can turn women on. We will also know *what* turns us on, and instead of men's ideas of what women want, we will produce our own erotic imagery. Meanwhile, young girls today still turn reverentially West, to Hollywood, for an image of sexuality.

At least, films fill the aching void. At worst, they give us an idea of woman and sex so overly romanticized that when it does come at last, we wonder why it doesn't feel the way it did when Robert Redford held Ann-Margret in his arms. We confuse sex with romance because we never see a sexual woman from a woman's point of view. Says film critic Molly Haskell: 'What we get instead are men's fantasies of women, that a woman is either a virgin or a whore. We used to get the pure girl next door – Debbie Reynolds, Doris Day, Grace Kelly. In the late '60s they tried to give us sexual women – Carrie Snodgress in *Diary of a Mad Housewife* and Jane Fonda in *Klute*. But these women were not a source of energy and imagination for women. They projected a kind of enervated, used-up feeling.' They were not the way we wanted to be.

Molly Haskell's general remarks are given poignant, individual meaning in an interview with a thirty-year-old woman. 'I used to go to the movies three times a day,' she tells me. 'I didn't have any sex activity in my early life at all, no sex play, never masturbated, no sex games with other kids, but I did have tremendous amounts of fantasy, based on what I saw in the movies. I used to get a tremendous amount of sexual feelings through watching them make love in the movies – though of course I didn't know then that was what I was feeling. Nobody had told me anything about my body. I just thought my crushes and movie nostalgia were romantic fantasies that adolescents were supposed to have. I had no idea that I was reacting not romantically to the people on the screen but sexually. I didn't know what to name these feelings, and since I'd never touched myself, and I never looked at myself – had in fact been discouraged to look at myself 'there' – I was just terrifically curious and confused about sex and romance most of my life. I resisted getting married. I was always afraid that if you lived with someone day to day, the "mystery" would go. He would see me as I really was, and not as the romantic sex queen I'd made myself after all those stars of the silver screen.'

Between mother's great No to sex and the false sexuality we see in the commercial world we live in, little wonder that one of the biggest jobs we have in adolescence is to establish that core of self which psychiatrists call 'gender identity'. It is a fascinating concept.

Gender identity can be defined as the way we see ourselves as either male or female – subjectively, not anatomically. And one of the measures of our lives is the degree of certainty we feel in this identity. Until recently, how a woman felt about her femaleness didn't matter. If her anatomical identity said she was female, there was a rigid set of personality and character traits she was expected to have, and they corresponded exactly with how others reacted to her. Today we are beginning to see that by strictly defining emotional or behavioral patterns as *masculine* or *feminine*, we put straitjackets on both sexes.

When I was fifteen and read Stendhal's *The Red and the Black*, I think I identified not with the Duchess but with the daring and courage of Julien Sorel, the hero who leaves home to seek fame and fortune (which is the storytelling way of saying goes off on the quest for identity). But my identification was a secret one. Twenty years ago it was unladylike to even think of acting 'like a man'. Because my identification was hidden and shameful to me, it was only partially nourishing. When instead of marrying like the girls I grew up with, I left home to go north, my allegiance to my role was only tentative. Because I could not be open about who and how I wanted to be, I was only half responsible for myself. I worked as ambitiously as Julien, but unlike him, when I succeeded and the top jobs were offered to me, I made excuses to turn them down. I slept with the men I wanted, but feared rejection constantly. My heroes, my models, the people who had attracted me in books and in real life were men. It was too confusing. I wanted to be a woman but I didn't want to be like other women. I had no models.

'Everyone has the potential to have the qualities we think of as masculine or feminine,' says Jessie Bernard. 'I would like to see both sexes have them – sons who are gentle and tender, daughters who can be strong and assertive. Perhaps with men becoming involved with the raising of children today we will see this happen.' The contemporary idea of gender definition is more complex and richer for women than it has ever been. Given a modicum of ease about her gender identity, a young girl in the process of formation will try to strengthen those feelings about herself she likes best, borrowing character traits from the most admirable female and male figures around her. She may choose to be a girl-girl, as pop lyrics put it, an old-fashioned, clinging creature; or she may take on the characteristics of a woman so contemporary she has not yet been given a pop-tune name – someone sexually giving, who possesses what used to be called masculine assertiveness. Or any mixture of the two. When I was nineteen, my authoritarian grandfather turned on me when I argued with him. 'Where did you learn to speak back like that?' he demanded. 'From you,' I told him. If we are secure in our gender identity, it never occurs to us to feel we are "wrong" to be the way we are. 'Since I am a woman,' a friend said to me recently, 'anything I do is womanly.'

But let me add an important caveat here. While I do believe notions of gender identity are changing to allow all of us to take in more of life's complexity, that change has not yet become a universal gut feeling. We live an almost schizoid sense of values. Right along with our assent to the latest manifesto on sexual freedom, says Dr Robertiello, 'we find that a woman's idea of her gender identity, her subjective feeling about herself as a woman, is much more connected with her concept of herself as a mother than it is with her concept of herself as a sexual person.

'For instance, say a woman is divorced and has a number of lovers. She still isn't going to be able to think of herself as an adequate woman if she isn't fulfilling her mothering functions with her child. Can you have good sex if you think of yourself as a bad woman? You might have a good time in bed, but you would put a pejorative connotation on it. Instead of saying, "Aren't I an exciting, sexual woman?" you would say, "I'm a bad person, I should be home taking care of my daughter."'

I would go even further than Dr Robertiello. We do not even have to be mothers to see our gender identity more connected with motherhood than sexuality. So long as we have not repeated the model of our mother's life, most of us will live with a suspicion of failure, of being incomplete.

For instance, I would have told you that I was totally committed to my decision not to have children; and yet when I was writing the first chapter of this book, my argument against the maternal instinct was so strong and out of proportion that I was almost unable to get past it. I could not give it logical emphasis – no more, no less – because I was defending myself. All the intellectualizing in the world hasn't yet convinced me that in going against my training I have not abandoned my true gender identity, true femininity.

Women I have interviewed who are fifteen years younger than I say it is easier for their generation to choose whatever life they want. To whatever degree this is true, I am sure it has to do with the models of other women's lives. Young women today have an unmistakable advantage over previous generations, and as they consolidate the gains made by the women who came before, they too will become models for those yet to come. When a woman can have sex with her husband or lover and feel as sure of herself in that role as when she holds a baby in her arms – that is a time worth working for.

In a fascinating study, sociologist Pauline Bart documents the damage done to the psyche when a woman substitutes *motherhood* – which is one possible element in gender identity – for *femaleness*, which is the whole. The study was based on hospital records of 550 depressed women in Los Angeles, in the age bracket forty to fifty-nine. 'I also did twenty interviews,' says Dr Bart. 'When I asked the women about sex, they would sort of avoid it. If I asked them to rank sex roles in order of importance – one of which was "Being a Sexual Partner to My Husband" – that was never chosen first or second, and only rarely did it even come in third.'

In another part of this test, Dr Bart showed women twelve simple but evocative pictures and asked the subjects to make up a story about the life of the women in the pictures – a well-tested and standard projective technique. In one of the pictures, the woman is seen in bed wearing a black lace nightgown, and with one leg raised. 'It was a very sexy picture,' Dr Bart says, 'but the subjects rejected the picture. If they did choose it, they denied the sexual content. They'd say something like, "This is a picture of a woman who has just put the baby down for a rest, and she's tired herself." ' The threatening idea of sex was immediately replaced with the safe association of motherhood. When Dr Bart asked why the picture was omitted, the reply she often got was, 'Oh, that picture is about a woman with not very good morals.'

'These women,' Dr Bart concludes, 'just could not deal with sex. They were very, very conventional, good, traditional, well-scripted women who followed the rules a hundred and fifty percent, and part of the script is that a woman is not sexual.' Can we doubt that the inability to connect femininity and sexuality is in part responsible for the depression suffered not only by the women interviewed by Dr Bart but by the female race as a whole?

While role models and identification figures help us separate from mother, surrogates play a different role in our lives. Child psychologists usually limit the meaning of the word 'surrogate' to those early substitutes for mother – often dimly remembered but almost mythically important people who fed us emotionally as well as physically. They were the nurses, housekeepers, grandmothers and older sisters who gave us warmth and intimacy when mother was physically or psychologically not available to us for any of a variety of reasons. In that dependent time of life, before we were ready to separate, and closeness to someone was all, surrogates taught us many of the emotional and personality traits we carry through life.

Theirs were the smiles we wanted and it was in their eyes we looked for the love and approval we needed. 'They are our psychological mothers,' says Betty Thompson, 'the ones who teach us our emotions. Many women who have unemotional, nondemonstrative biological mothers nevertheless grow up with the spontaneity, vitality, eye behavior or warm voice cadence of the surrogates who held them and responded to their needs when they were babies.'

'I actually call the woman who nursed me for six years "mother",' says Joan Shapiro, professor of social work at Smith College. 'I have her sense of humor, her gestures, her love of music, dancing, and out-of-doors. When my daughter went to visit her, she saw so much of me in her that she immediately called her "grandmother". My nurse's feelings about me as her oldest child are even now so strong that her own grown children are jealous.'

Given the developmental imperatives of adolescence, in which we need to experiment with freedom while never wanting to lose our bond to mother, the need for surrogates arises again. At twelve and fourteen we go through a replay of the *rapprochement – or refueling – phase*, experienced first at two or three. In adolescence, the person we find to substitute for mother in this experimentation with getting away is often a girl of our own age. We hold on to each other for safety even as we plan for the adventures ahead. These ardent crushes, even when there is homosexual activity, are usefully understood as a need for refuge and mutal mothering more than a desire for explicit sex. 'The first love one has,' says Betty Thompson, 'is usually a re-creation of the emotional relationship of Eden – the one that once existed between your mother and yourself.' Falling in love means falling in love either with a memory of that relationship, or with a fantasy of how you wish it had been. 'Even in those suffocating affairs,' adds Dr Thompson, 'where the girl cannot bear to be away from the boy for one moment – that's a re-creation of the infantile relationship. It is easy to see that the boy friend is playing the role of surrogate mother.'

Fortunate is the adolescent who has a relationship with someone she can admire, but who also loves her back. This other person combines the role of both surrogate and role model. It can be a girl's first taste of resolving the seeming contradictions of wanting freedom from mother but wanting to be close to someone too. One of the great advantages is that the surrogate is not so fearful for us, nor so locked on. The emotional intensity of the relationship is not so burning. Equally important, our fears of re-engulfment by mother are eased. With a surrogate, we have the old mothering security at our back, giving us the freedom to face into the future. If we are lucky, we will find this feeling with someone else once again later in life. This marvelous balancing act between two people can be a rehearsal for marriage.

'In my work, as well as in my own personal life,' says Professor Shapiro, 'I've found that when you have a good experience with an early mother surrogate, you tend to develop a nose for finding others along the way. You develop an appealing "needy" quality that potential surrogates pick up on. There are those who need mothering. There are those who enjoy giving it.'

There is a big difference between the surrogates of childhood and those we find during adolescence. It is choice – ours. Our nurses and older sisters who comforted and held us when we were babies did so by their choice. The surrogates of adolescence, the people whose bodies, approval, touch, and esteem become so vital to our continued growth, are chosen by us. *We pick them.* We are old enough by now, formed enough to have some notions of what we want. Our needs are more psychological than to be fed, held, and bathed. And yet both early and later surrogates often share a similar fate in the end: oblivion. We tend to forget them, to play down their importance.

'I had this nurse when I was little,' recalls a fifteen-year-old. 'I remember folding laundry with her. I loved that. I called her grandma, though she wasn't my grandmother. I still love folding laundry.' She also loves being close to someone and has an ability for intimacy her cool, unemotional mother doesn't understand. 'My daughter has this intense thing with her boy friend,' says the mother. 'I never went through that sort of thing. She's far more affectionate than I. I can't imagine where she gets it.' No one remembers where the girl learned her emotional behavior. A fondness for folding laundry is as close as the young woman allows herself to come to admitting her inheritance.

Another woman I interview speaks of the influence of a teacher in her life, but says she felt compelled to hide it. 'My English teacher when I was fourteen changed my life,' she says. 'She taught me to read and to value being intelligent. She was not pretty, which was what all the girls in my crowd prized. I am ashamed to say that I never told anybody how much I admired her. I just took what I wanted and ran. I never thanked her, never, and I've always been sorry about that.'

This odd ingratitude has nothing to do with intelligence or age. 'It was only recently, in my own group analysis,' says

Dr Robertiello, 'that I discovered this very important uncle of mine. He was nineteen when I was five, and was perhaps the most important man in my childhood. Even with all my years of psychoanalysis, he's just never before appeared on the scene in my conscious mind. Here I am today, fifty-one, and he's been completely repressed all these years.'

These are just three examples; again and again in researching this chapter, I come upon evidence of this denial. Even when directly asked if there isn't someone who mothered them, or with whom they identified while growing up, most people will pause, shrug, and say no, there was nobody. No surrogate, no heroine, no model: 'There wasn't anybody who mothered me (besides mother), or anyone I wanted to grow up to be like.' Are these women lying to me?

I don't think so. There is no anger or defensive heat in their dismissal of the subject. They are puzzled themselves — especially if they feel they have transcended the image their mother presented to them. How did they do it? 'I guess I just made myself up,' they shrug.

'I think this kind of forgetting,' says Dr Robertiello, 'may be a feeling it is disloyal to our parents to recognize how important these other people were. If only unconsciously, we realize that we owe the role models of our youth too much, and turn away. This is a kind of defense of our old notions of omnipotence. We may acknowledge that our parents were formative to us. After all, that's normal. But that we needed other people too? Oh, no!'

To admit even to ourselves that we once preferred someone else to our mother opens us to the awful self-accusation of being cold, selfish, and terrible people. We 'forget' because we are too guilty to remember. 'It is often the case,' says Dr Helene Deutsch, 'that if a woman cannot remember how important a nurse or housekeeper was to her emotional development as a child, it was because of guilt toward the mother, that she allowed herself to have these feelings of love toward another woman.'

It is a guilt born of symbiosis. To people who are attached, admitting there is someone else opens them to fear of the symbiotic partner's anger, retribution, and possible abandonment. We can no longer afford to live in this squeeze. Today, when mothers are involved in more than one job, children need more than one mother. Not just someone who sits with them as coldly as a television set, but a person to whom they feel free to turn, who will be there for them, and from whom they can openly take in warmth without feeling they are making mother jealous. Young women, particularly, are going through great changes in manners, mores, and expectancies; they need all the love they can find from as many different people as possible; they need access to a variety of role models other than mother.

But mother first must give up her illusory gains from symbiosis carried on too long. Perhaps the easiest person to whom she can cede at least part of mothering is her husband. Says Mio Fredland: 'It really doesn't matter what the gender of the mothering person is.' Some men are maternal. Some women are not. To the child, it does not matter where the warmth comes from. 'Motherhood is too important to leave to women,' says Jessie Bernard. 'It's got to be shared.'

There is no doubt however that most fathers have not yet learned to accept responsibility for children to the same degree as women. 'When I'm at work, I can't help worrying about whether he's given Susie her lunch,' one woman tells me. 'I know that when we're both at home and the baby cries, he sleeps on. It's me who hears it. How can I rely on him?'

How can she not? The fault is not entirely with men. So long as a mother feels her main value derives from being the only one who can be counted on to raise a child, she will never accept that anyone else can take care of and understand her daughter as she does. Never given full responsibility, father soon takes less than his half.

'In the modern family,' says Dr Betty Thompson, 'the mother-daughter relationship is going to be seriously altered. There is going to be more than one mothering person. Some men make marvelous mothers. If you have a father pinch-hitting for a mother, you have a surrogate relationship right there.' This idea is reinforced by Dr Fredland: 'I don't know what makes a woman maternal. I know women who have had terrible mothering from their biological mother but are very maternal anyway. Other women who had adequate mothering, aren't maternal at all. I think what it is, is that *somebody* has been very maternal to them. I don't think it has to be the mother, or even a woman. It could have been the father, or an uncle.'

Day-care centers and flexible work hours are not the subject of this book, but any scheme involving surrogate care will be undercut if mothers do not learn to give up some of the responsibility for what happens to everyone in the family. They cannot be total mother, total wage earner, total wife. Daughters of women like these pick up their mothers' anxieties and jealousies. Even if part of the surrogate is taken in, the gift will be poisoned by fear that the gain is a betrayal of mother's symbiotic emotions. The daughter gets the worst of two worlds. She suffers from her mother's absence, and struggles with her ambivalence at allowing herself to be warmed by the substitute.

'Freud said that very often life itself is the great healer,' says Dr Fredland. 'Certain experiences, people you come into contact with – they can undo early damage. A child is very plastic. Neurosis sets that plastic into a hard, distorted form. But if the child is lucky and has happy life experiences, for instance with a surrogate, the neurosis may be at least partially repaired, and the basic emotional structure given a chance to reset in healthier form.'

If in her heart mother knows she was as good a mother as she could be in the circumstances, she may come to terms with her daughter's need for other models in her life. 'But if she knows she was not a good mother,' says Dr Sanger, 'her guilt will make her furious. She will show terrific hostility to the very people who could have helped her daughter the most. How can she admit she was not all the mother society and her own mother taught she must be? Her own womanhood is at stake.'

Social workers report case after case where mothers want their freedom, but still want their child to be primarily tied to them. 'The worst mothers I've seen,' says Mio Fredland, 'the minute the child gets attached to a nurse or another person, they get rid of that person. They hate the child, they hate their role, they hate everything about it, but they can't stand that the child should be emotionally attached to somebody else.'

One mother will resent surrogates because she is symbiotically tied to her daughter and fears the break. Another resents surrogates because she doesn't really like her child, but fears that a surrogate reveals her lack of love. Either way, the daughter is the loser. When she becomes a mother herself, she will remember her mother's anxiety that to give a child over to someone else for love and care is to be a 'bad mother'. It will never feel right for her to do it with her own child – even if economic circumstances dictate that she must go out and find a job.

While many women today have to take on all the risks, fatigues, and drudgery of what used to be the male workaday world, they cannot give up any of the risks, fatigues, and drudgery of being a mother too. Says Jessie Bernard: 'A three-year-old boy will say, "I want to be an astronaut, a fireman and a soldier." We accept that as he grows up he will see that he can't be all those things, and that he will narrow his sights. But little girls are raised to live by a hidden agenda. On the surface we say, Yes, you have as much right as a boy to have a career, to be a doctor, a lawyer, but there is a hidden message: first, you are going to be a mother too. So the girl says, Yes, I'm going to be a lawyer, but I'm also going to have a family. No recognition is given to the fact that in our society it is structurally very difficult to be a mother and a lawyer too. It is like the little boy saying, "I'm going to be a fireman *and* an astronaut."'

Some women can combine full-time careers with being full-time mothers, but they are the superhumans among us, and you cannot base a rational society on all women being superpeople. It is too much to ask, and when we fail, we are in a rage – *but don't know why*. Other young women recognize they can combine marriage and a career, but decide they can't be mothers too. Says Professor Jean McFarland: 'I feel it's only fair to warn women that having a career and being a mother is worth the effort, but don't think for a second it is easy. Some of our best women are choosing not to become mothers, not because they don't want to, but because they recognize they can't do both jobs well. It's a tragic choice for women to have to make, and society will be sorry.'

During an interview, I ask a prominent sociologist if there were any important identification figures in her life. She pauses, then says, 'My mother admired Margaret Sanger and had a book about her that I read. On one level, my mother was just wonderful. I thought women social reformers were wonderful. I wanted to go out and change the world like them, to do good. I came from a very political family, but I didn't really have an identification figure. Maybe my aunt, she was a doctor. I'm furious at my family now. I was never presented with any alternative to marriage. Their plan was that I'd go to college to have something to fall back on, but I was never presented with the possibility of having a serious career. And we had a woman doctor in the family! They left me with the feeling I had to marry, so when that schmuck came along, I married him. I really got married to get out of the house, to get away. It was idiotic.'

This woman is divorced now. Her story opens up with Margaret Sanger's name, her MD aunt is mentioned, but her remarks close on the denial of any identification figures and a great deal of anger. One might think she could say today: 'It was because of Margaret Sanger and my aunt that I had courage and incentive to become a sociologist.' But instead of emphasizing the positive force these women may have been in her life, she dwells on her anger at her family, including her 'wonderful' mother. Isn't her real anger at the hidden agenda – the understanding conveyed to her by mother that Yes, she could have a career, but had to be a wife and have children first?

How destructive that anger at mother should take up so much of our adult lives. We may say, 'I'm not angry at my mother!' – but why do we go into such a rage when our daughter doesn't clean up her room, or our husband is late? The fury is not appropriate. It has been displaced from mother onto someone 'safer'. This is unfair and bewildering, leading to arguments that cannot be resolved because the real target for our furies is never named or even made conscious; to examine our unresolved angers even now would mean to reawaken those infantile emotions of loss and retribution we never outgrew.

The truth is that once faced, we could live with that anger today. Unfaced, it contaminates any real love we may have for our mother. As the models and images of independence and life we once found so attractive slip through our fingers, we find ourselves becoming more like the anxious, critical, sexually frightened woman we never intended to be. Anger at the person who inhibited our trust in any model but herself works on us in the disguise of passivity, conservatism, and resignation.

Says Dr Betty Thompson: 'Passivity in women can be humiliation, fear, lack of ego strength, terror that you're going to be found wanting. All too often it is anger.' Unlike men, who gets points for being tough and hot-headed, women have their anger termed unladylike. We start to get angry, but feel guilty about it, and tamp it down. The passive-aggressive personality is the result: someone who expresses her anger in a seemingly civilized disguise. 'Where do you want to go tonight, honey?' the husband says, not so much wanting to get the name of a restaurant from his wife, but wanting to hear in her emotional tone that she is pleased to be going out with him. 'Anyplace you want,' his wife says, depriving him of the real answer he hoped for but disguising her desire to frustrate and annoy him by seeming to comply with the overt question put to her. 'The passive-aggressive personality,' says Dr Thompson, 'is like a parked car that only backs up.' Such a person is a two-year-old who won't do what anybody wants. It makes her feel strong to say No. To withhold is reinforcing to her sense of self – even if she is merely being asked to go forward into growth. The natural desire is for life, and a child feels thwarted when growth is denied, no matter if she is doing it to herself.

Anger is negative, but still it is a tie. It retards separation because as long as we are angry at mother, she is uppermost in our thoughts, and we are still her daughter. 'OK, so you're angry, let it go,' a therapist might say. 'Let *her* go.' But no, we would rather have the anger than nothing.

One day when I was talking to Dr Robertiello, he said as an afterthought, 'Nancy, why can't you accept the fact that your mother doesn't love you?'

For a moment, I thought I was going to hit him. Instead, I went through one of those instantaneous, self-protective reflexes, and changed the subject. But his sentence thundered around in my head. For the first time in my professional discussions with Richard Robertiello, a subject had come up that I did not want to discuss.

For weeks I would think about it, wince, retreat, and then return to it again. How could he have said such a thing? It became a familiar pain, until one day, like a weight lifted. I felt relief. Of course she didn't love me! Not in the perfect, idealized way I'd wanted all my life, since I was a baby.

I couldn't wait to tell Dr Robertiello of the feeling of freedom that had come out of this understanding of his disturbing statement. 'But, Nancy,' he said, 'you've twisted my words. I didn't say your mother didn't love you "perfectly". From all you've told me about your relationship, I said she didn't love you, period.'

Every mother-daughter story has two versions, and Dr Robertiello knows only what I've told him. For the first time in writing this book, it has occurred to me that my version of my relationship with my mother is not just distorted by the absence of her voice, but by my own unfaced emotions.

Perhaps the reason I have always felt free to acknowledge the importance in my life of my nurse and my aunt was that my mother so easily accepted them. She has never hesitated to give them credit for what they gave me, never made any reluctant show of her gratitude to them. How many times have I heard her tell other people how much she owes them, how glad she is for me that I found them. Isn't this love?

The lunatic other side of the coin is that I am angry at her for not giving me herself what I found in them. It is the case of the woman with the too-liberal lover. She is grateful that he takes her back after he learns of the other man, but why didn't he throw her out? Did he value her so little?

I have never wanted to confront my mother with my anger. It would be to little avail. She wouldn't understand, and if she did, what could she do now? It is too late for nursery angers, but I will be left with them for all my life if I do not accept that they are there, and why. Otherwise I will be in the position of those people who, as Dr Sanger puts it, 'endlessly try to shake love out of their mothers by the lapel.'

The possibility that mothers may come not to resent but to welcome the necessity for role models and surrogates in their daughters' lives is a thrilling idea for the future. Equally remedial in raising the mother-daughter relationship to an adult level is to see our own lives become a model for mother. Says a twenty-eight-year-old divorcée: 'My mother is fifty-three. The last time I was home, she said to me, "I never in my life thought what it would be like to sleep with another man than your father . . . until I heard about your life."'

The reversal of roles in which the child teaches the parent seems to release both women from the fixed demands of anger and symbiosis. Even if we have outgrown her, we can forge a new and loving tie by becoming *her* role model. 'My mother worked from the time I was fourteen,' says a twenty-nine-year-old woman. 'Whatever my mother achieved was subordinated to make my father happy and seem successful. I married when I was a sophomore in college. I wanted a family, I expected to be a traditional wife, like my mother. The stereotype didn't work out that way. The man I married never found a career – he was just like my father. I followed my mother's model and did everything so this man could be successful. I got a part-time job, I went to graduate school, I wanted to be as strong as my mother in helping my father. Eventually I couldn't take it. I left him.

'I was glad to be out of a bad marriage. I found a good job, everything should have been rosy, but I felt this terrible anger in me. I thought it was at him. I soon realized how much of it was at my mother. I had been a good daughter, I had done everything she had trained me to do, and it hadn't worked. In a sense, she had lied to me about what life was all about.

'I'll tell you something that has helped relieve the anger. I have recently come to see how much my life has influenced my mother. She makes choices now she never could have before, without me. Like saying to my father, after thirty-three years of marriage, "You can do as you like, but I'm not going to turn down promotions because you'd feel like a failure. I'm going to go as far as I can in this career." She couldn't have said that without having watched what I've been through. I am proud of my mother when I see her growing and doing things she should have done years ago. It gives all those years she spent raising me significance and meaning. I am prouder of this than anything, that my life has given mother a second chance.'

If mother can believe in our new identity enough to trust her own weight on it, we can believe in it too. We have not lost her. The debt is paid.

CHAPTER EIGHT

Men the Mystery

To this day I make Ms. When I scribble while on the telephone or write in the sand, it's always Ms. M stands for Morgan, and Morgan stood for Man Incarnate, Man the Mystery, Man Unobtainable. From the beginning – around age thirteen – I focused on Morgan. I never took my eyes off him, though he never put his hands on me. Except to punch me. Whenever one of us girls teased him, pushed him too far, trying to get something (what?) out of him, he would haul off and give her a swift rabbit punch in the arm. He did it dispassionately and without words, as if she were a fly. It was a badge of honor to carry one of Morgan's bruises. We had been touched.

Morgan belonged to the crowd of boys our own age, the ones we girls started on. We went to dancing class together, and theirs were the photos we carried in our Genuine Leather wallets, along with the eighth-grade graduation head shots of one another autographed, Love ya', Mary Beth. Within a couple of years we would outgrow the local boys and graduate to the cadets at the Citadel – a military college for men in name, but in fact a repository for southern boys. But throughout all those years and beyond, I remained faithful to Morgan in fantasy. He stood for an idea of manliness, the person who would stand opposite me and make a woman of me. He was the promise of my sexuality, the white heat of my glandular fever, the ache I loved living with while I waited. I grew to love the waiting too, and was so in love with love that something in me still waits for Morgan. My husband knows I dream of Morgan at night, and smiles at what he calls my 'persistence of emotion'. How can I expect him to understand? He grew up in New York, that very unadolescent city, safe from the sexual heat of small southern towns, the drive-ins and drugstores, matriarchy and male supremacy. Besides, he is a man. Only women understand waiting, how years of it train you to dream, to never expect it *will* happen, or to recognize it if it should.

Occasionally I wonder what sort of man Morgan grew into; I imagine myself sitting opposite him, me grown splendid and sexual, Morgan now the one suffering from the white heat in the groin. But in this fantasy, we are not in some smart bar but in Schwettman's Drug Store, and while I look like one of those women in a vodka ad, Morgan is still fourteen. On those infrequent trips back to Charleston, I never seek him out. I do not choose to confront the old fantasy, to ruin it. How can you update a god? To me Morgan will always be slouched behind the wheel of his black Chevrolet, wearing a maroon windbreaker with the sleeves rolled up, and a tough look. Morgan never smiles.

When he chose one of my best friends as his girl, I kept right on dreaming about him. Nothing could touch what he stood for. It was about the time my mother quietly announced at the dinner table that she was going to remarry. I had no words for my anger. I left the table. It was my Aunt Kate who walked me to the Battery and sat with me on a park bench beside the cannon balls while I sulked and stared at Fort Sumter. She talked about her days at college and once again, in the light of her life, everything seemed possible.

I can't help wondering how relevant to my mother's decision to remarry was the emergence of all the women in our house into a time of sexuality. It would have been an unconscious pressure, of course, but timing is so much. There we were, four women: my mother, Aunt Kate, my sister, and I, each needing her own man, her own identity. My aunt married within a year of my mother. My reaction to the news of my mother's remarriage was childish but much less important than my own need to solve the mystery of men. In the end, I took the arrival of a man in our house as no more disturbing than Morgan's choice of another girl. My time would come. When I thought of Morgan, I simply x'd her out.

To be near Morgan I went out with his fat friend, a football player painfully shorter than I and from the wrong side of town. (Morgan had a taste for thugs.) I was sure Morgan realized my sacrifice and silently approved. I settled for Friday nights at the drive-ins with lesser mortals, all the while making Ms on the cover of my blue loose-leaf notebook and up and down the spines of Homer's *Iliad, Ivanhoe,* and *Basic Geometry.* I wrote other boys' names too but only to obscure the intensity of my desire, the portent that leapt out at me each time. I faced that sea of names and saw only one. Other boys held me, and eventually, in their arms, I reached that weightless state that enough kissing could arouse in me, but when I closed the library doors at home and put on my favorite records, the longing and the dying I willed to well up inside me was for Morgan.

Nothing really happened in those fantasies; Morgan didn't even have to materialize in them for me to reach the feeling I was after. But pushed to humanize these desires, to put a name to my wish on the first star at night, it was his. It wasn't sex, or life in a vine-covered cottage that I wanted with Morgan. It was to have his eyes on me, for him to see me, to make me whole, to want me so that all those desires that made moonlight painful could be consummated in one great crescendo of Tony Bennett's 'There's No Tomorrow.'

After we girls had cut our teeth on the mating grounds of Madame Larka's dancing class, we were ready for the more sophisticated sexual posturing that was traditional every Friday afternoon at the Citadel Parade Grounds. Like generations of young Charleston women before us, we instinctively knew it was our turn to move in the ritual procession of cars to the four o'clock dress parade. With neither instruction nor invitation, we lined up our cars along the edge of the parade grounds, bumpers to barracks, car hoods (with us perched prettily atop) aimed at the sea of blue that drilled smartly past for our inspection. Was it here I developed my keen eye for a well-turned ass, the poignant stab of pleasure at the sight of what I later learned in art history to call the classic S curve? Certainly no one said a word about the unnervingly tight zip-front jackets the cadets wore, or the heartbreak reversed parenthesis of the two dark lines down the back, tracing the curve of shoulder, waist, and hip. Nor did we even think about the real reason we came to these parades: to be on display ourselves. We were the ones who needed to be looked at, to have a man's eye on us; a very genteel southern meat rack, if you will. Somewhere in that army of men there was someone who would make us a pair, give us stature, significance, mobility. 'A woman alone is nothing.'

It is a message mothers give their daughters still. If my own didn't say it, I knew it well. I had not been trained to dream of a future without men, myself flourishing alone. Though I had no idea who a man was, I knew one was necessary. After the parade, it was dancing class all over again; gone were the drums and the bugles, the dreaming and watching. Here came reality, as hundreds of men broke rank and moved toward us, the waiting women, all of our future, our importance in their hands. How effortlessly they chose us, singling this one out, rejecting that one, most of them, I am sure, unaware of the very real power they had over us. For those girls who wore their men's company insignia on their cashmere sweaters, there was no tension; somebody wanted them. The rest of us sat and smiled as though it were the most inconsequential thing in the world whether or not a uniform would stand opposite us and give us life.

In time, I too had my share of cadets, loved one after another, went to Christmas hops and homecoming games, collected white dress gloves and other pieces of oversized male garments. In fact, I cannot remember not being in love. I could catalogue the past twenty years of loves by the take-me, make-me songs to which I loved them, each man to his own music. In time I would have jobs, wonderful work, but my emotional sustenance, the air I needed, came from what men breathed into me. If I owed my life to my aunt, I was my mother's daughter.

Being in love was a habit. Though I never wanted to marry, I had to believe each love was forever. I didn't want a husband, I didn't think of men as the fathers of my children. It was the promise of men, that around each corner there was yet another man, more wonderful than the last, that sustained me. You see, I had men confused with life. Since you couldn't count absolutely that one would never leave you, I loved each man of the moment with a kind of madness. His not telephoning reduced me to a zero. His presence, my sureness that he cared for me, enabled me to charm the world and even be nice to my sister. It was a religion of a god who gave and took away life, bringing peace so that I could go to school, sit at meals with my family, and not appear to the outside world like the deranged person I was inside. You can't get what I wanted from a man, not in this life. Morgan was and always will be unobtainable.

Growing up in the South is different. But only by degrees. The humidity simply reinforces the cultural priority: men first. When I went north to college, the first thing I wanted to share with my new roommate was my collection of pictures of Sam. By him she would know me. I talked of my summer in the sun with Sam, and showed her his class ring. She talked about her summer job. Oh, she talked about her man too, but I realized there were other things in her life. No one I knew ever had a summer job. What we did best in the heat was lie on the beach and hypnotize the boys with the sheen of our oiled bodies. Something in me responded like a drum to what I found in the North. I wanted men in my life, but I wanted to be free of my fear of their rejection. Intuitively and instinctively I knew that finding alternative sources of life, satisfactions in addition to those I knew with men, would free me – like a hypnotic freed from the spell.

Mine, however, is not one of those stories of the beauty and power of nature, the blade of grass growing through stone to reach the sun. Getting past those years of training in romantic delirium and need for men was like going against nature. It still is.

One night before I left for college, I found myself in the back seat of a car with Morgan. Emboldened by our steps away from the boys of our youth, my friend Kathy and I had telephoned Morgan and his friend Steve. The four of us went to a drive-in and suddenly there I was, lying across the back seat in Morgan's arms. He kissed me, and I began to give myself to what I believed would be as close to heaven as I would ever get. Now, I thought, would begin the evening of rapture, hours and hours of window steaming, holding and kissing. He put his hand between my legs. I pushed his hand away, burying my head in his chest and prayed against hope that like every other boy I had ever dated, he would agree to my rules. But Morgan was a god, and had not become one by acceding to women's rules.

'You see, Nancy, it wouldn't work with us. That's what I want and you don't.' He said it in the kindest way, with a man's certainty.

Until I met Bill, I never knew a man whose rules I respected as much as my own, who had absolute certainty about himself. I will probably make Ms for the rest of my life, but at least now I know why.

Sexuality is the great field of battle between biology and society. It is born long before we are deemed adult enough to play with its magnificent fire. Mother is the first regiment pressed into battle. The job comes with surprising suddenness. She is still young, not yet ready to limit her own sexuality in order to chaperone ours. No matter what the sacrifice costs her, whether she does it well or badly, angrily or gladly, we resent her for it. Do we thank our jailers?

When, as infants, we touch our genitals, her job begins. She takes our hand away. 'No,' she says. It is one of the crucial experiences in life, and starts mother's lifelong role as the eternal no-sayer in her daughter's eyes. Conversely, men are set up as her opposite, yea-sayers to sex, daring, and freedom. Men are not prim and proper prudes like mother. They are lusty rogues, sexy devils, and we yearn for our time with them to come. But we wait with mother's watchful eye upon us.

When mother takes our hand away from between our legs, when, as we grow older, she lets us know by look, tone of voice, attitude, and gesture, that it isn't nice, she is being what society considers a good mother. *The effect is to cut us off from our own bodies.* 'In our culture,' says Dr Robertiello, 'women are trained to expect that in some magical way, men will make them sexual people. They can't do it to themselves.' Little wonder then that men seem mysterious to us. Who can understand such powerful creatures that they can command sexuality itself? 'Invariably,' says Dr Schaefer, 'the way women put it is, "He gave me an orgasm." I tell them, "Someone doesn't give you an orgasm. You give yourself an orgasm."' Usually, words like these are treated as if they were merely semantic tricks, not to be taken seriously. A woman thinks she needs a man to bring her to life. Passivity is indoctrinated and reinforced.

'When a mother hinders or arrests a daughter's sexual activity, she is fulfilling a normal function whose lines are laid down by events in [her own] childhood, which has powerful, unconscious motives, and has received the sanction of society,' wrote Freud in 1915. 'It is the daughter's business to emancipate herself from this influence and to decide for herself on broad and rational grounds what her share of enjoyment or denial of sexual pleasure will be.'[1]

Freud's dictum seems to be fair enough. It lays the responsibility for our sexuality where it belongs – with us. But he is talking about the years when we are old enough to decide 'on broad and rational grounds' how much sexuality we should allow ourselves.

For most of us in our teens, that time is not yet. Mother's inhibitions of our sexuality re-creates in each of us the myth of Sleeping Beauty, and a complementary myth becomes our future: some day my prince will come, the knight in shining

armor who will awaken my dormant sexuality. Our parents
smile at our teen-age acned Lancelot, but in our eyes, they
arrive trailing clouds of glory. We become pinned to them,
braceleted, chained, and enslaved to how we feel when they
hold us in their arms. They release us for a time from prison,
from waiting, sleep, and passivity. When not in their arms, we
live on fantasies, until they hold and release us once more. I
am not talking of the release of orgasm, but of the release
from tension – the fear that no man will want us as much as
we need him. Of course this tension is sexualized, is itself part
of the rhythmic build to orgasm, but we learn to satisfy it
without the forbidden climax. We come to find more release
in the certainty that he will never leave us than in having him
inside us. *That certainty becomes more important than
orgasm ever can be.*

The real thing, the penis inside, for many women never
does live up to that early substitute: security. And tight
security – control – is the antithesis of orgasm – letting go.
After hours of fondling and kissing, young girls go to their
rooms with their pretty panties soaked through, but do not lie
awake in sexual frustration. We sleep sound in our virginal
beds because we have lain in his arms long enough to believe
again, at least for tonight, that 'everything will be all right,
I'll never leave you, I'll love you forever.' Who he is, what he
wants – *sex itself* – is never so important as the fantasy of
permanent security he gives us. Is it any wonder that after a
year or two of marriage, so many women wake up with a
stranger? 'Why did I ever marry him?'

'I was an only child growing up in a house full of women,'
says actress Elizabeth Ashley, 'So men were always mysterious
to me. My mother had been damaged, but, like so many
women of her generation, she felt impelled to hide her scars.
To show pain would have been a fall from dignity. She was
really an early and very private feminist, strong, idealistic,
and brave. Her mission was to raise me to be independent.
And she succeeded in that, but those mysterious men still had
this huge power.'

'In a way, men to us were like drugs are to this generation. The kids are told, "If you take them, you'll be addicted forever." Men were our "reefer madness". They became imbued with this mystical, dangerous, irresistible romance. And romance is, of course, the cornerstone of any addiction.'[2]

Young women today tend to have friendships with men where ten or twenty years ago there could only have been romantic love. It is a significant change. However, when sex does enter, the pregnancy and abortion rates among teenagers are frightening. Young girls still expect something wonderful, magical, mystical, and dreamy from their sexual partners. As much as any generation before them, they think love will make the lyrics to the songs come true. It is a hard-nosed axiom in the rock music business that for every girl singer who makes it, there are at least a dozen male superstars: girls dream to music, boys do not.

In a recent study, educator Patricia Schiller found that adolescent girls tended not to read pornographic books, nor were they aroused by the sight of men nude or in tight trousers. The major sexual stimulant among young girls of every socioeconomic group, she found, was music — especially the words to the songs.[3] It is not sex young girls dream of. It is this unknown and mysterious fulfillment that men will bring. For instance, a major manufacturer of vibrators tells me that when he advertises in college newspapers, the response is nil. Adult women may buy his product from adult magazines, but young girls yearn for the satisfaction of mysteries no vibrator can touch.

'Our lives as women,' says Dr Schaefer, 'are filled with fantasies. You have the fantasy of what you think your father is, and the fantasy of what your mother says he is. You have the fantasy of the kind of man you think you should marry and the fantasy of the kind of man you actually do marry. You have a fantasy of what life is going to be like. A lot of us end up not being able to cope with the reality we live because we always have that fantasy in our mind of what it should have been.' The cliché is that the wish is the father to the thought. Perhaps it would be more accurate to say the wish is mother of the thought.

'How will I know if it's really love?' a girl asks her mother. 'You'll know when it comes along,' mother says. And then one day, astoundingly, it turns out to be true. Being held in our lover's arms creates a feeling of warmth, love, and happiness we have never felt before – or have we? The odd thing is that it is almost familiar. We are pervaded by an eerie sense of having been here before. We have always known this feeling existed, and have merely been waiting for it to come along again. *It feels right.*

'The reason the feeling of love at these moments is so satisfying,' says Dr Robertiello, 'is that in a perfectly acceptable, heterosexual situation, the woman has re-created the intensity of satisfaction she once felt at being held like this. It was when she was a baby in her mother's arms.' Since this thought is vaguely unpleasant, somewhat threatening to our gender identity as women, it is repressed. For all their masculinity, men can give us moments in which they remind us so much of the love we once had with mother that we are afraid to recognize it. We cloud the feeling in mystery.

But they give us sex too! It is easy to be unconscious of the fact that the feelings of tenderness we find with men are rooted in our earliest experiences with mother, when our present, and equally real feelings of sexual excitement are rooted very much in the now – *this man, this* moment, *his* arms and body. The differences between the two ideas is important. It helps explain women's lives.

When both elements are present – the nurturing plus the explicitly sexual – the marriage or affair is said to be serious, and continues for some time. If the unconscious nurturing we learned to expect from mother is missing from a relationship, we say it is 'merely sexual', and it soon ends. The ultimate richness of life depends, in my experience, more often on satisfying our unconscious needs than meeting the demands of the physical.

'The whole emphasis in psychoanalytic thought in the past

ten years,' says Dr Schaefer, 'is to move to an earlier time than the years of the oedipal triangle. We used to be so focused on that; now we're beginning to concentrate on the earlier, mother-child dyad.' Whether we like it or not, in the vast majority of American families the major figure for the child – male or female – is the mother. Our entire pattern of relating to others is set up first with her. 'Whatever mother is,' says Dr Robertiello, 'that is what we learn. She is our first model on how to be a person. We not only learn how to deal with reality through her, but we also use her as a model of the kind of person we will want to be close to.'

Women who perceive that their mothers didn't like men in general or their father in particular suffer a devastating effect. 'If the girl does like her father,' says Dr Schaefer, 'mother's negativism sets up conflict in her. She doesn't feel free to like him if mother doesn't, if mother is always finding fault, nagging him. She may ally with her father, but it will be a guilty alliance. Her relationships with men often repeat the way her mother was with her father: nagging. Father didn't make enough money, he wasn't as smart as other people – that is how the daughter remembers family life.'

Dr Schaefer continues: 'Often we find that men rebel against these nagging wives. They act like naughty, contrary children. Although they are capable of doing better, they don't – just to spite the wife. A daughter in a family like this grows up seeing men not as strong people you can depend on but as irresponsible children up in arms against women.'

The reverse of this kind of daughter would seem to be those who call themselves *daddy's girl*. These women are adamant about denying any ties or similarities to mother. 'I was always closest to my father. He was stricter than my mother but never as petty.'

Of course not! He'd given over all the nasty, necessary jobs – including the titanic-even-if-forgotten struggle over toilet training – to mother. She got the shitty end of the stick – all puns intended.

Daddy is godlike, not just because he's distant and has this attractive sexual quality, but because like executives who let underlings deliver the bad news while they themselves announce promotions and raises, mother has had to do the day-by-day discipline, withholding allowances and pleasures when we are naughty, forcing us to eat and do things we don't like. When dad comes home from work, we may be at the end of our rope with mother. He enters with a clean slate. We are a bit of dessert at the end of his day. We argue less with him when he tells us to come home early because we don't have this long-standing battle with him over a hundred other things. 'I never talked to my mother when I was young,' a thirty-five-year-old woman says, 'It was my father who gave me my most important feelings about myself. With him, I felt this wonderful security. As soon as he left the room, that feeling went away.' I asked this woman if she spent a lot of time with her father. She tells me that he was away in the war until she was five. The most significant moment with him she can remember was, 'when he drove me to the train when I left home at sixteen. He said, "You must remember that not everyone is going to be as kind as they are at home." I think that was his way of referring to sex.' This oblique reference is her most significant memory of sex education and of what she calls her deep and significant relationship to her father.

'Women like these,' says Dr Robertiello, 'have the illusion of being closer to father than mother. Maybe they got more of the pure unadulterated loving stuff with him but there is no way they could have been closer to him. Ask any man, the fondest father, just how much time do you spend in direct communication with your daughter? It boils down to maybe ten minutes a week. A one-to-one, up-and-back system of intimate, meaningful, close communication between father and daughter? Very, very rare.' No wonder that in his silence, absence, and mystery, we can make dad the most wonderful man in the world. The absence of real data about him makes him the stuff of dreams.

The popular superstition is that daddy's girls get along

better with men when they are grown. They are 'a man's kind of woman', have affinities with the male sex that the rest of us are sorely lacking. The reality is that these women often have the hardest time finding a man who can live up to the idealized image of manhood they got from their father. Even if by some magic of time travel they could meet their father as he was twenty-five years ago, *he would not do*. He would not measure up to the fantasy.

All our real, nitty-gritty, personal interactions are with mother. It is with her that we work through the important issues on which our character and personality are based. Mother is the hammer, we are the anvil, and in our arguments and agreements on getting fed, being held and loved, getting toilet trained, getting disciplined, facing competition and reality, learning separation – our souls are forged.

If father is the ice cream of life, mother is the daily meat and potatoes. It is an issue of semantics: we may *like* him more, but we are *closer* to her. Mother doesn't have his glamour, but with her we know where we are. She is more familiar than anybody else we will ever meet. Later, when we run into anyone – man or woman – who arouses in us some of the feelings we once had with her, we will be attracted. Even if they are not nice people, even if they treat us badly, we will dismiss other people's injuctions against them and declare we find them 'simpatico,' taking the woman as a friend, the man as a lover. The illusion is that we are coming home.

'I meet a lot of women,' says Dr Robertiello, 'who will tell you how mad they were about their fathers, and that they even married men who looked like him. But when you get to know them better, you very often find that whatever he looks like, *inside* the husband has the personality of her mother. A girl whose mother was cold and narcissistic, but still gave her enough so that the girl has some positive feelings about her – she will often marry a man who is also cold and narcissistic. Just as she learned to have a high tolerance for these character traits, she will tolerate them in her husband also. She has unconscious ideas and fantasies that he cares about her in the same stupid, nutty way that she had fantasies of her mother caring for her behind that coldness and narcissism. Man or woman, our first marriage is often to someone with the personality of our mother. If your mother wasn't a nice person, you're in trouble.'

'What kind of man was my first husband?' a woman says. 'He was as cold as my mother. To this day my daughter calls her father The Machine. I had no reason to be allergic to this kind of man. My mother was my model so I was used to it. Like living in a part of the country where the soil is poor — you don't think about it because it's all you know.'

This kind of unconscious, usually self-defeating, behavior goes on even among women who think they dislike aspects of their mothers so much that they take her as a negative model . . . the way *not* to be. For instance, here is a twenty-seven-year-old woman who consciously laughs at her mother's disagreeable 'little sergeant' character, and therefore chooses to think she is more like her father. Even though she senses that her life and actions contradict this wishful thought, she is unable to grasp the full degree to which her mother's pattern still dominates her relations to other people:

'No, I'm not like my mother. I'm more like my father. All my friends look upon my parents as a model because they have such a solid marriage, but I know my mother is a bitch. We call her the little sergeant. She is fussy, and my father is patience itself. I can remember laughing at my mother's irritability because it was so irrational. But I have been the same irrational person with my oldest daughter — over a bobby pin. And I see my daughter calmly saying, "Really, mother," when I fly in all directions.'

This woman thinks of her one identification with her mother's way of reacting as a kind of aberration, an isolated 'funny' bit of business which really has nothing to do with the way she leads her life as a whole. But people like this repress a larger part of their models than they are aware. 'She will probably act like her mother in larger, more subtle patterns, but never be able to see it,' says Dr Robertiello. 'Her whole story is out-and-out repression. She practically comes right out and says she acts like her mother, whereas she consciously thinks she is like her father. Women don't want to think of themselves as those parts of their mother they hated most, but those are the very parts they take in. It's awful to think that everything you hated in your mother, you've become. But that is how it works. That is one of the biggest shocks in therapy.'

Since nagging is so abhorrent, but so many women find we do it anyway, let me once again try to illustrate its genesis. This time the story is about a young woman of sixteen, but the mechanism of repression works as powerfully in her as in any of the previous illustrations of wives or mothers. 'I hope I won't nag my husband the way mom nags dad,' she says. 'I used to hear myself doing it with my boy friend. Even though it was what I hated most in the relationship between my parents. I couldn't stop. My boy friend used to tell me, "You nag me just like your mother nags your father." It frightened me when he said that. My father and I are very close. He's far more supportive than my mother. One day he said to me that he hoped I would break the tradition of nagging women in our family.'

This is a classic story. The young woman says she is closer to her father, but the way she acts is like her mother. She's unable to stop nagging even though she says she hates it. Proximity, sexual identity, need for mother's protection – all kinds of forces work to make mother, not father, her model. She takes in both what she likes and what she does not.

Professionally successful women often consciously think they have modeled their lives on their adored successful fathers. They give as evidence of their closeness to him the fact of their success itself. A life in his footsteps. They are right to a point.

In Margaret Hennig's Harvard doctoral study of twenty-five high-level women executives, she found that every one indeed had had a strong attachment to and identification with her success-oriented father. Their mothers were usually conventional, non-competitive women with no great involvement in matters outside the home, and never loomed in the girls' lives as a giant figure who might cut them down in the rivalry for father's attention. Father had been theirs from the start.

These women were never seen as substitute sons; their fathers did not believe in sexual role-playing (at least as far as their daughters were concerned), and so their daughters did not confuse feminine gender identity with masculine notions that striving and achievement were for men only.[4]

And yet in my research, I have met one executive woman after another who, no matter how cool and competent she was in the office (like father), experienced a deep emotional change when she married or became seriously involved with a man. Often, the change was not apparent except in hindsight.

'I was always my dad's girl,' says a thirty-five-year-old professional woman. 'I thought he was the handsomest, smartest man in the world. When he was home I hung on him, and when he left the house, I was always two steps behind, waiting for an invitation to come along. He used to talk to me, not like a kid, but like an adult – stories about Don Quixote or how the Mormons settled Utah. I don't remember my mother having any opinion at all about my closeness to my dad. Her stand about the whole thing was kind of like we were invisible. She was a nice warm loving mom, but I didn't want to grow up to have her life. I got my good grades for my dad. Because I was more adventurous and wanted more than most of the girls I grew up with, I gave myself the phrase "my dad's girl". It was a way to think about myself, an acceptable category I could fit into. After college I continued my studies because I wanted a career, to teach like my dad. I always planned to get married. When I did five years ago everything began to change. I didn't notice because I was still working. Outwardly, everything looked the same, but on some level, my work had begun to take a back seat to my role as a wife. As the marriage progressed, I tended to slip into a position where my feelings about myself as a success, as a person, were far more attached to my role as a wife. I think a lot of it had to do with how my mother had been with my father.

'All my life I'd denied I was like her, but when I married, it was uncanny. For the first time in my life, the big thing with my father didn't come in handy. He couldn't be my model of how to be a wife. If you've always had a pretty clear idea of who you are and how you operate, it's startling to see how marriage changes you, how you suddenly find yourself slipping into the one role you said you'd never be in – the way your mother was with your father. This accelerates when you become a mother yourself. I'll tell you a funny thing that happened after my daughter was born. The bank called and asked why was I suddenly signing my checks Mrs Philip Henderson. I'd always signed them Sheila Henderson. It took me a long time to understand that when I became a mother, I had stopped being *me* and had become Karen's mother, my husband's wife, *Mrs Philip Henderson.*'

The different roles our parents played in our earliest life furnish a clue to why even successful, career-oriented women so often slip back into regressive roles when they marry: mother began to teach us how to be a woman and a wife long before dad came along to teach us how to be a success in the office. They way we are in our jobs and careers relates to patterns of behavior and feelings learned relatively late. These ideas are more conscious, can be handled more rationally, than needs picked up in our earliest relationship with mother. 'Father may be the model for how to behave in an office,' says Dr Robertiello, 'but how to behave with a man, at home, on a date, in the bedroom, anywhere basic emotions rule – the structure of that relationship is based on mother. Women take mother's life as the model of how to be with men in terms of how they perceived she was with father. *Or with them* – which was usually not so different.'

If mother was mousy and masochistic, we may be a tiger at work; in our intimate relationships we will suffer a man we would never hire at the office, or even give the time of day. If our mothers were domineering and/or symbiotic, then we are that way with men. 'You see it again and again,' says Dr Robertiello. 'A woman will tell you she identifies with and is looking for a man like her father. Then she marries someone who puts her in the same unconscious bind mother used to.'

This is an illustration of what Freud called the 'repetition compulsion.' It is a reluctance to let go of infantile omnipotence. Says Dr Robertiello: 'It centers around the unconscious conviction that you can go back and take a bad mother like the one you had and make her a good one today. The repetition is due to inability to accept that we failed with our mother . . . that she didn't love us enough, or the way we wanted. This time, it's going to be different.'

This mechanism explains the magnetic power of Mr Rat, those dreadful men who pretend to love us but do not. The nice guy who just plain loves us out and out – why does he seem so insignificant, his love so meaningless beside the chance to win the heart of Mr Wrong? Because the model of love our 'bad' mother once held out to us is reincarnated in Mr Wrong. With Mr Wrong, we get our second chance to win the love of our life – the one we failed to get the first time around. The love of that nice boy next door? It holds none of the glamour of a chance to succeed where once we failed.

Just who daddy is, is never quite so clear as what he does for mother . . . and by extension, for us. He is this mysterious outside force, he 'brings home the bacon', showers the family like Santa Claus with the goodies of life – the house, the car, the washing machine, summer vacations, money for that special pretty dress for a dreamed-of occasion. Even in those families where mother also works, she usually contributes less than he to the income. It is a feeling that she reinforces for her own reasons: most women need to feel that their husbands are the major providers, and this is the feeling they pass on to their daughters.

On the other hand, mother sits at the gate of all this wealth. She is the day-by-day administrator, giving us our allowance or withholding it. If we are 'good girls' we get extras – a form of behavior we have seen her practice on father. For us too, the reward of money conferred by a man soon has greater significance than any we earn on our own. 'I get my allowance from my husband,' says a woman who makes six figures annually. 'Money is sexy.'

Father is the source of generosity; mother is niggling over pennies. Mother scans the shopping pages of the newspaper to find the cornflakes sale so she can save three cents a box. When we want to go to an expensive summer camp, it is father who says the meaningful Yes. If we see a film in which Steve McQueen, when the waiter presents the check, carelessly puts some bills on the table and does not wait for the change, we respond with a sexual warmth. That's how men are, moving in a world so large nobody quibbles over the bill; when we have lunch with our girl friends, the pettiness is notorious: 'You had the extra cole slaw, and Sally had the glass of wine . . .'

Little wonder then that long before the question has arisen of how/whether mother should prepare us for the sexual experience of men, she has given us a picture of life in which they are indispensable. Like those photos in fashion magazines where the men are either out of focus, characterless, or homosexuals, *who* they are is never so important as what they give the women in the picture: stronger definition. The dress costs $200, but without a man, whole gaggles of men lolling at her feet or helping her out of the car, the image of the woman in that dress would be far less significant *to other women*.

The thrust of our development today is away from this; and yet the notion that men are absolutely vital to any value we may have is so woven into feminine reality that most women think to reject it would be like trying to reject the law of gravity. When I say women still need men 'to take care of us,' the idea sounds dated and old-fashioned. It is too easy to dismiss if taken only at its superficial meaning. Women do not need men to pay our bills or repel marauders. We need men to take care of us because we don't believe we are visible, that we exist, without one . . . much as we felt lost, abandoned, near death as infants if mother did not appear when we became frightened at being alone.

'No, I insist. I'll pay for myself,' says a young woman who has joined my husband and me at a restaurant table. But when she reaches into her wallet, she doesn't have enough money. If he can, a man usually goes out in the evening with more money than he thinks he will need. He knows emergencies may arise, and he wants to be prepared to cope. Women are trained to carry only 'mad money' – just enough for a taxi ride home. In her mind, this young woman who was offering to pay for herself was willing to be a contemporary and responsible person. Something deeper, inculcated into her since childhood, made sure she could not.

What makes this inability to take care of ourselves so maddening is that women are beginning to realize that the free ride men supposedly offer is not free at all. 'My boy friend doesn't have much money,' says a sixteen-year-old. 'I've told him I don't mind paying for myself, but he only likes that to a point. He's always going out with the boys – which admittedly doesn't cost much. But when he does, he expects me to stay home. Why can't he use the little money going out with the boys costs, and add my dutch treat money, and go out with me? No, I'm supposed to stay home when he's not in the mood to see me – because that's what it really means when he says he's broke. If I go out alone, or to a party without him, he's furious.' If the man only 'lets' you share expenses when it suits him, the independence that money offers is as false as the quality of the relationship.

By turning men into Father Christmas, mother deals an enormous blow to the problem of competition between us. Daddy isn't this sexual person, this attractive man we both want. He's really a nice, big, warm provider, as comfortable and nonerotic as a hot-water heater. What could be sexual about a person who works his way to an early heart attack, who comes home so tired and grumpy he barely has the strength to peck a kiss on Mommy's cheek? Mother further cements the alliance between us: Daddy is not the competitive prize we both want but a fuddy-duddy opponent whom we league together to fool: 'We'll tell him the dress only cost twenty-five dollars, not forty-five.'

There is an enigma in this nice, safe, domestic picture she is presenting. Here she is, telling us what a nice man daddy is, how hard he works for us, how much he loves her, what an ideal marriage they have. But why is she always up to these sly little manipulative tricks that make him look like an oaf? Doesn't she remember they just had that frightening quarrel last week? Doesn't father usually seem bored with her, spending more time than she likes away at the office or bowling with his friends? When she talks of the rewards of marriage (as opposed to the dangers of sex), we feel a loss of reality. Part of us does want to get married, but her own marriage turns us off. Something is missing. Sex is problematic, she's always telling us; brutish boys are only out for one thing. We may be young but we already know that life is not worth living without the excitement boys give us. How can we buy mother's promises? She presents boys in such a dangerously attractive light that sex becomes the one thing we are always thinking about too.

We accommodate ourselves to this fact of life by deciding that mother is good and we are bad. Little wonder then that daughters become puzzled and resentful if mother divorces and begins to bring home different men. These aren't nice, comfortable, rent-paying daddies. Can it really be that it is sex she wants – after spending all those years telling us it is bad, unnecessary, dangerous and that it must never come between us? She has broken the symbiotic bond: she is more attached to this new person than she is to us. 'I'm not competitive with my mother,' says a fifteen-year-old whose mother has brought her lover to live in the house. 'I'm competitive with him – when she pays more attention to him than me. When I grow up, I'd rather be married to someone, not just live with him. I don't want my mother's life.' In this girl's circle of friends, she has the reputation of being naïve and antisexual.

Marriage and divorce counselor Dr Sonya Friedman speaks of a case where a live-in lover brought about an opposite reaction. 'When her thirty-five-year-old mother brought this man to live with them, the daughter was so embarrassed that she wouldn't invite her friends in. They would ask, "Who is that man? He's not your father. Why is he sleeping in your mother's bedroom?" The daughter couldn't stand that. Children have a very narrowly defined sense of morality, of right and wrong. I was not surprised when it turned out that the daughter soon entered into some pretty wild sexual experimentation of her own.'

When mother reveals that her interest in men is not merely cozy and domestic, as she had always promised us, she robs men of their mystery. They are sexual, and we want what she has. The flood gates of competition suddenly open. Daughter's anger is often expressed by finding as explicitly sexual a man as she can to flaunt at mother, to get back at her.

Mother did not deliberately lie. She wishes us to repeat her life because thus she is validated herself. She keeps life a mystery because if we knew the little she knew, we might not repeat the cycle; if we reject her choices, she would feel anxious and guilty. 'Where did I go wrong?'

Once again, the wish is mother to the thought. As Dr Schaefer says, mother actually does have the fantasy that her marriage is, if not perfect, well, then, better than most. If it isn't, why has she sacrificed so much for it? Gladys McKenney, who teaches in a high school in suburban Michigan:

'Daughters are only too aware of the inconsistencies going on in many marriages – mother saying one thing about the beauty of marriage, and all the while living this unhappy relationship. It's hard to admit to a child, "Dad and I haven't always been too happy together." In the families I see of above-average socioeconomic status – which means most families in the place where I teach – there is a great deal of anger between husband and wife that doesn't get expressed. The kids are aware of it, but it is hidden, suppressed.' A double message is being sent out: sometimes we hate each other but it is better to call it love.

The mystery grows.

Says Dr Schaefer: 'The only way for a mother to prepare her daughter for the reality of living with a man is by being honest about her life with her husband. If you try to tell your daughter one thing, but you are living something else, the split creates the biggest hardship. It is what I like to call The Big Lie – to be caught between what our parents say and what our parents really feel.' We want to believe life with father is as nice as mother says, but in our heart we know it just isn't so. We are left with her rosy picture of him, but with no idea of how to reach this ideal goal. All we know in the meantime is that any man who does not make us feel this idealized emotion is not Mr Right. That is how we will recognize him when he comes along at last. He will transport us into this magical place that mother is always talking about.

Mothers raise their daughters as fools because they believe in the divinity of innocence. Sexually, all mothers are Catholic. They pray for their daughters' innocence while simultaneously praying for a man for their untutored, unblemished girls. The keepers of the vestal virgins guarded their purity, knowing sex would be their doom. Our mothers keep us pure and dumb, knowing that even if sex is our future, it will also be our doom. In the light of such inevitability, rational, intelligent thinking fails. A pious belief that the innocent shall be spared prevails. In case after case where I have interviewed both mother and daughter, the mother will say, 'Oh, my daughter knows it all, she picks it up at school, from her friends, in the street. I don't have to tell her.' But when I interview the fourteen-, fifteen-, sixteen-year-old daughter, her knowledge is piecemeal. What she doesn't want to know – the whole truth about her body, contraception – is frightening. Where does she get her reluctance to know about herself in a world that has never before had so much sexual information available?

Our difficulty begins with mother's ambivalence. If it is hard for her to say, it is impossible for us to listen. 'Nobody tells you about the feelings you will have when you get close to someone,' says Dr Schaefer. 'In fairness to mother, how can anybody prepare you for the enormity of orgasm? Many women are so unprepared they don't want it. They resist it. It is not that they can't reach orgasm, they just can't handle all those feelings.'

Dr Schaefer continues: 'Take the problem facing a mother if she tries to get specific with her daughter. Just because the older woman can accept certain sexual ideas – even welcome them – doesn't mean thy don't frighten the hell out of her when she thinks of them in connection with her daughter. Now the boy friend has come around to pick up the daughter in a car. The mother knows that they'll park sooner or later tonight. She knows her daughter's fantasies are about the good feelings she gets from kissing. But she also knows that the boy's fantasies are about the girl touching his cock. How does she explain that to her girl if she is still guilty about sex herself?'

'A lot of women are objective about a man until they go to bed with him,' says Sonya Friedman. 'Then they literally get all screwed up. They become inappropriately bonded to him. He assumes an emotional importance out of all proportion. Here is this woman, so calm and rational yesterday, agreeing with the man that it is just a little flirtation, a roll in the hay, a limited affair . . . and today she's crying, "I want him, I want him, I'll die without him!" I hope this kind of thinking is dying out. It was awful in my generation where we had a little hanky panky, a lot of guilt and/or the terrific "want" of him. Above all, the imperative notion that if you wanted him sexually you had to marry him.

'One of the things that happens as you mature,' continues Dr Friedman, 'is that you gain the ego strength to remain intact. You can enjoy someone physically and emotionally without becoming bonded to him, sitting beside the telephone waiting for it to ring. This is what I hope my daughter is learning, that if she has some significant skills, a good opinion of herself as someone all by herself, she won't have to trade that off for a relationship dominated by the notion that she can't live without him.'

We expect marriage to liberate us from this sexual guilt. The contradiction is that while the wife wants the man to be strongly erotic and magically male, to awaken us sexually, we want him to do this within the emotional framework of warmth, nurturing, cuddling, affection. 'No, don't touch me there!' we exclaim when something he does threatens to take all tenderness out of the erotic. The man is bewildered: if she doesn't think that's sexy, what the hell does she want? We have kept our hands off our body for the past twenty years. How can we tell him what we want, when we have never been allowed to explore the idea ourselves?

What is puzzling and frightening is when mother says in one breath that men are bad, they aren't trustworthy, they're children who will selfishly let you down – and then in the next breath tells us of the marvelous future we will have married to one of them! In our culture, a good mother never, never admits to her daughter that she may not marry, or that it may not be the best idea in the world. The fear and distrust of men that some mothers lay on their daughters is later projected on each man in the girl's life as he comes along. The love affair, the marriage is doomed before it starts. The girl is often angry at all men for what one man did to her mother, or what mother *said* he did.

Women justifiably make the complaint about Don Juans that the specific girl doesn't count: 'He'll go to bed with anyone.' Men return the compliment when they say about a woman, 'She'll marry anyone in pants.' We wake up like sleepwalkers and say, 'I didn't make a choice. It was simply part of the picture. You got married, and had two children, and then you got the dog and the summer house . . .'

At fifteen we of course are no less a mystery to boys. But

they are edgy, only too aware of how close to female dominance and entanglement they still are: mother is always around. And although young men may want closeness and love as much as we do, they don't want all that other business females (mother) stand for: rules, dependence, and control. Both boy and girl see in each other an escape from mother – an alliance that will separate us for good from her – but in mutual ignorance of any relationship between men and women except the symbiotic one we have seen at home, we proceed to set up the same thing between ourselves. 'Going steady' gives both boy and girl what they feel is security. More often it is like two drowning swimmers, clutching each other by the throat. Men are usually the ones who break the death grip first. Their major advantage is that they have alternatives, experience in walking away: they don't need to 'buy' a relationship at any price. Their cry of suffocation – just before they slam out the door – is famous. What is little commented upon in these situations is that the woman too must have felt suffocated. But she would have paid that price – anything to keep the relationship going.

When the romance and fantasy fade, when we see men defrocked and their great mystery turns out to be that they are merely human like us, we grow angry. When we are fifteen, mother seemed archaic; we were sexual heroines, breaking ground that would have terrified her had she known. What happened? Suddenly, the glow has left our lives and we realize we have gone no further than she did. *We are just like her!*

This explains the inappropriate anger we feel when our men say, 'You're just like your mother.' We may feel it is disloyal to take that as an accusation, but even stronger is our fear that he means we are as asexual as we perceive her to be. 'How does it feel to be a woman?' my mother asked the day my first period started. A conventional enough question, but I was embarrassed. I didn't feel like a woman, and any discussion of womanliness/sexuality between women made me feel awkward. It would be men – not menstruation, not my mother, not other women – who would define and help me understand my womanliness. Writing this book has confirmed something my body and soul understood long before I did: to play the passive spectator to the life of our own body is a choice we make or not. Women are beginning to see that sexuality cannot be conferred by anyone else. If men remain a mystery it is because of their intrinsic 'differences', not because of some magical power they have over us. Women today are mysterious to our mothers because we have become active agents in our own sexuality.

CHAPTER NINE

The Loss of Virginity

My Aunt Kate was expecting her first child the summer of my
freshman year at college, and because my family had moved
north that winter, I was staying with her in Charleston. We
were painting the new nursery, and talking about my best
friend's wedding in which I was to be a bridesmaid, when she
casually remarked she had been a virgin when she married.
Given this atmosphere – my aunt's pregnancy, the wedding,
my mother being far away – you might think a discussion of
sex and contraception would follow. It did not.

I asked no question, not thinking of myself as sexual; she
had given me as much as she was able, comfortably, to say on
the subject. Except that she did add how much her virginity
had meant to her husband. The conversation was easy and
nonmoralistic, parenthetically slipped in between pale pink
brush strokes – my aunt's loving way of giving me something
meaningful from her life. Her comment meshed easily with
my romantic visions of what lay ahead and I promptly
'forgot' it. Looking back now, I can see her message etched
itself on my brain.

If, unlike my aunt, I wasn't a virgin when I married, it
doesn't lessen my indebtedness to her. I had gone north to
college, like her; and was to become an actress and then a
writer, like her. These were things I wanted to do but I had
taken over the idea of them from her. Without the model of
her life to help me out of that warm southern bath I'd grown
up in, I might have married as young as all my friends. The
way she was, the picture of her, allowed me to become sexual
in my own time and without guilt. This is what I owe her ...
not a rule or command that held me back but a model of

restraint I could use while I needed it. The best our heroines can do is give us a hand up and then let us go; the way we thank them is to grow into ourselves – not them. Whenever I drew the seventh virginal veil in my current lover's face – after helping him part the first six – it wasn't because I heard my aunt's words thundering like doomsday: *save it!* I simply wasn't ready. The example of her life was all the reason I needed. My body had experienced everything but the final penetration; in my mind I remained a virgin. The night I did lose my virginity was as meaningful and memorable as the ritual nuptials of any maiden raised by nuns.

One sunny afternoon during my junior year at college, I happened to open a medical textbook left on a table by a friend's date. A paragraph informed that you can get pregnant without penetration. It said that highly active sperm can wiggle up a warm moist vagina on their own even if you were only doing what Steve and I had been doing in his car the night before. While I read, I was counting on my fingers the days since my last period. I knew the next one would not come.

It was destiny that that book fell open to that page, one of those accidental bulletins that were to mark my life. I searched the text for reassurance but quickly ran into a sea of medical jargon. The Great Curtain had briefly parted to give me a message and, as quickly closed again. I was pregnant. I was certain of it, and that there was no one to whom I could turn. I'd never known a girl who'd become pregnant. I had never heard abortion discussed. I was madly in love with Steve but marriage was out of the question. I had too many things to do. Unable to face either alternative, I was left with panic.

It never occurred to me to call my mother. Mother was someone to whom I went when I was on top of the world. I couldn't bear to see anxiety in my mother; my remedy was for her never to see it in me. I circled the college infirmary on the hill, desperate to know the truth, but unable even to form the sentence in my head: 'I think I'm pregnant, help!' Me? – president of my freshman class, secretary of student government? What would people say when I was revealed as a split personality, a person who wanted to spend her life with a man's cock between her legs, who would take it anywhere, in cars, on sandy beaches, any dark secluded place out of sight (but just barely) of others? I would be expelled, shunned; I was immobilized.

I telephoned Steve but his reassurances weakened as the days passed and my own anxieties increased. The chances of impregnation were a million to one, he told me. I was the one millionth. I was six days late. On the seventh day I woke to find a beautiful red spot on the sheet and I shared a religious moment with my God: 'Dear God, thank you, thank you, I will never do it again.'

That Friday I signed out for a weekend, and Saturday morning Steve and I were naked in each other's arms in his roommate's sister's canopied bed on Beacon Hill, his cock moving between my legs, my vagina hot and moist as the intrepid sperm once again tried for that one chance in a million. Is there anyone as stupid as an eighteen-year-old virgin?

Recently I had lunch with a man I hadn't seen since I was nineteen. He had read one of my books and when I heard his voice on the telephone, I smiled, remembering those days in the big feather bed in Kitzbühl, the wine, the après-ski massages we gave each other, the days we never skied at all. I had loved him madly, but when he talked of marriage and slipped me a copy of St Thomas Aquinas our last night (he was Catholic), I let him carve his initials in my arm instead. I still could not think of marriage: I was just beginning. But I wanted to give him something, and so I gave him my arm. We were in bed, drunk on wine and good-byes, and where we got the idea of his autographing me midway between elbow and wrist, I don't know. It is what I remember most of Kitzbühl and him – the act was so unlike me.

What he remembered, he told me at lunch, was that, 'I almost took your virginity. You are what we used to call a *professional virgin*,' he said over our Bloody Marys. 'Don't you remember that last night? I almost had it in. If I hadn't said, "Nancy, do you realize what you are doing . . .?"'

'But you didn't put it in,' I said. 'It takes two to keep a virgin. You are what we virgins called a professional virgin-keeper.'

My mother came to visit me before I flew down to San Juan, Puerto Rico, to begin my first job on an English-language newspaper. She came with my stepfather and two friends to the summer playhouse on Cape Cod where I had been an apprentice my last three summers at college. I had reserved them the best rooms at the best hotel. The best table at the best restaurant and had, of course, gotten them the best seats in the house for that night's performance. I was proud of my mother. She was pretty, young, and she never criticized me.

'You know,' she said, admiring my summer setup, my friends, my perfect life, 'Susie would love to be doing something like this. But she's so irresponsible.' My older sister was still living at home. My mother's preoccupation with the difficulties of my sister's life faded as she turned to me. 'Oh, Nancy,' she smiled, putting a hand on my shoulder, 'you've always been able to take care of yourself. I've never had to worry about you.'

I don't know when my mother and I had agreed on that bargain. It seems it had always been that way. I never took the bad news home. Certainly, by the time I was twenty, my mother and I had further refined the deal: since she did not worry, she wouldn't interfere either. I would take care of myself. That night at dinner I brought along another of the men I was always madly in love with, this time a bad actor. I mentioned that he was driving me to New York, where we would have a night before my flight to San Juan. My mother never asked where I would be staying in New York, whether I had enough money for my ticket, or what I was doing with such a disreputable fellow, one who obviously had neither the background nor manners for the country club. Instead, she smiled shyly at him, and gave me a neatly folded check for twenty-five dollars.

'Now let me know if there's anything you need,' she said, knowing I would not. Suddenly, at the last minute, her face collapsed into that sad wistful look she always had when we parted. 'Oh, Nance,' she began, and reached for me tentatively. I returned her embrace with less warmth than I would have liked, hating myself for not being able to give my mother what she wanted. Why did these good-byes always fill me with such guilt? I waved them out of sight, then drove to New York with my actor. My grandfather had told me I could use his suite at the Plaza. Never a word of caution, even from him. The sign around my neck told the world: Nancy can take care of herself. That night, the actor and I did everything but.

I shared an apartment in San Juan with two other girls, virgins all. The night of our housewarming party, someone brought us a palm tree from which hung three hollowed eggs, symbols of fertility. We laughed and planted ivy in the bidet.

By the end of that year, each had lost her virginity, each in her own time. Not a word about contraception. Not a diaphragm in the house. I had been awakened one night by noise on the terrace and had sat up in bed to see my one roommate making love to a man I had never seen before, and she would never see again. My turn came soon afterward. Riding down Ponce de Leon Avenue on the bus the next morning, I remember my surprise that the freckles on my suntanned arm were still there. I hadn't changed.

From the primitive to the most sophisticated cultures, the unconscious wisdom of the race has seen the need for young men to be confirmed in the assumption of manhood through puberty rites, Bar Mitzvahs, hunting ordeals, etc. Today you are a man. In complex civilization, sex may still be delayed a few years. Nevertheless the youngster has been signaled: it is time for you to put away childish ways and begin to separate from your family. He has looked forward to this ceremony of separation for so long that when it comes he has no doubt of its value. His mother weeps for joy, his father is proud, he himself knows he has reached life's next lofty step. When sex comes, it is the inevitable outgrowth of the rest.

There is almost nothing comparable for girls. There is no ritual, no step-by-step training for womanhood. No celebration of our sexuality. Our one symbolic act is loss of virginity, which is done in secret and without applause. Should we wait until we are married, the act of sex like marriage itself is meant to accomplish what should take years of process and preparation. What should be an act of separation becomes but another form of symbiosis: now that he's 'taken' our virginity, will he love us forever, call us tomorrow, leave us for another woman? Instead of making us free, curious, experimental about the future, sex fills us with regressive, postcoital anxiety. 'Hold me, love only me as I will love only you, forever. Promise.'

Everyone remembers the first time. What we were wearing, the lighting fixture in the ceiling, the feel of the car upholstery. It is set apart in an airtight compartment of memory. The initiation rite has been experienced. One act that says we are children no more, and have pushed aside mother's rules. We are adult, grownup, sexual – synonyms for separate. Except we are not.

More than in any other area of our lives we expect sex to grow us up. Much as mother may not have wanted us to leave home or take a career, she forbade nothing so much as she did sex. We are right to think of it as a step away from her, but it cannot do the job alone. 'Because women have no other formal preparation for sexuality,' says Dr Robertiello, 'the act of losing your virginity comes to bear an impossible load. It just cannot accomplish what people think it will. Separation is not a physical act, like breaking the hymen. It is an emotional one. It must begin during the first years of life and be progressively strengthened all during development. It's no wonder so many women grow disappointed and lose interest in sex. They have feared it so long and then expected it to do so much in one fell swoop. Nothing makes you independent all at once.' Separation is not something that 'happens' to you one night in the back seat of a car or is given to you by a husband in a honeymoon suite.

What a blessing if women could be relieved of their virginity at birth. One simple act to get rid of a label which more than anything else confounds our thinking about sexuality; the marketplace for virgin brides wiped out once and for all, mothers relieved of an anxiety that has nothing to do with their daughters' essential heart, soul, and character. Instead of cops, they could function more easily as loving nurturers. Instead of thinking that in one night we 'lose' some mysterious treasure between our legs, we might come to understand that our sexuality lies between our ears and is won by us alone.

Every free act, every victory over fear and inhibition, leaves an increment of courage, making it easier to try again the next time. Therefore, let's imagine an area of development in which a young person *could* practice her sexuality and learn to feel separate from her mother. Ideally, it should be safe, cheap, quiet, private, and hurt nobody's feelings. It should be self-motivated and self-performed – a self-satisfying pleasure with no possible consequences to anyone but yourself: masturbation. Nature is cunning.

And yet, Kinsey reported in the early '50s that 'No other type of sexual acitivity has worried so many women as masturbation.'[1] In 1964 Dr Schaefer found every woman in her study on female sexuality – which included some who were professionally trained psychotherapists – felt anxiety about masturbation.[2] Nor did the sexual revolution of the last decade profoundly change our ideas. According to Robert Sorenson's 1974 research, women today may masturbate more, but still describe what they feel as 'defensiveness and discomfort.'[3]

The topic itself continues to be anxiety-laden, whether women do or do not masturbate. Why? Says Dr Schaefer: 'The anxiety is connected to an unwillingness to be responsible for one's own pleasure – one's own fantasies – even to be responsible for one's own orgasms.'

If we do not understand why we do not masturbate, we cannot understand why we do not ask for what we want in bed. If we do not feel free to touch ourselves, how can we open ourselves to pleasure with another person? When mother began to take our hand away from between our legs when we were infants, we didn't persist because we were symbiotic with her; whatever she wanted, we wanted.

'When I was six,' says an eighteen-year-old college sophomore, 'I never connected masturbation or childhood sex games with intercourse. I remember lying on my stomach, spreading my legs and wiggling until what I called "the good feelings" came. I felt no guilt about it and even tried to turn my friends onto it. The guilt only started when my mother caught me and I was scolded. I didn't connect the pleasure I gave myself with sex. I thought sex was a very fast maneuver when you wanted a child. I'm still too tense to use Tampax. Last year I fell in love with a smooth talker who finally talked me into going to bed with him. My God, but it hurt! The only thing I enjoyed was being close to him. He went into the army and I never heard from him again. I haven't let myself get close to anyone since.'

This young woman enjoyed masturbation until her mother connected it with sex and told her it was bad. She continued to masturbate but she feels so uneasy about that part of her body that she can't even use tampons. If she doesn't like to touch herself, how can she believe anyone else enjoys it? What chance did she have of actively choosing a partner for sex? He chose her, he smooth-talked her into it, he hurt her, he deserted her. A 'good girl' to the end, she sounds as if she were hardly there at all. 'The only thing I enjoyed was being close to him.' Symbiosis.

'I can't live without him!' cries the abandoned wife. Is that the cry of a woman or baby? Is it lack of sex she is dying of, or lack of someone to be dependent upon?

Little wonder then that most women do not think of entering into sexuality as a break with the symbiotic patterns of childhood; it becomes instead a search for that old togetherness, even if in a new, sexual mode. 'I'm glad I saved myself for Steven,' a young woman says. 'My first time was wonderful. It made me feel part of him.' These are beautiful sentiments, sincerely felt. But there is a confusion of two important ideas here. Closeness and sex are not synonymous. As long as we mesh one with the other, we jeopardize our chance of having the best of either.

I believe that sex is an absolute, an end in itself. If 'making love' does that for you, it is a bonus, not the *raison d'être* of sex. Sex with love is marvelous, but sex can be exciting without love or closeness. If we enter into it only to heighten the symbiotic union, we soon find we have been using sex for a function it cannot perform well. Sex gets its energy from connecting two people; the spark needs a gap to jump. If it is used as a kind of treacle syrup to hold together two people already meshed like a layer cake, you may stay together, but the sex is smothered in sweetness.

In spite of our training, many of us do feel at least a momentary thrill of separation. 'I had a great feeling of power after that first night,' one woman says. 'I felt exhilarated, relieved of a burden,' says another. 'It was wonderful!' says a third. 'I'd arrived; I was a woman at last!' Despite the commonplace phrases, these words have terrific emotion; they give us the sense of people living in their authentic selves if only for the moment, doing what they wanted, walking into the den of fear they had been warned against and finding it instead a fountain of pleasure. They were living in their own experience, not mother's.

But this sudden confirmation of self is unsettling. The experience of reveling in this body, this skin, these breasts, my vagina – an awareness of an inner life that is ours alone – is joyous but scary too. Nothing says you can make it on your own more clearly than a shot of sexuality. Good as it feels, we retreat instinctively. It is too foreign to the only identity we have been taught is acceptable for women: I am a nice girl, not really sexual at all.

'After I lost my virginity, I felt free,' says a twenty-eight-year-old woman. 'I felt more attractive, but it didn't change my sexual pattern. I went out with the next man for nine months before I went to bed with him. I still didn't think sex was nice. In my head, I was still a virgin. I'd had sex with one man but that didn't mean you shouldn't wait until you were married.'

If you've smiled with recognition at what this woman says, you will understand the rest. Part of her had agreed to go to bed with a man, but a more important part had not. She still wanted to be nice, to obey mother's rules, to be loved for not entering sexuality. We want to be women. We want to remain daughters too. In this split we live. Sex has failed to do its magic thing.

The world sees us as women; we have the sexual experience of the female race. Why don't we feel it? Why aren't we the sexually mature people we dreamed of becoming when we were still virgins, saving ourselves for this glorious event? We hasten to confirm the legitimacy of our title of woman. Props are hauled in, a stage production is being born. Who are you? Are you that little girl you fear you still are? No, I am the woman everyone envies for having that wonderful man, this fantastic house, those tickets-around-the-world, six lovers, sixteen Halston gowns, a Christmas card family. Some of us use men and sex like props too, piling up numbers to bolster our subjective fears that we are a sham. Is there anything missing from your sex life? No, I am the woman who had four orgasms last night and seventeen different men in the past month. And yet late at night – even though we lie beside a beloved man and count our blessings and tell ourselves we have everything a woman could ask for – the doubts go on. Is this all? We decide that sex is overrated. We do not realize that by trying to make it function as a form of symbiosis we never gave sex a chance.

The beginning of menstruation and the loss of virginity are doors into the adult world. 'Menstruation,' says Dr Schaefer, 'is stepping into it biologically, while loss of virginity should be the emotional step into adulthood.' Menstruation is something over which we have no control. Sex, when it happens, where, with whom and whether we take responsibility – these are things we can choose to control. Most of us do not.

I am not saying that outwardly we do not say yes, nor that the man rapes us. On an overt level, we do consent, but a distinction must be made between consent that is the signal of active choice, and consent that is hesitant, passive or no choice at all: 'I don't know what I want, do with me what you will.' To the camera eye, the woman chooses the man, decides to uncross her legs. Subjectively, from the inside, we don't look at it that way: we want to feel carried away. Do we want him to touch our breasts? Not a word is breathed. Do we wish he would move more rapidly or slowly? More silence. We communicate with our lover by hope and by prayer. Would we like him to kiss us between the legs? The thought is so unsettling we aren't sure we do want it. Better to let the moment take us where it will, let him push our body here, put our leg there. He did it, not me.

'If women could subjectively say, "I choose to do it and this is what I want" – and mean it – they would make a developmental jump,' says Dr Robertiello. 'But this would increase their separation, and that is frightening.' When we were mother's little girl and living under her roof, it was appropriate to be aware of her strictures. How appropriate is it for a woman old enough to be in bed with a man still to be bound by rules to the point where she hesitates to do and ask for what she wants?

The next morning we question the mirror: Am I now a woman? We go over that first time like an unsolved mystery: what was missing? It was our sense of choice. We did not choose to enter sex. The experience was not *ours*. We just let it happen.

'What a letdown after all those years of waiting,' a woman recalls. 'I'd been expecting an earthquake. I didn't even get a tremor.' After years of saying No, we decide to go! In one jump we go – but stop too. It's like being shot from a cannon and falling down a foot or two from the cannon's mouth. A big decision to go nowhere.

Who are the men we choose for this momentous occasion? We choose a nice boy. A boy who has a familiar feel; who is, in fact, like us, not too experienced. Should we by some chance choose a sexy devil, you can be sure that either he or we are just passing through town: he won't be around tomorrow to remind us of our secret indiscretion, to suggest to our friends, or mother, that we are anything less than good girls.

Ostensibly what we want is a sexual experience, but we choose men who are good at relationships, good providers, men who are serious about their work, who will take care of us. These are reasons perhaps for liking someone, loving him, marrying him, if that is what you want. But they cannot be said to be criteria for a sexual partner. These are men mother would approve of. In fact, they are often male versions of mother. No wonder they are so popular with her. They do not arouse in her the dangerous idea of sex she warned us about and would prefer not to think about herself. Women proudly say, 'Of all the women in the world, he chose me.' We close our eyes to the fact that we had certain reasons of our own for choosing him.

'You always hear about men who are out for only one thing,' says a thirty-five-year-old woman. 'I never met them. I must have had a sign around my neck. They knew I was untouched and untouchable, so they never even tried. Even after college, men still didn't try to get me into bed. I was always the one they wanted to marry. I guess I was the only full-fledged virgin they'd ever run into.'

Certainly there are men who want virgins, just as there are men who don't. But this woman makes it sound as if it were only pure luck that sent her the first kind, never the second.

She takes a passive stance – these nonsexual, marrying-type men merely happened to be attracted to her; she didn't actively choose them. The truth is that she chose to 'see' only them. She sent out signals by the way she dressed, the people she moved among, her body poses, clothes, language, attitudes. If ever a scoundrel of the other kind approached, you may be sure her choice became less passive and more active: 'No!' she would say if he asked her out. All of those is forgotten now. But her story takes an interesting turn as she continues:

'In the end, I began to get a bit curious. I *wanted* sex. Finally, I met Pete. But I didn't have an orgasm. You know what that bastard called me? He said I was frigid! What a rat!' When she finally chose a man, she picked one who called her asexual. She may call him a bastard today, but he gave her a satisfaction so deep she cannot acknowledge it: he told her that she maintained her psychological virginity so deeply, he had been unable to touch it.

'If only somebody had told me what I intend to tell my daughters,' this woman goes on. 'I'm going to tell them to pretend orgasm. Yes, it perpetuates dishonesty for women, but it would have made my marriage very different. I'm going to say, "Look, if he's the kind of man to whom it is terribly important that you come, learn to fake it." ' Never a word about learning to tell a man what you like so that you might actually reach orgasm instead of lying about it; certainly not even a suspicion of the truth that your sexuality, your orgasm, is your responsibility, not his. It is a chilling story from a very well meaning mother who has learned nothing in the past twenty years.

We decide to let a man touch our breasts. For years we have felt ashamed of our bodies. We have been taught to cover them up. Our breasts aren't right, too big, too small. We expect that his hand will now give us a magically different feeling about them than we ever had. Stupidity. A man enters our vagina, the battleground of our emotional lives; we expect what we feel to have nothing to do with toilet training, masturbation, menstruation. Arrogance. Seductive as is its promise of pleasure, our vagina has also been the source of our greatest humiliations and anxiety. It is over this very part of our body that we almost lost mother. Fear of that loss made us introject her notions that the vagina, far from being a source of pleasure, is indeed a source of anxiety and unpleasantness. It was a painful victory over ourselves but it won us her love. It cost us so much, how can we choose to give it all away now? We try to compromise: we will let him touch our vagina, but we won't enjoy it.

We will go to bed with him, but won't come.

A moment's introspection tells us that his reality has begun to blur. We are turning him into a shadowy figure, a projection. He is more 'mother' than lover. We are afraid that if we showed him we had those 'dirty' sexual appetites and desires mother disliked, he would reject us. Mother did – until we hid them from her.

We explain all this to ourselves as 'guilt' – that catchall word that merely gives a negative name to what we feel but explains nothing. 'What is important,' says Dr Robertiello, 'is the feeling behind the "guilt". The real anxiety is the woman's fear that the sexual act has made her separate, on her own, cut off from her upbringing and so having to take responsibility for the course of her life. To do the traditional thing is always easiest. To strike out on a new road, to try to be independent, is difficult. To most people, facing the fact that they are still tied to their baby needs is the most shameful thing in the world. So the word "guilt" is brought in. It gives a serious, grown-up sound to the childish anxiety.'

It is not guilt we feel, but fear – fear of having made the break from the girl that mother wanted us to be. Fear that if she finds out, she will angrily widen the break, and we will not be able to go back. Fear of separation.

For instance, when you secretly had sex or went too far and felt 'guilty', didn't you feel better when you got home and found mother washing the dishes as if nothing had happened? The turmoil was due to your unseparated self being *sure* mother would know. How could she? When you were a baby, she knew when you were hungry, when you were wet – she was so tuned in to you that she could 'read' your mind. The unseparated self fears she still can.

To continue: when you had sex a second and third time didn't the 'guilt' diminish? The first time, sex gave us a feeling of separation from mother. We lived through it. We got used to it. It wasn't so bad. In fact, the pleasures of sex were so nice that it was worth it. When we have sex a second and third time it doesn't increase our degree of separation. We are simply repeating at the same level, and so we don't feel so guilty.

But let's say we introduce a new element, and conduct two affairs at the same time. Once again we feel that old stab of 'guilt'. Once again we are relieved when we get home and find that our lover/husband is sitting there reading the paper as if nothing has happened. Our degree of separation has been stepped up by having sex of a more 'forbidden' nature than before; once again we are reassured when we find the world has not come to an end. It is not postcoital guilt from which we suffer, but postcoital anxiety. Sex has cut us off from being the nice girl mother once loved. Because the fear is free-floating, we may not associate it with the loss of the early, all-approving mother. In fact we will most likely connect it with fear of loss of the man, loss of self-respect, loss of our women friends or roommate (should we have been too sexually explicit) . . . but it's loss, loss, loss.

What is being discussed here is not the morality of sex or even the wisdom of conducting two affairs at the same time. That is private business. What is common to most of us is fear of loss of the beloved because of the notion that in some uncanny way what we are up to is no secret. True guilt resides in the conscience, and you feel it whether or not anyone else knows what you've done. Nonseparated anxiety means you are afraid that your partner *knows*. 'He'll see it in my eyes.' You are afraid you'll lose him.

In a study conducted by sociologist Ira Reiss from the

University of Minnesotta, a nineteen-year-old woman says, 'I'm not doing as much as I would intellectually allow myself, and yet I feel guilty anyway. I believe in my head that it's OK to have intercourse before marriage, but I haven't done it yet. I get these guilt feelings even when I pet.'⁴ In another study at the University of Minnesota, Dr Reiss found fascinating similarities between the approach to premarital and extra-marital sex: 'You would think you'd get technical virgins only in the premarital affair – females who say, "I'll do anything *but*" and still consider themselves virgins. But we find we're getting the same thing in extramarital groups, where women say, "Yes, I pet and kiss extramaritally, but I don't have intercourse." We even find women who say, "I have oral sex but I'm faithful to my husband because I haven't had intercourse."'⁵

Even now, in the final quarter of the twentieth century, the act of intercourse remains a very powerful symbol. It puts you in a new category. It implies a break, loss, separation. That is its thrill and its fear.

When we were learning to walk, mother helped us practice, and her confidence in our success encouraged us to keep trying. When it came to sex, her emotions became communicated to us too; this time what we learned from her was anxiety and failure. Our practice in masturbating, sexual fantasy, pleasure in our body became secret, repressed. Since mother had always denied there could be competition between us, we have not learned through experience that we can win ground that she did not want to yield to us, and that the battle will not destroy her or us.

A nineteen-year-old is talking about her motheer. They are very close, but like most of us she cannot put her finger on what is wrong between them. 'When I was eleven,' she says, 'I wanted a bra. All my friends had one, but mother wouldn't let me. One night we were having dinner with friends and she started saying in front of all those people how ridiculous it was that someone my age should want a bra. I was so ashamed.' Later in the same interview, she says, 'My mother is the kind of person who talks a great deal. In a group, she is always the center of attention. When I bring a guy home who is older than me, for instance, she'll just take over. I can't get a word in. It really disturbs me.'

In the daughter's mind there is no link between these incidents that happened eight years apart. The idea of competition between her and mother is unthinkable. It has never occurred to her that her burgeoning sexuality may make mother feel older. The mother would not like to think that she becomes seductive when her daughter's date comes in the room – a man twenty years younger than she! If you told this mother she was acting competitively with her daughter, she would deny it. Her major criticism of her daughter's behavior is, 'She is not responsible enough.'

How could she be? Every time the young woman has tried to be separate, to be sexual, her mother has interfered – all the while denying interference. With no practice in seeing herself as a woman, in finding she can be sexual and still keep her mother's love, the girl avoids competition, by being irresponsible. She tells me that when she lost her virginity, she did not use any contraceptive. 'See, mother,' this kind of act says, 'I don't understand about all that. I may be entering sex, but only timidly. I don't have your expertise. Don't be mad at me. I'm still a little girl.'

The authentic self is not born. It is won. Regression into fear ever beckons. If you let some childhood limit keep you from doing something you know is your right, you are diminished. Our old infantile needs for symbiosis creep up again and again like jungle underbrush; you have to fight to keep clear what you won last week, last month, last year. Sex does not make a woman of you. It is your reward for having made a woman of yourself first.

And yet, some people who do not have sex are marked by that very fact as autonomous. 'If a girl feels she is still too young to handle sex,' says Dr Robertiello, 'and says no – that is very self-confirming. She is more separated than her friends who get into sex because everyone else is.' If we choose to remain a virgin until marriage, not because mother or society wouldn't approve but because chastity until marriage is one of the principles of our inner value system, that is an act of independence – much more so than is the case with girls who leap into bed for fear of losing the man.

Autonomy enables a girl to say *No* as meaningfully as *Yes*. 'Very often,' says Gladys McKenney, 'the girls who don't have sex in high school are the ones who have well thought-out goals, like going to college. They're not ready for sex yet, and they resist all peer pressures to get into it because everyone else is doing it. They will look at the other girls and maybe they wonder what these girls are doing, but they don't condemn it. You don't get the feeling they are holding back from sex because they are frightened of it. They just don't want it for themselves yet.'

To ask, 'What will he think of me tomorrow?' is to put the power into someone else's hands. The right question is, What will I think of myself tomorrow? Autonomy is making up our minds, not accepting the values or timetables of other people.

We tend to think that girl friends, the men in our lives, our school, college, or job are paths away from mother, alternatives and sources of support for our independence. Sometimes they are. Often they are not. Society, other people, and institutions reinforce what mother taught, adding their pressures to the unconscious residue of her we carry in our minds, making our tries for selfhood that much more difficult.

My emphasis has been on mother as the dominant force in the daughter's behavior but mother's rules would not have their heavy weight without public sanction. In fact, she is the prime agent charged by society for acculturating us to its norms. When we leave home and try to establish a moral framework of our own, the boss, the corporation, people at the office, our girl friends and lovers often compound our conflicts. They seem to be saying: here is your job, your apartment, here is friendship, here is sex; it is nobody else's business what you do. What is confusing is that behind it all we hear the old familiar double message.

Take men, for instance. We think they are as different from mother as possible. Haven't they always been talking us into sex, encouraging us to break mother's rules? And yet what are *their* rules? 'The boys know how far girls will go,' says a sixteen-year-old. 'You have to know when to say stop. Otherwise, a guy may suddenly say, "I love you, but I can't see you any more." The girl can't understand why. She's done what he's been begging her to do, but instead of committing himself to her more, suddenly he's backing off.'

The pattern is familiar enough. It might be said the boy needs more time to study, to pursue his career. He may talk about being suffocated, tied down by the relationship. We know he means something else, and we have already condemned ourselves. He has told us, *I love you but you have broken one of my secret rules so I'm not going to love you any more*. We went too far.

Despite all he said, what he really wanted was someone who was less threatening to his socially indoctrinated role, a nice girl. 'When I was single and men were always trying to get me into bed,' says one woman who speaks for hundreds, 'no matter how much a guy pleaded and persisted, I would refuse. I always knew that if he and I became a serious item, he would end up protecting and loving that virginity of mine more than I. What if I'd given in? I can't help wondering. What do men really want, a virgin, or a good lay?'

By putting us into double binds like these, just as mother did, men hinder our efforts to find our own direction at a time when we are experimenting with sexuality, and, hence, most vulnerable.

In a campus survey at the University of Iowa, Dr Reiss found that a third of the girls interviewed said they intellectually accepted the idea of sex before marriage but had not yet put this notion into practice. The boys they met and liked were too double standard. Says Dr Reiss: 'These girls thought that if the man had sex, he could not do it without prejudice. He would think less of her and they would break up.'⁶ If we intuit this about our boy friend, little wonder we postpone sex.

Most sociologists I interview agree that young men today are more amenable than their fathers to women being independent and assertive – traits once deemed for men only. This is an important change. But it does not follow that these same young men are prepared to grant equality in sexual experience to their women. In her recent study of college men, *Dilemmas of Masculinity,* Professor Mirra Komarovsky found most men still felt more comfortable when they were the more experienced partner. 'Making love to someone more experienced frightens the hell out of me . . .' said one of her respondents. Another student reported 'he'd feel funny, less masculine, making love to a more experienced girl.' Professor Komarovsky sums up: 'The great majority would not demand virginity in their future mates, though they would reject "promiscuous" girls.'⁷

The definition of promiscuous, nevertheless, continues to run along lines of the old double standard: 'While you're dating,' says a nineteen-year-old woman, 'men tell you they don't care if you're a virgin or not. But when they find the girl they want, then it's important to them. Most guys could tolerate it if you weren't a virgin, but they'd rather pretend that they were *the* one.'

The media message goes out to women: 'It's a great big, free, sexual world out there!' The real one is: 'But you better not believe it.' Says a very attractive divorcée of thirty-three:

'I met this man and he told me at dinner how much he liked my style, my independence. When we got back to his apartment, I thought, well, this is today, not the Victorian era. So what if it's the first date? I let him know I was willing to go to bed with him. After all, he'd admiringly called me "an upfront woman". As soon as we were in bed, I knew I'd done the wrong thing. It was awful.'

I asked several sex therapists if this story was uncommon. 'I'm always floored when this kind of thing comes up in group therapy,' says Dr Schaefer. 'A man will relate the kind of experience you just mentioned. "What kind of woman is it," he asks, "who carries her diaphragm around in her purse just in case?" He's half embarrassed but he means it, and the other men nod sympathetically. "We don't ask that she be a virgin," they explain, *"but . . ."'*

Society too sits in for mother. Gladys McKenney is not allowed by Michigan law to teach birth control in her high school Marriage and Family classes. 'I can only answer their questions,' she says. 'The kids know the law is outmoded and that way of offering information is a kind of hypocrisy.'

Despite the youth explosion, things are not all that much better on college campuses. 'There was no gynecologist or birth control clinic on campus and none in town,' says a young woman who goes to college in a western state. 'A friend and I went to the administration and asked that a gynecologist be appointed. The trustees finally agreed to hire one part-time, but stipulated that no contraceptives could be prescribed.' This kind of story was repeated to me in several variations, in a dozen states.

Young women can't even get full support from their peers. They are as divided as anyone by parental and cultural norms. 'I'm on the Commission on the Status of Women at my college,' says a nineteen-year-old. 'There is no birth control clinic on campus and you have to be twenty-one or have a note from your parents to go to a gynecologist in town. I get calls from girls who say, "I have this problem, but I can't tell you what it is." As for venereal disease, they can't even bring themselves to say the words. I wanted my girl friend to come work with me in the clinic but she said, "Oh, I can't! Everyone would know I'm on the pill!"'

Is it any wonder that even when we 'choose' to have sex our lifelong internalized *No* is still with us? We can make our bodies do this or that, but our minds and emotional consent lag behind. And so there is this absolutely uncanny, almost suicidally foolish manner in which women enter sex. What it says is that the solution to our problem is not to have to face it at all. It is the great Swept Away phenomenon.

'You don't want to be ready for it,' says an eighteen-year-old. 'You just want it to take over and happen, especially the first time. You want it to be spontaneous. You want to get carried away. There's a free clinic in town, where you can get advice and your first contraceptive free, but if you plan – that takes all the romance out of it.'

Swept Away: it is not merely a phenomenon of the very young. Women of all ages give it – unblinkingly! – as rationalization. 'I couldn't help myself,' they smile, as if you must agree that they have satisfactorily explained everything. You're a woman too, aren't you? 'Of course I didn't want to get pregnant,' explains a thirty-five-year-old divorced mother who recently had an abortion. 'Look, it was so great, this guy was so fantastic, I just didn't want to think about it. Besides, I was safe. How could it have happened? My period had ended four days before.' When I told her she had probably been entering her most fertile period, she said, 'I thought you began counting from the end of your period.'

There are songs for women like this: 'You Made Me love You, (I Didn't Want to Do It)' . . . 'I Got Lost in His Arms' . . . 'Don't Blame Me.' . . . The underlying message is always the same: I don't usually do that kind of thing. I'm not that kind of girl. I had no choice. I was just carried away.

Even our daydreams – the safest possible playground to toy with new ideas – are written along symbiotic lines. In over seven years of research on women's sexual fantasies, the most prevalent themes I found were rape, domination, and force. Good girls to the end, we make the other person *do it* to us.

I want to say this emphatically: not a single woman I ever talked to said she did want to be raped in actuality. What is wanted is something only in the imagination, release from the responsibility of sex. Only the terrible force of the brute can free us from the fear of wanting the sexuality he represents. 'Women are almost as strong as men,' says Dr Sonya Friedman, 'or at least, they could be. But they like to make the disparity seem enormous. Their feeling of almost total helplessness is used to keep themselves children, not responsible, needing to be taken care of.' It wasn't our fault. If we hadn't drunk so much, if things hadn't gotten out of hand, if the moonlight hadn't been so bright . . . *He made me do it!*

How many women lose their virginity or have their most abandoned moments with a stranger, the steward on the cruise ship, the handsome translator in Rome? 'These women are compartmentalized,' says Dr Schaefer. 'They go to Europe and have all sorts of adventures, and then they come back home and are back to being good little girls. They may not have sex again for months. They've said, Europe is not reality, it's fairyland, it doesn't count. What counts is when I'm home in my mother's domain, and here I am a "nice girl". Yes, they've done better than the ones who never have sex, but they've only allowed it because it was in a place that let them keep the all-important tie to mother.'

Young women today are more likely to have their first sex with someone they are emotionally involved with. Vera Plaskon works with teen-agers in the Family Planning and Gynecological Clinic at Roosevelt Hospital. She is twenty-nine but remembers only too well how girls lost their virginity when she was growing up. It was usually 'on vacation', she says, 'with some stranger, rather than with the boy back home. Today, kids have sex within the important relationship. There is more caring with sex. That doesn't mean however that they are more responsible. The feelings don't get translated into actions. It's so rare that I will get a young woman who will say to me, "I'm planning to have sex, tell me what to use." They prefer to let it come without thinking about it in advance, to be swept off their feet.'

Even the scientific organization SIECUS (Sex Information and Education Council of the US) cites the Swept Away phenomenon as a seemingly valid reason so many reject using a diaphragm or the pill. '. . . they cannot conceive of themselves as being prepared for coitus all the time. They must be emotionally carried away for coitus to occur.'[8]

Incredible! Never before in the history of the world has so much contraceptive information been available to young women. And yet the rate of premarital pregnancies is higher today than twenty-five years ago. In the '50s, Kinsey found that 20 percent of the women who had sex before marriage became pregnant. In more recent studies a full generation later, Zelnik and Kantner found 30 percent of such women got pregnant.[9] That is a full 50 percent increase in rate of unwanted pregnancies!

'Every woman knows about contraception, or could if she wanted to,' says anthropologist Lionel Tiger. 'In our book *The Imperial Animal,* Robin Fox and I compared the drugstore cosmetic counter with the contraceptive counter. Young women seem perfectly capable of understanding the 25,000 different items on the cosmetic counter, which can be used in millions of permutations and combinations on many different parts of their bodies. But they very often appear not to know how to – or be willing to – manage the contraceptive counter, though it involves a quite simple business. When one looks at this behavior, one must say there is something strong driving these people to do what is often far removed from their rational plans.'

There are many explanations, of course. Each one a logical, seemingly sufficient reason for a young woman's lack of decision or skill in using contraception. 'If you are raised to be a passive partner,' says educator Jessie Potter, 'you do not get fitted for a diaphragm. If you raise girls not to touch themselves, they make rotten contraceptors. If you teach them to think sex is beautiful only when the right man comes along and does it to you, then you are raising them to wait, to avoid taking responsibility for themselves.' Other explanations for not using contraception include rebellion, religion, getting pregnant in order to get the man to marry you, or to prove to yourself that you are capable of getting pregnant. Boys promise girls that they can control it, withdraw in time. Many women have a phobic avoidance of contraceptives. Dr Helen Kaplan, a psychiatrist at the Payne

Whitney Clinic, says women have a deep, unconscious wish to be impregnated by a man they care about. The list grows with every authority I interview. The fact is that all these explanations fit right into, and work along with, the need to be Swept Away – a need every professional worker in sexuality mentioned in addition to any other specific reason he/she gave.

'To sum up the terrific power and longing that being Swept Away holds for women,' says Dr Robertiello, 'you have to understand that it is *a method for avoiding separation*. If the woman feels there are forces which took her over, she is confirmed in her role of dependency. If she had no power, then it isn't her fault that mother's rules were broken; therefore mother should still love her. Swept Away is an escape from freedom. It tells the girl that even if she did have sex, it wasn't her fault. She didn't want to go against mother. She had no choice.'

From the day we are born there is a bit of what society calls *male* in all of us. It is our lust. Mother did her best to keep it in check. As we grew older she passed the job on to us. To be sexual was to be 'out of control', like an animal, like a man. Badgered to be 'feminine', we grew up afraid of our lust. We learned control instead, iron control – of ourselves, of him, of the situation.

It is hard for men to understand women's problems with control. A young boy is baffled by a girl's fear of being touched, her reluctance to touch him back. 'Girls in the sixth grade are horrified that a boy wants to finger-fuck,' says Jessie Potter. 'I try to explain to the boy, "Look, she hasn't even allowed *herself* to put her finger there." He can't understand that because he's touched his penis every time he pees and a lot of other times besides. Boys masturbate in front of each other, but there is no "show-and-tell" for girls. He expects her to be as eager to touch him as he is to touch her. I say to her that she must understand that his desires don't say anything judgmental about her or him, he is not "gross" to have these wishes. Because he wants to do it to her, she isn't any less the nice girl she wants to be. They meet like two strange people from different planets. When he wants to touch her breasts, he has no way of understanding her feeling about this encroachment on the body she has been taught to keep so private. So he perceives himself as being rejected and unlovable. In self-defense, to gain back some of his lost ego, he decides she must be frigid. She, not understanding how she was taught to withhold, frequently sees herself as unloving.'

Many young women have a tremendous fear that if we allow ourselves to become sexual, we will become promiscuous, whores. Why else would society/mother put on these ten-ton chains if sex weren't so titanically strong and dangerous? If we once let the barrier down, we will become sex addicts. 'We have a whole cultural fix,' says Dr Robertiello, 'about how sexuality is such a powerful urge that it overcomes all other forces. Men aren't afraid of this sexual force or of loss of control; they get points for being sexual. Women do not.'

A controlling relationship is what we know best. We may say we want the man to be stronger, brighter, taller, and that we want to be dominated in bed. That doesn't mean we don't want to control him. What we know about intimacy, how to gain and keep it, is how mother was with father – and with us. Mother's control proved she cared. Some men don't mind our moving in with ideas of eternal togetherness, others jump like rabbits. To be fair to both sexes, many women aren't aware of the manipulation involved in control. It comes disguised as love. 'If you really cared for me' we say . . . Guiltily, he does what we ask.

Perhaps mother was a quiet, retiring person. She may have claimed to know nothing about money, leaving it all to dad. But we knew she had a way of getting what she wanted and getting him to do what she wanted too. It had to do with the very fact of her seeming lack of power, her womanliness. *Already we know that as long as we are virgins, we have a form of control and power ourselves.*

'I was afraid of having sex,' says a college senior. 'Afraid that once I went all the way, that I would have no more leverage with him. If I couldn't hold out on him any more, I'd have no more control. Once you have sex, you never know if it's you or the conquest that was important; when you're growing up, ninety percent of the time it's the conquest.'

Increased experience does not lessen our fear of the overwhelming power of sex. 'Oh, no, the adolescent rules didn't affect my later sexual life,' says a woman of twenty-eight. 'When I started I really started. But I've always been monogamous. It is a kind of self-protection. The only way you can protect yourself is to mind your behavior . . . or it just slips away.'

As we move out of mother's area of control, and the man is gradually allowed to enter our vagina in the one-step-at-a-time ritual loss of virginity, we make a trade. We construct with him the kind of bargain we had with her: if I allow you to touch me there, promise you will never leave me. If I reject mother's laws for your sake, and give up my once-in-a-lifetime power as a virgin, promise nothing bad will happen and that you will take care of me as she did.

The man is being made to assume the protective stance of the absent mother. Symbiosis is continued. Forbidden sex, the source of anger for as long as we can remember, need not destroy us after all! We thought men were so powerful, so self-sufficient, but we can use sex to control them. 'With-holding sex,' says Sonya Friedman, 'is women's greatest source of power.'

'My first lover stayed with me for a year and a half,' says a thirty-year-old woman. 'I didn't want to marry him, but I didn't want him to leave me. Sex gave me the power to keep him. I'd always felt so powerless before. Now, with sex, here was something that I was good at. Maybe not good at, but that didn't matter. I had it. Men stay with you because of it.'

The price to the woman is high. To preserve our bargaining position, we must control our own desire first, hoarding lust like a miser, never spending it on pleasure. 'When I'm with a guy for the weekend,' says a twenty-seven-year-old woman, 'it's heaven while I'm there, while you're in bed. But Monday morning when I go to work, the good feeling fades and I get this funny idea I've lost something. I'm in a weaker position with him, and I can't help myself . . . I begin these maneuvers about when am I going to see him again. I hate myself for it, but I have to do it.' The bitter irony is that having got rid of mother's control, we are unhappy without it. We long to set it up with the man. Under these circumstances, we are not taking on a lover. We just switch mothers.

My own sexual ideas are different from what they were ten or fifteen years ago, and so I expected to find dramatic changes in behavior and attitudes toward virginity in young women today. Even my mother's attitude – unswerving for all of my life – has been affected by what she has seen and read, and perhaps most of all, by her neighbors' attitudes – those whose children have come of sexual age in the sixties. 'When your child runs away to San Francisco,' says Dr Sidney Q. Cohlan, 'or becomes pregnant, or marries a hippie or goes on drugs, you must accept some of the changes in the life-style of her generation if you want to keep a relationship with her. You may not like these changes, but it is easier for you to accept them nowadays because you find your neighbors are accepting them too.'

Surely if I lost my virginity today, instead of in the sex-taboo fifties, I'd do it differently. 'In 1963, only twenty percent of adults said it was OK to have intercourse in some circumstances before marriage,' Dr Ira Reiss tells me. 'That was a national sample. By 1970, it had jumped to fifty percent. If we took a new national sample today, I'm sure we'd get more than half the parents saying it was OK under some circumstances.'

Therefore I am not surprised when gynecologist Sherwin A. Kaufman tells me that the mothers who consult him today are not so concerned with their daughter's loss of virginity as they are afraid of her becoming pregnant. 'They have come to accept that a girl who goes off to college,' he says, 'may not graduate without sexual experience. It's an idea they didn't want to think about ten years ago.' And though Dr Kaufman is quick to add that the New York women who consult him are a special subculture, I wonder if these liberal mothers aren't in tune with what college girls in their teens and early twenties are feeling all across America. They are a special subculture too.

'What *has* changed are attitudes,' says Wardell Pomeroy. 'The real change is more in approach than practice. A lot of people talk a bigger game than they play. From this big change in attitude will come later changes in behavior, in what people do (and not what they say they do). But it really hasn't shown up yet with statistical significance. People just don't change that rapidly. They develop certain norms and ideas, but it takes more than a film or book to change their behavior. It is a gradual process. Change usually comes between generations, not within one.'

Statistics must be read in context. There are over 200 million people in the US today, double the number fifty years ago. When twice as many people do something, we are prone to believe 'everybody' is doing it, that something new is going on. It is merely more visible. We are changing, but not all that rapidly. There is more talk and general acceptance of sex today. Nonvirgins used to keep it a secret. Today, they go on TV talk shows. 'Everything is different nowadays,' we tell each other.

Gladys McKenney recalls that not too many years ago a high school girl would never admit she had lost her virginity. 'Of course some had, but they would tell me privately,' she says. 'They couldn't be honest in class. They didn't want the judgment of their peers on them. It's almost a reverse of that in the higher grades now. Last semester I had a class in which there was a group talking very openly about how they enjoyed sex and wouldn't consider marrying a boy they hadn't slept with. But there was another group of girls who I know hadn't even dated much. They didn't say a word because they didn't want to reveal their inexperience. What has changed, you see, is the openness of those who have sex. There is no longer a stigma attached to losing your virginity.

But that doesn't mean it is not still a very important event.'

'What is important about losing your virginity,' says a nineteen-year-old, 'is that you keep it important. That you don't have sex casually.'

We want so badly to be easier about sex. As mothers, we don't want our children to grow up with our sexual inhibitions. We change *our* attitudes and think that will change *their* lives. We look at them behaving far more guiltlessly than we'd dreamed ten years ago, and identify more with their generation than the one we grew up in. We talk of multiorgasms and bisexuality and glibly think something as primary and emotive as loss of virginity is old-fashioned, tame stuff. But for all our new attitudes, the liberated poses we strike, our children don't believe us. They are still uncomfortable when we bring up sex. We are hurt. Haven't we made enormous efforts to understand their world? Haven't we met them more than halfway?

A parent who asks these questions is being as sincere as she knows, but once again is confusing the difference between attitude and gut feeling. Children may listen to mother's words; what they really take in is how mother feels on the deepest level. Our ideas about our bodies, our eroticism, our sexual limits, are so much a basic part of us that we may not be aware how they determine the things we *say* to our daughters. We got them from our mothers; she got them from hers. When we talk to our daughters about sex, or when we have sex – what we feel is a mixture of the old and new, of what our mothers felt about it, and what we would like to feel.

In a study on parent-child perception and behavior at Illinois State University, low correlation was found between what parents said were their sex attitudes and what their children said they were. But there was a high correlation between how the children *perceived* their parents, and how the children behaved. For instance, if a seventeen-year-old girl said, 'My parents are very low on permissiveness,' she was often wrong, but the girl herself was more likely to be low on permissiveness. And if an eighteen-year-old said, 'My parents are very high on permissiveness,' again, she might be wrong, but she was more likely to be high on permissiveness herself. The conclusion was that the *perception* of one's parents' permissiveness is more important in predicting the child's behavior than are the actual words of the parents.[10] Clearly, if a daughter thinks her mother – no matter what she says – is permissive about premarital sex, the daughter is more likely to be permissive herself.

If mother has sincerely tried to change her attitude, it gives the daughter a certain freedom to experiment, to see just how much mother really does mean what she says. If the girl is courageous, lucky, and gets enough societal and peer approval, she can make a start on discarding the old sexual inhibitions. In time, reality will come to reinforce her new ideas: it's easier, happier to live this way. Then whatever ground is gained can be passed on to the daughter's children. This is the work done 'between generations' that Dr Pomeroy mentions.

Some mothers can do it. For most it is not easy. When we take the lag Pomeroy speaks of – the distance at which *behavior* follows *talk* of sexual freedom – and then add the even greater lag in our gut about whether what we are doing is *right* – it is evident that very few mothers are so integrated on all three levels that they can send their daughter a message behind which the girl will not hear older, more familiar overtones of anxiety; if these ideas make my mother nervous, where may I put my full weight? On what she says, or on what she feels? For instance:

Two girls both know about the pill. One takes it methodically, in advance of sex. When, sooner or later, she enters the bedroom, it will be with the fear of pregnancy (at least) diminished. The other girl doesn't take it, or does so sporadically. Statistics say neither is a virgin, and that both are members of the liberated seventies. But the quality of their sexual experience is totally different. Why? Because the first girl's attitude toward sex, her behavior and gut feelings, acted together. Faced with no conflicting double message, she felt free to choose the pill. All too often girls in therapeutic counseling sessions for unwed mothers know about the pill but do not use it or use it incorrectly. They have one attitude in their head about sex. In their gut, they are entirely different, much more judgmental.

'In their hearts, the parents of girls who come to the Family Planning Clinic,' says Vera Plaskon, 'are against early sexual activity. At the same time, they are middle class, they want to be IN. So these mothers re-run their own fantasies of what they would have liked to have done – or what they would do if they were their daughters today. They push these fantasies onto their kids before they are ready. "Just let me know when you want the pill," they tell their thirteen-year-old. They don't stop to think maybe the girl is not ready to hear this. It can be a lot more subtle. The mother may be fully unaware that by buying her daughter the latest seductive clothes and make-up, she is pushing her into what *she* would have liked to have done when she was young, before the sexual revolution. Once she has the girl living out her fantasy, there is also the mother's competition with the girl, *plus* her own guilt at what she has done. It may be unconscious, but it is very confusing to the daughter. Recently I was talking to a girl who is very sophisticated for her fifteen years. She laughingly said her mother always told her that if and when she needed birth control, to come to her. "But you should have seen her face when I actually did!" she said. Most girls are not so sophisticated, and they don't laugh about it. They don't know what to do. And finally, there are many girls who really wish their mothers would say, No, *and mean it*. They can't handle all this freedom at fifteen or seventeen – their own growing up, and often their mother's as well. The girl doesn't know what the mother wants from her. The mother doesn't know herself. In the gut of the liberated Manhattan mother you very often find the same doubts and anxieties I see in women who have just arrived from Central and South America, from the heart of the macho culture. Feelings she hasn't really dealt with. So she sends out the contradictory message to her daughter: "This is the modern age, do what you like!' But when the girl comes home at three in the morning, the mother screams at her that she is acting like a whore.'

'It's very unconscious,' says Dr Robertiello, 'a mother's unexpressed desire for a girl to have a sexuality she never had. Often there is a specific admonishment against it, which is like a reverse suggestion to do it. For example a girl will come in and talk about the date she's been on, and how she almost had sex. The mother will smile – giving the nonverbal message of approval – even while she gives her holy hell and tells the girl she will break her neck if she ever does it.'

A double message like this undermines our reasoning powers and gives us no clear-cut line of separation. In our muddle, not knowing which way to go, we surrender our will. Either we allow ourselves to be swept away by the man, or we turn back to mother. Neither is an autonomous choice. It is just a need to depend on someone. We listen to mother's contradictory commands, and in true symbiotic fashion, act out both halves of mother's conflict. One day we are 'good', and say No to the boy. The next day we are 'bad' and become pregnant. What more could mother want?

I ask Dr Robertiello how a mother could possibly be sending out a message for her daughter to get pregnant. 'Pregnancy and intercourse,' he said, 'are often confused and tied together in people's minds. Getting pregnant is proof of getting laid. If you are thirty-five and married and six months pregnant, that is not a sexual idea. But if a girl has a friend, let's say, who get pregnant at fifteen, she can read the light in her mother's eyes: Boy, that is a sexy, bad girl.'

If mother tells us that she is not certain that 2 and 2 are 4, we smile and say we have no doubts ourselves. In the area of arithmetic, at least, we are separate from her. If her words about our pregnant fifteen-year-old friend are negative, but we see that excited light in her eyes, we respond to her excitement. Despite all our own real fears and attitudes about getting pregnant, down deep we don't think it is so bad at all. We have taken in mother's unconscious wishes and act on them as if they are our own.

In a survey of girls who went to a campus contraceptive clinic versus those who did not, Ira Reiss found the clinic girls believed they were attractive to men twice as frequently as nonclinic girls. The clinic girls also more frequently felt they had as much right as men to initiate sex. 'What the pill does,' says Dr Reiss, 'is put choice in the hands of the female. It tells her, "Look, if you don't want to have intercourse, that's your right, but you have to have a different reason to say No than fear of pregnancy. That can be taken care of. You are going to have to make up your mind without pretenses."'[11]

Choosing to use the pill is evidence of a good deal of integration. The clinic girls are saying by their behavior that they are entitled to sex. By acting on what they say, and going to the clinic to be prepared for the consequences of their actions, they show their behavior, attitude, and gut reactions are in line.

To my mind, their autonomy is illustrated in another area in which most women usually betray great insecurity: *they did not wait for a man to tell them they were sexually attractive.* Their actions tell me that they made their own evaluation of their looks and bodies, and, having decided they were attractive, decided to reap the reward for it by getting into sex.

I would emphasize however that it was not going to the clinic that made them more autonomous than the girls who did not. That is reverse reasoning, confusing cause with effect. They were more separate *before* they went. That is *why* they went. The pill did not make them autonomous. Their autonomy enabled them to decide to use the pill.

Psychoanalytic theory used to say that if a girl entered into premarital sex, especially if it were an unhappy experience or ended with pregnancy, it was an expression of rebellion. Sex was seen by the girl as a way of getting back at the restrictor, doing exactly the opposite of what mother wanted. That is still often the case, but nowadays psychiatrists have come to see that rebellion is one of the symptoms, not the complete statement of the overall problem – which is lack of separation.

Rebellion should not be mistaken for separation. As long as

the effort to break away is seen not as a blow for ourselves but as a reaction to the parent, it is still a symbiotic proceeding. Rebellion becomes separation when the goal is self-fulfillment, not mere frustration of something the parent wants us to do. Says Dr Robertiello, 'Rebellion within the family is often a sign of how much we are still tied to the family – fighting someone from whom we should have been separated a long time ago.'

The difficulty in understanding rebellion begins with the romantic glow that folklore has given the world. To researchers in human development, it has a very specific time-related meaning. When we are two, rebellion is appropriate. This is the No-saying stage children go through. Another rebellious period comes in adolescence, but by this time, just saying No is not enough. Certain moves toward autonomy have to accompany the sixteen-year-old's rebelliousness or it is inauthentic, a sign of attachment. We may have more sex than we really want, or drink too much, but at the same time, if we are meeting our academic requirements, handling money responsibly, it can be said that the rebellious elements are in the service of separation.

But at twenty-five, thirty-five, the time for rebellion should have been long over. If we are not taking care of ourselves, not paying our bills, turning up late for work, having a lot of sex without really enjoying it, then rebellion is immaturity. The rebellious person who must always put a minus sign where she is asked to put a plus is merely reacting to somebody else. She is not free to go her own way, to choose not to argue. She is ever tied, ever waiting. Give me something to say No to.

We look at the very young today and envy them their sexual ease and apparent lack of guilt. Despite all that has been written, said, experienced, and thought in the past decade, most of us have not reached the kind of free-flowing sexuality young people seem to have been born with. They seem to be so accepting of their sexuality; the word used for them is 'liberated' – which is another way of saying they are separated.

It is the old philosophical problem of appearance and reality. To the outside eye, they may indeed seem free. They appear to have won the rebellion against those antisexual rules which cost us so much. In our fight for autonomy, sexuality was the one battlefield above all others. To have won any degree of freedom there was more difficult than anywhere else.

For those of us raised before the sixties, the rules were hard and fast – especially about sex. Mother made no bones about wanting to repress and inhibit our sexuality – or our retaliatory anger. *No* was the clear message her attitude gave us. *No* was reinforced by her behavior. *No* came to us from her gut reaction. She was all of a piece: we could either conform to mother's ideas, or gather up our strength and say, 'The hell with you, Mom. I'll do it my way.' She gave us firm ground on which to plant our defiant feet. In the anger and quarreling, separation between mother and ourselves gains definition; we may not have attained autonomy, but at least we knew where she stood.

If we've been raised in too permissive a manner, separation can become difficult. The rules are vague and elastic. Rarely is the permissively raised child out-and-out forbidden to do this or that. We were merely presented with more attractive alternatives. In this way our own desires were manipulated and used against us. We weren't told not to play with that nasty little boy next door. Whenever he appeared on the horizon, mother took us to the drugstore for an ice cream instead. If we got kicked out of college, that was unfortunate, but a new school was found which was more tolerant of our special temperament. If we broke the parental rule about sex (if there was one), it was not the end of the world. Even if we insisted on a fight, wanting to clarify the difference (separation) between us, mom once again quickly shifted ground, to join us. 'Oh, I'm so glad you feel free to express anger at me! What a healthy thing to do!' How do you separate from somebody so glued to you with admiration? Anger is not allowed to do one of its principal jobs: separate me from you. You never get a clear-cut No; no firm ground is offered from which to push yourself off.

It is difficult. We love mother, but there she is, *surrounding* us. We want to separate from her (even if we don't use the word) but we can't get a fix on the problem. If we want to run away to India, she'll pay for the ticket and remind us to phone collect when we want to come home. Never having been let go of, we can't let go ourselves. Permissively reared people have had no experience of separate relationships, and so never look for them. We gravitate to what we know. Permissive girls choose permissive boys, and they glom together.

On the surface, relationships like this seem freer, easier than those between sharply defined people. If one partner wants to go to a movie and the other wants to go to a ball game, neither insists on dominance; it needs hardly any discussion to decide to compromise and go ice skating. This is not the first choice of either, but the relationship has not been roiled, even for a moment. Everything is soft, blurred, hazy, friendly. Even sex becomes nondifferentiated. (It is no coincidence that the permissive era is the Unisex era.) Young people do not regard each other today across the differences of sex as if the other were from Mars. They have been raised to relate to other people without fuss, without fighting *without separation*. Sweetness, gentleness, amiability are all.

'Thank God,' says the mother of seventeen- and eighteen-year-old daughters, 'the young people I meet nowadays are not so hassled by sex as I was. They seem to have found a natural relationship with one another. My girls connect with boys in a friendly manner. Young people have much closer, deeper relationships today. This whole nightmare thing of sex doesn't seem to arise like it did in my generation. Sex doesn't play a huge part in their lives.'

As far as friendliness and lack of fear goes, this is certainly an advance. But this woman says one thing that is perhaps more important than she is aware. She says sex doesn't play a huge part in her daughters' lives – a fact which relieves her anxiety. What she intuitively understands is that being closer, caring deeply about someone of the opposite sex doesn't necessarily mean you see him in a sexual light. If you are afraid of, or envy, your daughters' sexuality, you think these 'friendly' developments are positive.

People who come out of a background of being coddled, who are not allowed to develop separately, indeed often do have sex – but it doesn't mean they are autonomous. It can mean the opposite: that they are using sex – which is one of nature's methods of helping us grow up – to remain childish instead, to create a nice, warm relationship with this other person which is similar to that one they once had with mother, which they never had to outgrow, and which is all they know. Proof of this is that such 'sexual' relationships between young people often cease to be sexual at all; they soon become fond and fondling palships. Or maybe they were that all along: 'I slept with a lot of guys before I lost my virginity,' many young women tell me. 'We didn't have sex. We just liked each other and were good friends.' Is being 'free' of sex such an unqualified good?

Says Dr Schaefer: 'The kind of symbiotic union you see today in kids who at thirteen and fourteen are already going steady delays separation . . . is a defense against separation. You see them together, day and night. They tend to have low-energy relationships. Symbiosis drains them of interest in anything outside the little womb they've built. They sit side by side in a room, silent, polite, friendly; just being together is their choice against all the variety that life can offer.' It can hardly be said to be a real choice if they did not feel the freedom to explore the alternatives first.

Some sociologists have gone so far as to suggest the days of the double standard may be coming to an end. That too is a gain, but if monogamy is settled on without choice, where is freedom? 'It used to be that only girls were like this,' says Betty Thompson, 'but today we see boys acting the same way, refusing even to look at another girl.' On the surface it may look like love and fidelity. In a few years, we may see it differently. That is when symbiosis has so killed off whatever degree of sexuality there was between them that they flood the divorce courts, crying, 'I need my own space!' Freedom to have sex together has been bought at the price of never giving each other air to breathe.

If people raised in nonpermissive times envy the freedom from sexual guilt of young people today, Spock-reared people seem to have lost their elders' ability to work toward well-defined goals and aims in life. 'The rebellion of the permissive generation is aborted almost from the start,' said Dr Robertiello. 'They often have a hard time finding what they want. They are looking for the rose garden that mother promised them.' Their freedom is illusory since they reject reality to look for what does not exist.

Says Betty Thompson: 'When you are indulged, when everything is done for you, you do not grow up with a recognition of the realities of life. You break your bicycle, and mother says, "Don't worry, we'll buy you a new one." If mother and father saw to it that you got everything you wanted, there just hasn't been any practice in being responsible for yourself. What is not available is a recognition that everything in the world cannot be bought. When a girl says, "I don't want to carry a diaphragm when I go on dates," it is an evasion of responsibility, it is regressive in the sense of character development. It is not romantic, it is not being separate and adult. It is babyishness.' Carelessness, lack of forethought, and disorder may masquerade as freedom to the outside eye. But they tie us with chains of consequence.

At seventeen our problems with autonomy arise from one direction; at thirty-seven they come at us from another. Lack of separation is where both lines meet. Autonomy is the declaration and affirmation of the self; sex is one of its expressions. 'I am a woman and this is my body and my life. I will do what I want with both because that is what I want, not because I want to get back at you.'

It took me twenty-one years to give up my virginity. In some similar manner I am unable to let go of this chapter. Unanswered questions run endlessly through my head like ticker tape: how does the daughter's loss of virginity affect her relationship to her mother? Shouldn't she wait until she has left home to lose her virginity so that her mother won't be involved? Doesn't the fact that a girl hasn't yet left home mean she is not yet ready to have sex?

It is August. Everyone is at the beach but me and, luckily, Richard Robertiello. Once more I trudge past the baseball players in Central Park to see him. Dr Robertiello hears me out. 'Nancy,' he says, 'you are asking the wrong questions. They show you are still trying to protect some false structure. You are trying to place the issue of a woman's sexuality within the framework of her relationship to her mother. Sex, more than anything else, should have nothing to do with mother. Why should losing her virginity have anything to do with what goes on between her and her mother? You talk as if the mother *knows* the girl is having sex, that she is inside the girl's head, the way she was when the girl was a baby and thought mother could read her mind. *That is symbiotic thinking.* So what if someone has sex while she is still living at home? Privacy and secrecy do in fact aid separation. Your questions, the inability to finish this chapter, are all about how to continue the tie to mother while being a sexual person. No wonder you can't answer them. There are no answers – you can't be sexual and symbiotic with mother at the same time.'

That is preposterous. My sexuality has always been my badge of separation, my identity. Richard Robertiello has failed me. I storm out of his office.

In a dream last night I am back in London where I once lived. I am at the printers, watching illustrations being laid out for a book I have written on economics, a subject I know nothing about. Soon I will be exposed as a fraud! Suddenly an even more terrible anxiety hits me: I haven't telephoned my mother. There is no way in the dream I can get to a phone. I wake up in terror.

In reality, months may go by without my talking to my mother. It is no accident that wrestling with ideas of loss of virginity immediately bring me to a dream of losing my mother. This chapter has revealed a split in me. Intellectually, I think of myself as a sexual person, just as I had intellectually been able to put my ideas for this chapter down on paper.

Subjectively, I don't want to face what I have written: that the declaration of full sexual independence is the declaration of separation from my mother. As long as I don't finish this chapter, as long as I don't let myself understand the implications of what I've written, I can maintain the illusion, at least, that I can be sexual and have my mother's love and approval too.

The shame of still needing, still wanting to be tied to mama even after we're grown, is universal. 'I feel it myself,' Dr Robertiello once told me. 'I'm always pointing to my sexuality as proof of my autonomy.' Separation is a process nobody completely attains. We can only keep trying. Gone are my illusions that I am an individual person who has this terrific sexual identity. How humiliating! At least Richard Robertiello isn't separate either.

CHAPTER TEN

The Single Years

Even as a child I had a great respect for money. Other little girls didn't share my passion. When I was ten I held rummage sales. My mother smiled nervously. When I was thirteen I blushed when they teased me about the glass bank on my desk, but as much as I hated being different, I wanted money more. I saved my allowance, along with coins I filched from coat pockets in the hall closet or won from my sister in Monopoly. Susie couldn't save money any more than she could win a game.

The glass bank was shaped like the world, and as I saw the lower half of Africa disappear behind my stash, I had a good feeling. But there was no one I could share it with. The only person who seemed to enjoy money as much as I was my grandfather. He had a great deal of it, and what I admired most was his ease with money. Unlike my mother, he treated money without apology. This is how you move around the world, his manner said with great logic, as he paid restaurant bills and bought himself and other people beautiful things. Handling money made my mother anxious, and she raised me never to discuss the price of anything. Her attitude baffled me since clearly you couldn't even buy groceries without money. Why was money so secret and distasteful?

I grew to associate the dirtiness of money with the vile part of me. Except for my allowance, I never asked my mother for money; something more than cash, I realized, was being exchanged. If I wanted something badly enough, I often stole it. Meanwhile, my mother sighed at how my sister 'let money slip through her fingers,' her words more a girlish lament for the two of them than a criticism: this is how women are. I understood it was nicer to be like them than like me. It was a dreadful dilemma: how could I have what money gave my grandfather if I grew up like my mother, dependent on him? But if I grew up like him – unfeminine – who would want to take care of me?

As I grew into my teens, I hid my secret interest in money as I hid my growth by bending my knees when I danced. Surely someone would take care of me if I were littler and poorer. The bent knees made for painful spinal problems in my thirties. But the need to put my head on somebody's shoulder, when dance partners were running two to three inches shorter than I, outweighed everything. When it became the fad to pry the heels off our loafers, I was thrilled: another inch lost. 'You are ruining your skin,' my mother said as I baked in the Carolina sun. Tan was less prominent than white. 'Wait until you're thirty,' she warned. She might as well have told me to wait until I was dead. My only problem was getting through being fifteen.

When I was nineteen and told my mother I wanted to go to Europe, the idea was so far-fetched she agreed to match whatever money I could save, just to close the discussion. She could no more imagine me saving that kind of money than she could picture a daughter of hers so far away from home. She had never left the East Coast, and when in her early thirties she had to travel alone by train from Charleston to Buffalo, her father had given her an elaborate typed itinerary of people she should telephone at checkpoints along the way. To be fair to her, she didn't hedge when I produced my half of the money for my trip. And though I had outrageously underestimated the cost, I never cabled home for more. Nor did she offer. The bargain had been struck between us: it is one thing for a little girl to save money in a glass bank of the world, but when she breaks the bank and leaves home for a world the mother never knew, she has changed the relationship for good. In the game of who-takes-care-of-whom, the last chips had changed hands. 'Not enough to live on, too much to die on,' was how my husband described young women's allowances from home in one of his novels.

I was right not to ask for more; you cannot take money without strings. I couldn't afford to be angry at her stinginess then; I still needed her. I am wrong to be angry at her now, not that right and wrong have anything to do with nursery angers. There are two sides to any mother-daughter story of separation; on my side, I wanted to leave home for a bigger world. On her side, I was leaving her. What neither of us could say was that I wanted more than she had, to become more than she was.

Her abdication made it easy for me to go, but even when you want the territory, it always comes too fast; you never understand that leaving her means being by yourself. As much as I wanted independence, as hard as I tried for security in the woman I made myself into, I have always missed her, missed being tied to her. I have always been afraid that my self-confidence made me less feminine, less like her, and so less liable to find the connection with men I wanted so desperately. I was the one who had left her, but my emotions said I had been abandoned. Unfairly, I blamed her for letting me go, for making me so dependent on men for what she could never give me and for which money was never a substitute.

I never trusted my looks. In the Persian fairy tales, the genie locked in the bottle swears for the first thousand years to reward his liberator. During the second thousand, he vows to take revenge on whoever lets him out. By the time my looks came I had already wished for them too long. Raised to believe in the power of beauty – but in other people – I had long compensated with personality. I smiled even in my sleep. Who could resist me, failed at beauty though I was? Then, in the middle of my first job, I acquired the fine curve of an ass. I saw a face in the mirror people turned to look at. But it was never more than that, a reflection that might disappear. What I believed in was the old, smiling, charming but funny face I had grown up with. My too-late looks were like sudden riches that buy you entrée to a world into which everyone but you was born; you never trust them. I learned to wear my skirts tapered and ass-tight, and to cross my legs with a finesse beyond my years. I loved the compliments and worked to get them, but it was as though they were meant for someone standing behind me.

I went at my first job with a fervor. When the praise came for the amount of advertising space I sold, I winced with embarrassment. I could not take it in either. Though there was some reality here. It is disturbing to be praised for the wrong skill and I knew selling newspaper advertising space wasn't my real work. I wanted to be a writer, to say things in a way that allowed Nancy Friday to be perceived. I wanted to do something that was really my own so that I might believe in the praise I was starved for. But when writing assignments came up, I made excuses, ran in the opposite direction, doubled and tripled the hated advertising that was a cinch to sell with my new ass and my old personality. I did only the most rudimentary reporting. Why? I would ask myself. It was a terrible puzzle because I had never failed at anything. I would take any dare. What was I afraid of?

I compromised. Instead of success I could believe in, I went after success other people believed in. I got my reward from other people's opinion of me rather than my opinion of myself. It was like getting food after it had been chewed, with all the flavor and nutriment removed. Superficially it worked. Men pursued me, better jobs were offered, I had an identity in the eyes of the world. My boss fell in love with me; for a moment I thought I could take it in that he had seen me, and what he had seen was what he loved. But the excitement of conquest soon turned – as always – to the fear of loss. I knew he loved not me, but the marvelous and meretricious portrait I had projected. One unguarded moment, and he would see the jealous, insecure child beneath, who needed to hang on to him for dear life; one glimpse and he would run away. All my signals told the world I was a successful, sexual, professional woman. I knew my shabby secret: I had never tried what mattered most.

* * *

I took my men and my jobs home to mother. I think I enjoyed them most there. In her home they acquired a final polish, and gave my history with her definition it had not had before. I never understood women who took their anxieties home; I only went there in triumph. I don't know what I liked more, my mother's admiration of my single life, or my own feeling of added life when I experienced my world in her house. In my twenties it seemed I had been given the magic opportunity to rewrite our lives together. No longer was home the place I had to leave, but the place I chose to come to. No longer was I wicked for wanting to leave her; now I came home bearing gifts, stories, successes, and people I could share with her. And at last there was something she could give me.

I was proud of my mother. You could put her in a barn and by the way she placed a chair it would become hers. Once I left her I could love her. Distance gave value to all the things around her I had grown up with: the golds and greens and white of her living room, the flowers, the silver cigarette boxes, the white wicker furniture on the lawn, all were dear to me as they had never been when it had all been mine, when it was all I had. Even her anxiety and shyness that had so upset me as a child were now lovable; they were rallying emotions for all of us. We would follow her into the big comfortable kitchen with our martinis before dinner, as though we didn't want her out of our sight, as though to protect her. She would lay elegant tables, prepare wonderful food with an effortlessness I hadn't remembered she had. I began to see talents in my mother I wanted for myself. 'I don't know why we always end up in the kitchen,' she would blush and smile at this new man I had brought home, and I would touch her and say, 'But, Mom, this is where we want to be,' loving her now that I hadn't become like her.

I warmed, I softened, I lost my nervous edge in her house. Men seemed to love me more there. I brought them to her, knowing she was on my side. One night in her pretty four-poster guest room and, as in a fairy tale, they were mine for life. What was it about her that drew them to me? I would go out of my way to give them time with her alone. After growing up feeling everyone but me had something with their mothers, now when all my friends were at odds with their families, my mother and I were in bloom. We had things to exchange: she enjoyed my life, and when my lovers saw me with her, it seemed I gained a missing dimension in their eyes: I was a single, sexual person who could take care of herself, but surely they must see that the daughter of a woman as feminine as this must also be a woman herself.

Fascinated by my life as she was, my mother didn't want the details. She never asked why I didn't marry one of the men or pursue any one of the careers instead of hopscotching around the world. And I never offered the information. Neither of us wanted her anxiety. I learned to put my arm around her, to tease her about her red hair and her naiveté with jokes. I began to call her Rusty, a childhood name no one else used. Occasionally I tried to be alone with her. But when the merriment and the men were absent, I would sense the old sadness in her – of what? – and the old guilt in me – but of what?

Very late one night after my stepfather had gone up to bed, she launched into the old refrain. 'I never have to worry about Nancy,' she said to the man beside me. 'She could always take care of herself.' So long as I was living at home, these words had aroused a kind of pride in me. Now that I was on my own, I realized how false they were. A well of anger rushed up in me so fierce I wanted to strike out at her. 'Is something wrong, darling?' my mother said. 'No, nothing at all,' I replied. My words were like ice.

In fairness today, I can see it was almost impossible for my mother to understand my anger. What was there she could do for me? I had my apartment waiting in the city, my job in my pocket, my man beside me. I was more self-sufficient, less in need of her than ever. No matter. Without another word, I went up to bed.

By morning, the incident had been forgotten. But I knew the anger at her was there now and I grew to fear another outburst the way an epileptic fears a seizure. I didn't want to hurt her, but even more, I did not want to know there was something in me totally unaffected by grown-up success, that I could control no more than an infant can control its crying.

I tried to make up for everything with men. To get the nourishment of a lifetime from them. There was such a vast supply of energy and love, I never wanted to marry. Why stop when around each corner there was yet another man who would enlarge my life? From different men I learned about literature, theater, art, and politics. It never occurred to me that I could get from my work what men did.

My jobs were important to me and I worked hard at them but there was a built-in catch to success. If I stayed with any job long enough, my super-responsible approach to work would lead to promotions and higher salaries — jeopardizing what I needed from men. They would see the aggressive, 'unfeminine' person who had always hidden inside me, showing herself to the outside world only as charming, industrious, but essentially nonambitious. I could be lovable only as long as I wasn't handed too much authority, and so turned down jobs that might lead to vice-presidencies; and worked even harder at my glamorous but short-term projects to show I was nevertheless serious. I was convinced that only men could feed me. When they didn't call I died a little; when we argued I couldn't keep my mind on my work and when I sniffed rejection in the air, total paralysis took over. But I never telephoned home with anything but good news. Even when I was down, I honestly believed only men could save me.

Ben is the one man in my life I am not proud of. I met him at a party and had he asked me to marry him right then and there, I would not have considered the proposal any less keenly than I did in the months that followed. He was a total throwback, as beautiful and dumb as the Unobtainable Prom Kings of my adolescence. He was everything my family wanted for me: he belonged to the right clubs, knew all the right people, and he smelled good. While every reasonable, valued, and intellectual instinct in me rejected him, some old forgotten me cried, 'Take me, make me!'

I sat at his feet and filled his pipe while he read Edgar Guest. I lowered my hemlines and groveled to please his friends grown dull and quarrelsome on too much money and no work. As I undid myself for him, I saw the rejection coming and lay beside him, unable to sleep; for the first time in my life, unable to leave him. I told myself I wouldn't marry him, but I already knew he wouldn't ask. Ultimately I made it come true by convincing myself I couldn't live without him. 'Suffocation,' he said.

I called my mother. Her voice greeted me, free of the usual anxiety she felt for my sister. I did not tell her Ben and I were finished, I wanted to reverse the bargain, undo the shift in responsibility made so long ago when I had become sharer in my mother's guilts, protector of her timidities. I wanted to be her child again. 'Why do you always treat me as if I could take care of myself?' I asked her. 'Why don't you ever worry about me?' My mother's voice faded.

She had no way of dealing with this anger from a daughter whose jobs and men shone with power and mastery over a world she had never known. 'Oh, Nancy,' she said, 'one day you'll settle down with someone nice, you'll be ready to build your nest.' It wasn't what I wanted to hear. The desperate me that needed someone to take care of her – who needed a mother – had finally emerged and declared her fear. My mother was calmly passing the job on to a man who was running away from me. I knew in that terrible moment of regression, with all my glittering defenses down, that she had never wanted the job of being my mother in the first place. It had been a false bargain all along: I had never left her. Like Ben, she had left me. I had always said, 'I quit' to avoid the humiliating knowledge that I had been fired.

She had always silently warned me that while men were alluring, the answer to all of life's problems, they were somehow dangerous too. She had turned out to be right. I could not go on alone. I wanted someone. I needed a mother. I needed to let her know she had never been a good one.

These things were unspeakable. I wanted to hurt her, to arouse her at last to worry about me, to provoke that profound anxiety in her which was the counterpart to what I was feeling myself. Hadn't she been left by my father? Reunited with her at last in a symbiosis of terror and grief over lost men, I would not be alone. All the fear I had spared her during all my life had not been spared at all. I had merely saved it up and presented it to her in one big bill. I wanted to gain my revenge because she had left me so weak. Oh, I did. I surely did.

Our single years! The first time on our own, our second chance to form ourselves. Total self-reliance, sure sense of value may never be won, but they are goals to try for. Our single years begin one of our great rites of passage. Life becomes more fluid and malleable, old forms and structures are shattered, new ones emerge. This is our chance to outgrow mother's training in passivity, her fear that without someone to lean on, we are nothing.

'I think it's important for a woman to have time on her own after high school or college, and before she marries,' says an eighteen-year-old. 'You can find out that you can support yourself. That you don't have to have a man to survive. So many girls get married right away. It's frightening never to find out you are able to take care of yourself. You think you must always depend on somebody else.'

Imminent independence and separation give this young woman a sense of adventure and power. Life with all its options is about to unfold. At eighteen, we feel we can do anything. 'I'd love to have my own apartment,' she continues. 'My brother left home at seventeen, but my mother doesn't think I can handle it.' With every step forward we have to fight mother's legacy of fear.

Here's the other end of the spectrum:

'I love my marriage,' says a thirty-two-year-old woman, 'and yet it has made me more frightened than when I was single. Without my husband and children, who am I?' Neither her husband's arms around her nor her child's head on her shoulder can ease the anxiety: what would she do when/if they leave her? She has attained the goal her training promised would end all insecurity, but it hasn't. When this woman's daughter grows up, how can she be expected to encourage the girl to leave?

In poignant form, these two women recapitulate different stages of our early drama of separation from mother. At first we are hungry for a life of our own, for freedom, no strings, to go our own way. Behind our youthful vigor and eagerness to explore, a lifelong anxiety waits for us. Children and a husband are a fulfillment, but they are also hostages to fortune. We regress; we grow as dependent on them as once we were on mother. Pop radio is filled with songs about girls aching with loneliness, but statistics show that never-married young women with college educations, earning decent salaries, are the least depressed segment of population. On the other hand, TV commercials show us smiling young mothers, supposedly secure in their marriage, home and family – but the same statistics say that married women with small children in the household are among the most depressed people of all.[1]

The eighteen-year-old rushes into life. Who is to say she will not end up with the thirty-two-year-old's hopelessness?

The fear of freedom – which we dress up and call the need for security – is rooted in the unresolved half of us which is still a child, still looking for a man to replace the mother we never successfully left. So long as we have our need for symbiosis, we will not believe we can make it on our own. The child thinks that if she becomes too 'strong', too independent, mother will decide she can make it on her own and neglect her. We keep ourselves little. It means we must continue to live as a child: powerless.

Love puts the child in us back to sleep. When we doubt love, lose love, or become inappropriately afraid that in a world of 4 billion people we will never find love again – we must learn to look back to that little girl. The fear is hers – which is why it baffles us so. Rather than railing at fate or the perfidy of men – which is easy but not the real issue – it would be better to re-examine the relationship of that child to her mother of long ago. 'I'm sorry, I wasn't myself,' we explain when our rage gets out of hand, when in the throes of lost love we've spied on him jealously, when the fury is not proportionate even to the vile hurtful thing he has done. Of course we weren't ourselves: that was the rage of the frightened child who still sees the threat of desertion as imminent death.

'The pervasive problem for many women,' says sociologist Cynthia Fuchs Epstein, 'is their basic low opinion of themselves.' If so many of us are dependent, helpless, anxious creatures, how can we believe that men may love us? Of course they will wise up and get out sooner or later. The work of our single years is to turn this opinion around.

The first job is to prove to ourselves that we are agents in our own lives, not passive patients forever operated on by other people. Marriage may be beautiful, but all too often it is a call back into symbiosis: the desire to merge and lose our identities in someone 'stronger', more valuable than ourselves. Attaching ourselves to him for life itself, without him we fear we will die. What does it matter if he says, 'I love you'? Words are easy to say, compared to the importance they hold for the symbiotic child within.

'My wife is extraordinary,' a man tells me with genuine pride. 'She is a wonderful mother, cook, and when I look at all the trouble some of my friends are having with their wives, I get down on my knees and thank God I have such a terrific woman.' This man wouldn't think of leaving his wife. But she tells me privately that she lives in the fear that he will meet another woman. 'A brilliant man like him,' she says. 'What does he see in me?' Having no feeling of self – outside him – she does not exist in her own eyes.

Says Dr Schaefer: 'Women's desire to subordinate them-selves to the man is the pattern of dependency learned from mother. To escape the feeling that she may be ornamental but nevertheless fundamentally valueless, she becomes the "woman who is behind the successful man." She will not try on her own. But even as she succeeds, even as she makes the man more successful, more valuable, her own feelings of self-worth diminish. The bigger he gets, the more frightened she becomes that he will leave her, a nobody.'

Until our single years, we lived by other people's rules. It is salutary now to find the sky does not fall if we question them. The childhood need to be 100 percent safe 100 percent of the time is the biggest danger to life of all. If we do not have time on our own to test the ground, we will remain as afraid for ourselves as mother was. Along with the money we make goes the right to spend it as we like. If mother pays the rent, she has a voice in where we live. *New York Magazine* quoted a twenty-one-year-old girl who was asked to make a political commercial. She agreed because her family would like it. 'As long as I live with them,' she said, 'I'm expected to be a Republican.'[2]

In our single years we have our first chance to act so that the existential evidence of our lives tells us that we are new — helpless children no more. If we can successfully make the break away from home and discover we can live without the immediate emotional backup of mother and family; if we choose friends who reinforce our individuality rather than because they are 'nice' or live nearby; if we meet men with whom we can explore pleasures mother never allowed; let the experiences of life happen and find in even the painful ones that there is an excitement in knowing an existence larger than we dreamed possible; and get a job which not only delivers the thrill of economic self-sufficiency but builds up our self-esteem because we do it well — we have set up a bank account in our own name on which to draw for the rest of our lives. *I enjoyed living by myself once. If I have to, I can do it again. My world does not stop if other people leave. Their going will sadden me. It will not finish me.*

Our anxieties seduce us by coming up disguised as politeness, common sense, 'safety first' — even as strengths. I used to think I made myself up. I hear the same phrase so often from young women I interview today. Our lives are so different from our mothers'. And yet I know that no matter how much I accomplish in my work and marriage, a frightened part of me remains untouched by success. I wasn't born with this fear, these constant needs for reassurance of love. 'I'm a very independent woman, very ambitious,' a twenty-seven-year-old woman tells me. 'I don't have a man in my life now because I can't find a man who treats me as an equal – but also makes me feel like a woman, taken care of.' In her mind, there is no conflict between being 'equal' and being 'taken care of'. 'The reason I turned down the promotion I was offered,' says another young woman, 'is that I want to enjoy my freedom, the variety of life. I love my work and I work hard at it, but I don't want it to be all I care about. I don't want to be like a man.'

It is a sentiment I shared when I was single. But I know now freedom was the last thing I wanted, the true freedom that comes from being my own, self-sustaining woman. The freedom I was preserving by not working 'like a man' was a stance to show anyone I cared about that while I was successful, I was not too successful. I needed him. How could I take on the responsibility for a really big job when at any moment I might have to rush out to the airport to persuade my lover not to fly to Paris without me? How could any job be worth the danger that I might not be able to go with him? To the symbiotic self, separation is not freedom but mortal danger.

Leah Schaefer was recently asked to write an article for a national magazine. She tried, but couldn't, and finally resigned the assignment. 'I told them I didn't have the time, but I realized it had something to do with the amount of recognition the article would bring. I can handle success on a one-to-one basis, in the privacy, almost secrecy, of a therapeutic situation. The amount of recognition I'd get in a magazine that millions of people would read froze me. I'm still working on my separation from my mother.' Dr Schaefer's mother died five years ago.

In our single years, we have a powerful ally in the fight to separate and grow up. It is our sexuality. It makes us take chances, pulls us here and there, brings us into a world larger than the family, fills our life with excitement, dangers, pleasures, and disappointments that make us grow even as we learn to handle them. That is why mother's house now seems too small for the two of us. So long as we live with her, we must do so by her rules. It is almost impossible for her to give us more space within the same rooms, under the same roof, where she protected and ordered us about for eighteen or twenty years. 'I think there are some women who are comfortable in their own sexuality,' says Sonya Friedman, 'but I know they are not comfortable in their daughter's. The daughter at eighteen is at the peak of what the American culture calls her sexuality, while her mother is considered nearly over the hill. *Vogue* magazine may assure their forty-year-old readers that life begins at forty, but these women grew up on ludicrous songs like, "You're Sixteen, You're Lovely, and You're Mine".'

The moment it was born in us, mother singled out sex as her greatest enemy. More than anything else, she knew sex would separate us from her. She could not even call it by its right name. Instead she would say, 'You're so irresponsible,' 'Don't talk back to me.' 'Why must you close your bedroom door, wear those tight sweaters, those high heels,' etc. Now when we want to leave, to have a place of our own, we too cannot say it has anything to do with sex. We are her daughter and lust is not ladylike.

'My mother couldn't come out and say it, but I knew when I left home she was thinking. "You want to move out so you can sleep around!" What she said was, "Why do you want to move out? You have a nice home here."' The speaker is a twenty-six-year-old woman who is writing her master's thesis on the difficulties women find in leaving home. 'Even though I'd moved out when I got married, when I got divorced and went back to school to get my postgraduate degree, I moved back in with my parents. I lived at home for two years, until I could support myself. When I began to look for an apartment of my own it was treated like a tragedy, on the level of a virgin going out into the bad, dangerous, sexual world. The fact that I'd been married made no difference to my mother. But I knew I had to go.'

When her daughter leaves, mother is often caught between what she knows and what she feels. The graduate student continues: 'Of the forty women I interviewed for my thesis, every single one had trouble leaving unless it was to get married. The women's movement hasn't really reached all that many people, even in a supposedly liberal place like New York. The great majority of mothers who responded to my questionnaire equated the daughter's moving out with rejection. A typical mother said, "I can understand a person needing to live alone." *A person*. Not her daughter. These mothers don't want to act the way they do but they are driven to it.'

This study included only forty women of various educational and economic classes, but my own research shows that even highly educated, liberal, career-oriented mothers feel anxiety about the daughter leaving. Says a forty-five-year-old woman who manages a staff of fifteen people at her office: 'I raised three daughters and worked the whole time they were growing up. But when the youngest was eighteen and leaving, I went through hell. I just didn't want to let go, even though, intellectually, I knew I had to. I had a husband and a job I loved, but that didn't help. I felt rejected.'

According to the US Census Bureau, 40 percent of women aged twenty to twenty-four were single in 1975, almost double the number for 1960. These figures seem to suggest a revolution. In terms of real estate, they may be: an apartment of our own gives the illusion of separation. Emotionally, how independent are we? We may feel a kind of emotional blackmail from mother when we leave home, or she may help us furnish the new one-room apartment and cheerily wave bon voyage as we pull away to a new life. Either way, we pack her anxiety along with our suitcases. Says Mio Fredland: 'Daughters know their mother's true feelings like they know the inside of their pockets.'

With mother's fears roiling uneasily beneath our surface, it is not surprising that the revolution so far is mostly skin deep. Once she's left home, the daughter is delighted to have a job and money of her own, but when she's offered a promotion, she hesitates. She doesn't want to become so career-minded men will feel they have little to offer her. She experiments with sex, but still wants to be swept away: she is contraceptively unprepared almost a third of the time. When she is with her friends, she is the brave new person she always wanted to be. When she goes home, she reverts to the dutiful daughter she wanted to leave behind. (She even speaks differently.) When she meets new people, she tells them what she thinks they want to hear, not what she feels. At a party, she does not think, Who is there here who interests me? Instead, she wonders, What do these people think of me? The morning after a satisfying date or a good sexual experience, the pleasures of the night before have turned to anxiety: will he call again?

Do any of these describe you?

We talk a brave game of independence and make a point of lighting our own cigarettes. Underneath, we still doubt the authenticity of what we project. Mother may have talked a good game too. Underneath she is afraid her daughter cannot make it on her own. (She never was good at it herself, when she was single.) We live not with mother's official declarations of confidence but with her inarticulated fears.

'More girls may be living on their own today,' says Sonya Friedman, 'but the umbilical cord is still there. It is the telephone.' To relieve our 'guilt' we phone mother. The cure is never complete because what we feel is not guilt. After all, we have not committed some dread crime. What the symbolically tied daughter calls *guilt* is really *fear* – fear that with every step toward independence, every step away from mother, we have lost her.

'What arouses the most guilt in you?' I asked a woman.

'My mother.'

'What is the worst thing you can imagine?'

'A phone call in the night telling me she died.'

I had a chance to interview this young woman's mother.

From *her* side, the story runs this way: 'I know my daughter feels guilty about not coming home for Christmas. I felt the same when I was her age. So this year, I went and spent Christmas with her. I love to see her, but I felt underfoot at her place. I'd really rather stay home with my friends. I love my daughter and I'd have felt guilty if I left early, so I stayed till the end of the holidays.' So much *guilt*, so much *love*. The semantic confusion is only surpassed by the emotional confusion in which mother and daughter place one another.

We disguise our attachment to mother with the miles put between us, and with the evidence of our new job, a sexual life. For instance, before she returned to college to get her PhD, and become a therapist, Leah Schaefer pursued a successful career as a jazz singer. She moved around the country, supported herself, and had sexual relationships with men – a life that seemed as different from her mother's as possible. Who could say she was not independent?

When she was twenty-four, she decided to have plastic surgery. 'I was living in Hollywood,' she says. 'If I hadn't been in show business, I don't think I could have had the narcissism and courage to do it. On my father's side, they have these perfect noses, like I have now. But I had a long Roman nose, like my mother. The kind with a hook in it. During the nose operation I had a local anaesthetic. I was able to hear what was going on. There was this terrific crack. The doctor said, "The hook is gone." I had this sudden wild feeling of having lost something.

'I thought I hadn't told my mother about the operation so as not to worry her. The real reason was because I was changing a feature on my face that was like hers. In fact, when I got rid of this hook in my nose, it was a real emotional separation – *the first time I'd unhooked myself from her*. Gradually I began to believe in my attractiveness. Since adolescence I'd been crazy about boys, but this nose was the bane of my existence. When I sang in a trio, I was sure people weren't saying, "Don't they sing great" but, "Isn't that an ugly girl with a terrible nose?" Suddenly I had boy friends, dozens of them. I thought it was because my nose was better. Later I realized that until I'd had that operation, I'd never thought of myself as different, separate from my mother. My mother was a person who denied her sexuality, denied it was an important thing. So I had denied it too. I used to think it was the physical act of changing my appearance that separated me from my mother. My real separation was the emotional one of beginning to think of myself as sexual. It wasn't how I looked but how I felt about myself that attracted the men.'

Our sexuality is running in the right direction. Before we marry, for the first time in our lives a bond is being formed which can be more powerful than the one we had with mother. It is the bond with men. 'It used to be a bit of folk wisdom,' says Dr Robertiello, 'that men should try out all sorts of sexual experiences before they married. The same now applies to women. Sexual experience doesn't have to be unbridled. If you are Catholic or Southern Baptist, for instance, you will have stricter limits than others. If you don't let yourself do anything else, then at least go to church where you can sit opposite or near a man. Women should try to give themselves experience *vis-à-vis* a number of men so that the male sex becomes less frightening and remote – so that the woman can learn she is able to attract and interest a man. For some people this might mean holding hands ... for others, a series of orgies. The single years are the time to be as experimental as possible.'

The single years are the time to enlarge and reinforce whatever degree of separation has been so far achieved. Otherwise, we will make our new ties with men into a form of regressive symbiosis, and sexual excitement will give way to safety. What we have with him will no longer be electric and powerful, but at best warm and friendly; at worst, merely a bargain in mutual control and dependence.

Good experiences build our desire for more autonomy. Bad ones hurt but teach us we can survive. Life is not so frightening on our own. With the beginning of self-confidence, some of the poisons of feminine life can begin to diminish. We get over the fear that if someone we love goes away we will never find another. Our need to grapple lovers with hoops of steel is eased, lessening the chances that they will cry suffocation (symbiosis) and go. We learn the ways in which we are our own enemy.

Experimenting with a number of men, different relationships, helps put the finger on what is 'always' going wrong. Men hurt us. Men leave us. At least half the fault must be ours: *we chose them.* 'Even if you have a psychological compulsion to make it only with bad guys who do you in,' says Dr Robertiello, 'it is better to go through it ten times than not to get involved with men at all for fear of being hurt. That way, you will at least get a feeling of the location of your problem, and look around for ways to solve it.' In the privacy of our single years we have time and opportunity to begin the work.

Privacy aids separation. For the first time in our lives, nobody knows what we are doing. Unless we tell them. 'My husband and I always told our daughter Katie that some things are private,' says Leah Schaefer. 'Not hidden or denied, but private. Now she understands when we close our door. Sometimes she locks her own door and says, "I want some privacy."'

Without practice in privacy when we are very young, we are ever after uncomfortable with it. If our closed bedroom door was meaningless, if mother was always 'straightening' our bureau drawers, asking questions about our friends and telephone calls, we grow up with the uneasy feeling that privacy is a guilty idea. We suspect no secret of ours is safe, that someone always knows what we are thinking. We feel 'guilty' when we do something mother wouldn't like; we can't be sure there is no way for her to find out. As if in reaction, some women rush to tell their mothers everything. We may say that sharing our lives with mother, keeping closely in touch with her, is gratitude, paying her back for all she did when we were little. And yet, under the guise of being dutiful and loving, aren't we forestalling the fear that mother might find out? Aren't we asking her to be a collaborator and condoner of our sexuality?

'Has my mother asked if I'm still a virgin?' says a twenty-two-year-old. 'I told her I was, but I lied. I'm not. When she asked if I would tell her when I did have sex, I said No, it was my own business.' This young woman only lives a few blocks away from her mother; she is shy, self-effacing, and has not been much involved with men. But her degree of separation, her efforts to establish it, are superior to another woman who travels constantly around the world and has sex frequently with many different men: 'My mother and I are really great friends, though we're very different women. We talk constantly on the phone. I even called her from France the first time I had sex. Recently, I had bad luck and got pregnant, I called her and said I had to have an abortion. She was sweet about it, but she didn't give me the feeling of support I really wanted. It was a downer. I wanted her to call me three times a day, or even get on a plane and come take care of me.'

This woman wants it both ways, to tell her mother about her sex life, to be a buddy, and to have her mother take care of her too — as her mother did when she was a child. 'Sex should be something you do on your own,' says Dr Schaefer, 'and for which you take responsibility. Telling our mother about your sexual life respects neither her privacy nor your own. It opens you up to her influence, one way or the other. You are giving her too much power to comment, to give or withhold approval, in an area in which she doesn't belong.'

It is a difficult issue for both parents and children. Says Dr Robertiello: 'I'm not against my daughter having sex. That is her separate decision to make. But if she brings the boy home to spend the night with her, that's different. She's invading *my* privacy, bringing me into a situation I don't want to be part of. Liberal parents who don't like kids to bring their lovers home are often called hypocrites. I don't believe they are. If it bothers parents, they have the right to say, "Don't do it in front of me. It's not my business." Children have a right to their sexuality, but parents have a right not to be made party to it.'

Some mothers want their daughters' sexual lives to be private, because it gives them a freedom too. 'Sometimes my daughter tells me more than I want to hear,' says the mother of a twenty-four-year-old. 'All the excruciating details of her romances. When she was nineteen, she asked me to go with her to get a diaphragm. I said no. It seemed *too* intimate. She knew I didn't disapprove, but I thought some of her life as a woman has to be her life. If you aren't prepared to go without your mommy to get a diaphragm, then you're too young to be getting one.'

A twenty-five-year-old woman tells me that she doesn't mind her boyfriend sleeping over at her apartment, but she is nervous if her mother calls while he is there. 'I have this uncanny feeling she can see over the telephone, and knows he is naked in my bed while I'm talking to her. I don't want her to know. I guess I have a real double standard.' This young woman has turned a healthy situation around and criticized herself for keeping her sexual life private from her mother. She should keep it private. And yet, if she is still so symbiotically tied that, like a child, she feels her mother can read her mind over the telephone, it is not surprising that the experience is filled with anxiety. Dr Schaefer's comment is that she is doing the right thing. 'In time, simple repetition of the experience will rid her of this anxiety.'

Like everything in life, the more we do something, the more expert we become, the less inhibition is felt. You can't get there without practice. The idea is so simple, and yet, without having been given any practice in being independent, young women of eighteen and twenty are plunked down in new lives. Problems of separation, never having been worked out at the appropriate age, suddenly come at us now in a chilling manner. We are unprepared, having been rewarded all our lives for *not* being self-reliant. The first time we go to a party without a man, we do it in fear and trembling. After the fifth time, it is easier. Practice is everything. Little boys got it. We did not.

Meeting and knowing a variety of men in our single years can help us see our capacity for life was greater than we ever dared think. One man, grabbed on to too soon, can ground us in the way we've always been. The symbiotic dependency of most marriages does not allow women to grow. The divorcée or widow finds herself alone again the world at age thirty or fifty, dealing with men as if she were a teen-ager. 'If he leaves me, I'll die!'

Most of us will marry. No one can promise it will last. Our love may be in other people. Our security is in ourselves. If we goof our way through our single years, not paying our bills, losing our keys, writing home for the rent money, our days filled with little more than waiting for Mr Right, basing our value not on achievement but on the men who didn't work out – we will have established an ominous memory of ourselves. Mother was right: we are too frail to survive on our own.

The irony is, our drifting, irresponsible behavior was half expected. Given our training, you might even say we have succeeded. 'That's how women are,' people sigh, half exasperated, half charmed – and they proceed to write a check to bail us out, offer shoulders for us to cry on when we are fired for being chronically late, when we can't recover from yet another broken heart. That is *not* how women are. It is how we become.

Things seem to be changing. The single woman looks down at us from every billboard – the symbol of our time. Pop heroines on TV, in films, and magazines make unmarried life seem so glamorous and easy. If you can't make it, baby – these successful, on-the-job creatures seem to be saying – there's something wrong with you. Everybody else is. Pseudo-role models like the *Cosmo* girl promise us the single life in all its glory, just for the price of a magazine. Reach out, and success, love, independence, and freedom too – they can all be yours.

And yet there is a built-in lie to the single girl as heroine. It is the hidden agenda – habits of dependence we have been trained to think of as our central feminine core. A way of rating ourselves lives on, deep within our value system. It is based on our first role model and is backed up by the entire culture. It says the single woman is 'unfinished'.

When Helene Deutsch entered the university, her mother 'thought it was a blemish on our whole family that I was going to study medicine. She wanted me to marry, to be like other girls. Was she proud of my success? Proud is not the word, though I supported my parents with the profession she did not want me to enter. When I eventually married, we had two witnesses. After the marriage, the first thing they did was to contact my mother. It was only then that my mother felt I had given her something solid.'

Helene Deutsch is ninety-three. But when I interview a woman sixty years younger, I hear the same refrain: 'My mother was pleased at my success in my job. After all, she'd wanted me to go to college. But among her friends, she is the only mother whose daughter hasn't married. Finally when I got promoted and a story about me appeared in the hometown paper, she had something to show them. I was pleased that she was proud of me, but it hurt a little too that her neighbors' opinions are so important. I know the best thing I can ever give my mother will be my marriage . . . if I ever do.'

Says Dr Deutsch: 'Mothers today may want their daughters to become doctors and lawyers, but first they want them to marry. Why not? It is better for a woman to be married. Perhaps if the daughter is a big success in her career, then the mother won't be disappointed that she didn't marry. A mother would rather see her daughter married and a mother than anything else, but if she is famous enough in her work, that can satisfy the mother's narcissism, the normal narcissism.'

Work rewards for young women even today come so slowly. 'The only people who seem to really want them,' says Jessie Bernard, 'are men. It's difficult for young women to find a spot in the world equal to their talents.' In most jobs you begin at the bottom. Getting married, you begin as a success. It seems such an easy solution.

Many men today have begun to say they believe women have a destiny outside the nursery and kitchen. They may even smile at their father's chauvinism in saying he prefers women who are 'feminine' and 'non-aggressive'. *But when they become serious about a girl of their own, these are the qualities they look for.* Sociologist Mirra Komarovsky points out in her book *Dilemmas of Masculinity* that the same liberal male who says he believes in the women's movement often wants to marry a woman who will stay home and keep house for him. He can't see why she can't pursue a career and run a perfect home too. As one student in Komarovsky's study put it, it is all right if the mother of a pre-school child take a full-time job, 'provided, of course, that the home was run smoothly, the children did not suffer and the wife's job did not interfere with her husband's career.'[8]

And yet I would like to add a word here in men's defense. One of the great cries of our time is that women are held back because 'men won't let us'. Sometimes this is true. Very often it is neither men nor society which holds us back. We do it ourselves. If the goal for women is self-reliance, we must understand why we succeed or fail in terms of ourselves − without the convenient catchall excuse of male malevolence.

'Even though I tell you I want to be a lawyer,' says a twenty-year-old, 'there is something in me that works against my independence. It comes out in my relationships with men. My boy friend says he believes in my career, but when he tells me, "I don't want you to do this or that," I hear myself automatically saying, "OK, I won't do it." It's like being hypnotized. It's frightening to know this can happen to you.' She has heard the voice of the symbiotic child within herself talking. A man did not put that child there.

Says Smith College economics professor Jeanne McFarland: 'We send young women ambivalent signals. We give them this terrific education so they can compete. On the other hand, we say − what you really need is to find a husband. So go slow on competition. Men don't like women who compete. Men like their women on the pedestal − goddesses of nurturing and socialization and all the other "good" things men don't have time to be. It's a mixed signal: compete, but don't do it too well.' Can we be surprised if despite all the current talk about women making it, down deep we are afraid? We have more to lose than to gain from autonomy.

Here's a twenty-nine-year-old, highly successful woman

journalist: 'Last weekend, I spent the whole time in bed with my new boy friend. I hadn't taken that time out with a man in almost a year. Imagine! We just locked the doors and made love and talked and it was wonderful. All the tension went away. I forgot about my work. Monday, I went back to the office and Tuesday night I saw him again. I had these feelings of hostility even in the taxi before I met him. I was difficult with him, hostile, from the first minute. "Shit," I thought to myself, "I've blown it, it's dead with him." But in a couple of hours we'd got it back. I don't think I can keep it up with him, though, because I work so hard and my work's so important to me. It's as though I can't afford these weekends. I want them but they frighten me. It took me a day to get back into my work, and then when I did see him, I was hostile again.'

Women like the journalist in the story above, to whom work is important, are often afraid of getting involved with a man for fear they will lose their juice and incentive to work. Having tasted the pleasures of autonomy, she pushes the man off because of fear she will be sucked back into a dependent relationship. The real addiction of course is her unresolved symbiotic needs. She is afraid, once the door is open to her old, denied, baby feelings, that they will come rushing back to grab her. The intensity of the desire to be dependent is vividly seen in the hostility she shows the man who inadvertently tempts her back into it.

The reverse of the coin is seen in the story of a thirty-four-year-old woman whose fears were aroused, not by the man getting too close, but because success threatened to cut her off from him. A fashion merchandiser, her work keeps her traveling from New York to California. Off and on for the past eight years, she has been living with an actor whose work keeps him traveling too. 'That was fine with both of us,' she tells me. 'We discussed marriage but everything was going so well, we both said, Not yet. I'd miss him, but when we got together, it was very intense, wonderful. Last year I was promoted to vice-president, the first woman in my company. I'd arrived. Suddenly, I was on the telephone to him all the time, crying,

"Why aren't you here? I need you," I'd wail. "I want your arms around me!" I was weeping all the time, accusing him of desertion, feeling lonely when I should have been on top of the world.' As a result of these new demands she began to make, the affair ended. A relationship that might not have been every woman's choice but was exactly what these two people wanted foundered in the face of the anxiety her success in work brought with it.

For most of us, the end of the single years comes none too soon. They are like a hectic trip to Paris. Exciting, but, 'Gee, it's good to be home!' And home, of course, is marriage. It is the pattern we know best. Even if we had a broken or unhappy home, we still have at least the fantasy of family life. 'What are your goals in life?' asks the American Council of Life Insurance in its annual national survey: 'A happy family life? Making a lot of money? A fulfilling career? The chance to develop as an individual?' In 1975, a full 80 percent of the respondents, male and female, eighteen years old and over, chose a happy family life. *This does not mean they had one.*

We have an unforgettable model of how to be a wife, patterned not just on how mother was with father but, more significantly, on how we were with her. We are the couple – mother and me – that we will try to re-establish with others. The more we needed her, the more she rewarded us. When we are grown, dependency is still the norm ever held before us. It is like holding a martini in front of the alcoholic. 'What happens,' says Dr Robertiello, 'is that the cultural idea of women's dependency reinforces the women's own childhood training. This is the single greatest trap held out to women. It might be called *the* feminine option.'

Like many traps, it is baited with honey.

This option says that any time a woman wants, she can give up on herself and find a man to take care of her – so why struggle to establish herself in the first place? This supposed privilege is so deeply planted in our psyche that we are often not aware that we use it as our ace in the hole. 'Men are so competitive. I don't see the point in working so hard.' Of course society applauds the woman who feels this way, who just marks time until she takes the option. She is one less competitor to worry about, someone who will take on all the unpaid work of housekeeping, etc., that men don't like to do. Dropping out on ourselves, giving responsibility for our life to a man, is not the mark of a woman but of a child.

Nearly three out of five first brides (57.9 percent) are twenty years or under.[4] For many young women, the height of bliss is still to marry on graduation day. Only eighteen and she has achieved lifelong security! The divorce courts are filled with people who discovered too late the meretricious glamour of that promise.

Says sociologist Cynthia Fuchs Epstein: 'Most women don't think they have any alternative to being a wife and mother. They just don't think success is possible for them. It's not in their spectrum of expectations. Not until they get into the marketplace and get decent jobs do they see there is some possibility for success.'

Often, it takes the experience of a failed marriage for a woman to realize that the supposed lifelong security of having a husband can be a painful myth. 'Women like these,' continues Dr Epstein, 'often become very career-oriented. They don't necessarily stop seeing men, but their anger at a shattered illusion has opened their eyes. They learn they can't look to men to be their sole gratification.'

Work-oriented women, however, face problems that men do not. Says Dr Epstein: 'There are few supports for women to say to a man, "I can't see you tonight, I have to work late." Women aren't used to thinking of themselves as plunging totally into work. This is not to say we couldn't. It is just not a resource we have developed yet.'

Faced with pressures like these, many career-oriented women choose not to marry early. In a study done by Professor Elizabeth Tidball on women achievers selected at random from *Who's Who of American Women,* she found that among 1,500 prominent women, only about one-half were married.[5] They had postponed marriage an average of seven years after their bachelor degrees so that they could give full attention to their careers. In Margaret Hennig's study on twenty-five high-level women executives, *all* began by feeling that marriage and career were an either/or choice.[6] When they were about twenty-five, in Dr Hennig's words, they 'stored their femininity away for future consideration.' Around age thirty-five, they reassessed their lives, got in touch with their shelved femininity, and about half of them married.

We don't know how angry these women were at having to play down their sexual lives in order to get ahead. I would have been. All of us have seen the anger of women who did make this choice – women without men. Someone or something – men, society, the structure of work in our culture – has let them down. There are exceptions, women on their own, living happily and wholly without men. Part of the respect they engender is due to perception of how few women ever solve this problem: to live without men without anger.

For the vast majority who have not solved the problem, it might be said that the logical place for their anger to be directed would be at the anachronistic training which linked femininity with dependence – but that would mean turning anger back, onto mother. The anger goes forward instead, to the prince who has not presented himself, in a kind of generalized bitterness toward all men.

Says Dr Cynthia Fuchs Epstein: 'Women are very torn in work situations. They have to make a whole set of decisions based on different priority systems – including love, friendship, marriage and children – not all of which co-ordinate.' If a woman becomes involved with her career, she's afraid love will suffer. If she gives too much time to her love life, she is afraid it will be at the expense of her career.

I feel these pressures myself: walking past a mirror today, I saw my mother. On my face was the expression of hers I like least: anxiety. The harder I work, the less womanly I feel.

'Nancy, I hear your questions, but you haven't taken in my answer.' The speaker is a psychoanalyst. I have been asking her why women laugh off these feelings of value that come with success. Her reply runs from my mind like water. I have to phone her again in the evening to get her to repeat what she said. I plan a dinner party so that I may at least hear some praise for my feminine accomplishment at cooking, but I am working so hard at writing that I cancel it – feeling more depressed, less womanly than ever. My husband and I have a terrible row and I bury myself in the papers on my desk, depriving myself of his company. Why? The repression lifts for a moment: I am leaving him before he leaves me – a game I first played with mother when I was six.

Madness.

Do not think that because I have written this down that I can make it work for me. I have already forgotten it. Freud was disappointed at first that his patients' new self-knowledge did not immediately ameliorate their condition when he made them aware of their unconscious conflicts. It was as if he had lit a lamp in a cartoon for his patient. 'I see it!' the patient would cry. And then the lamp would go out, the patient would 'forget' once more, the conscious ground not won at all, dark repression closing in.

Psychoanalysts have long become accustomed to the necessity of *working through* these bits of insight, making patients aware of the repressed connections again and again before they are truly grasped – the liberating, emotional truth integrated for good. Practice, once again. We women resist knowledge of ourselves and our mothers. We prefer our fantasy relationship and so we cannot put to work what we know about the two of us.

A psychiatrist with whom I have conferred shows the chapter on competition in this book to his wife. They have a fourteen-year-old daughter. The girl's mother reads it, commenting all the while, 'Yes, yes, that's interesting, but it doesn't apply to me.' An hour later, she bursts into tears. 'In a week or two,' he tells me, 'she may want to talk about it. Didn't you also deny that certain material we've discussed was relevant to your life until months, maybe a year later?'

Repression is an unconscious process. It has nothing to do

with intellect or how smart we are. We may remember every fact ever learned and have an IQ of 160, and still resist 'knowing' the facts of our relationship to mother – and how they are played out with different people in our lives.

The fear of losing mother doesn't even require having had an emotionally nourishing relationship with her in the first place. Some women openly dislike their mothers, others cannot recall a gesture of warmth, a moment of closeness. It is not necessary to have loved your mother, even for her to have been there for you, for the symbiotic need to exist. Sometimes, in fact, the hardest mother-daughter relationship to face is the one that is only a wish-fulfillment fantasy.

For women like this, the culturally idealized mother-daughter relationship is more important than reality. As children we miss the symbiosis we didn't have so acutely that we are perhaps even more desperate for it than women who were less deprived. It is too painful, too humiliating to admit. Casually, we say, 'I simply wasn't close to my mother,' or with relief, 'Thank God, my mother didn't smother me the way she did my sister.' Another defense is angry dismissal: 'When my daughter was born, I was determined she wouldn't grow up as I did.' Verbal formulas that are like cosmetics hiding our scars.

'My parents are very uptight about sex,' says a twenty-nine-year-old single woman. 'I don't want sex always to have to be part of some big, emotional intimacy, some ongoing relationship. I like to be able to have sex without strings. Recently I met a guy I liked a lot and went to bed with him the first night. It bothered me that he didn't call again. When I did get a note from him he didn't even refer to that night.' When I suggested that it had been a humiliating experience, she protested adamantly. 'No, no, it wasn't humiliating. It's just that I haven't wanted to see other guys since.' At the end of the interview when I am leaving, she stops me: 'Goddamnit, I did feel humiliated.' The curtain of repression had lifted for a minute. Will she ever be able to integrate her attitude – wanting sex with no strings – with her gut reaction of despair when a man takes her up on it?

'When a woman goes to bed with a man and he doesn't call,' says Dr Robertiello, 'she feels humiliated. It's like being used, duped, conned. It goes back to that early feeling of betrayal and loss of that first person who led you to believe that if you "gave" to her, she would always be there for you.' In her conscious mind, this woman has made a personal, rational decision about men. On the unconscious level she is still reacting to them as if they were her mother.

Men don't share our conflict. The more successful he is, the more a man feels he can get the best women, sex, and love. Where the sexes differ is that *we get involved with men symbiotically* – displacing our need for mother onto our husband or lover. No wonder we have more difficulties apportioning our time – so much for love, so much for work – than men do. In symbiotic love, the need is so great it swallows all time and nothing is left over for anything else.

'I always believed I could have love and work,' says Dr Schaefer, 'and therefore I did have them. I was brought up with this belief because both of my parents loved to work. It just seemed natural to love *and* to work. Men used to say, "If you married me, I would let you work." I used to say, "*Let* me work?" I didn't need their permission. It is their training that makes women think they must exclude men from their lives if they want interesting work. What we believe is what we make happen.'

Though the work we do and the reward we get may tell the world we are equal to the man, women live with a special day-to-day risk most men don't know. 'It's so unfair,' a woman tells me. 'On every level I am his equal, except I know he has the ability to walk out. He won't be happy, but still he can go to a bar and drink, see his friends. He'll probably work harder and get his mind off me. I'm mesmerized until he telephones. I resent it.'

It is like an intermittent disease: we are only as professional as the last assurance he still loves us. The power of the emotion we feel as the man walks out the door began with our fear, as a child, of being left. We never outgrew it. With no practice in being alone, we think we cannot survive it. Men respond to our fear. It makes them feel powerful. This reinforces an old, sad lesson: our weakness is our strength.

In terms of work that builds independence, there is no reason to think of jobs merely in snobbish or elitist terms. The woman who can run a switchboard gets a feeling of mastery and competence. If we can do small repair jobs around the apartment – unplug a drain or fix a blown fuse – it is one more area in which we have learned to dominate the nitty-gritty details of life, without depending on a man. The woman who is proud of her position as an irreplaceable secretary gets as much feeling of value from her job as does the woman vice-president. The world may put different monetary or status value on what they do, but as far as helping to confirm feelings of autonomy, both are equally desirable.

While the value of earning a paycheck that supports you cannot be overestimated, some women find that their most emotionally nourishing work lies outside an office. They may paint or write on weekends, go into politics or put in time with the Red Cross. This doesn't say, however, that the self-esteem of the dilettante or Sunday painter is automatically reinforced. The activity must be important enough to be worth the sacrifice of extra time, labor, and social activities. Otherwise, it isn't emotionally valuable enough for us to gain feelings of autonomy. Without real commitment, it is only a game. If it doesn't matter if you lose, you gain little if you win.

Today's cry is freedom; none cry it more loudly than the single woman who demands it even while she is out finding someone to surrender it to. 'Why can't I find a man to take care of me?' is a common complaint, even among Leah Schaefer's women patients who have jobs or careers. 'I tell them,' Dr Schaefer says, 'that the world is filled with men who feel more manly by taking care of women. But there is a payment you must make; you can't expect a man to take care of you, and also tell him what to do. The way you pay for being taken care of when you are little is to be the kind of person mother wants you to be. The same price must be paid to a man. Many women want it both ways. There is nothing wrong with wanting to be taken care of, I tell them, just as long as you know the price of what you are getting.'

Women accuse men of being afraid of closeness, being unable to love, etc. It may be that the man is responding to the unspoken half of the female message of love: 'Take care of me.' He may indeed love her. What frightens him off is not the closeness, the intimacy, but his fear of the burden. Even if the men we meet in our single years have been trained to feel that carrying the woman is the mark of a man, they may be too young, still too far down the financial ladder to be able to do it. Perhaps they are not yet ready to give up their freedom. 'The problem for the woman,' says Dr Schaefer, 'is that this idea, in which love means somebody to take care of her, is so deeply rooted, she herself doesn't realize she's laying it on the man. All she thinks is that he's cold, awful, unfeeling, he's rejected her. The idea of loving her, and taking care of her too – they are so intertwined, she can't tell one from the other. Wasn't that how her mother's love was?'

Martina Horner wrote her doctoral thesis on women's 'motivation to avoid success' in 1968.[7] By the early 1970s her ideas had become part of folk wisdom. What she said spoke universally and immediately to women in an area we had never been able to explain to ourselves. Never mind that other sociologists argued her findings were incomplete, that they were based on a study of only ninety women at one university. 'Of course!' we exclaimed, 'that explains my anxiety, my failures, my ambivalence about work. I am a woman just like any other. I have the feminine fear of success!' Our fears were not biological but socially conditioned. What was learned could be unlearned. Besides, it was all the fault of the paternalistic society anyway.

I sometimes wonder if Dr Horner's conclusions haven't done women more harm than good. Having the zippy phrase – fear of success – in advance of trying, it becomes a self-fulfilling prophecy. We recognize failure as an old friend, the very mark of our womanliness. We make the same mistake in reading certain feminist fiction. Eager for identification with other women, we recognize ourselves in the heroines – beaten down, harrassed, often humorous even if self-deprecatingly so. It is nice to know we aren't the only ones who feel uncontrollable rage when our husband comes home late, loss of identity if he doesn't come home at all. It doesn't follow, however, that identification with someone else's failures makes us better equipped to overcome our own.

Nevertheless, I feel Dr Horner was right. We do fear success; but the phrase is useless unless we see it in context. Fear of success used to be explained with emphasis on oedipal retribution: if you beat mommy out for daddy, she will seek her revenge. I think this is true of both sexes, but women do not fear mother's rivalry and anger as much as her loss. There is a shading of emphasis here that runs along sexual lines. Our problems of separation are not parallel to men's. A man doesn't have to leave another man to gain his independence. A boy can be a rival to his father and/or use him as a model – but in either case, continue to get love and support from mother. A daughter, however, often feels she must choose a field distant from mother's in order to reinforce separation. For many women, competition with men is much easier to face than competition with another woman.

'In developing strategies for winning, women have much quicker understanding than men,' says George Peabody, who is a doctor of Applied Behavioral Science. He invented The Powerplay Game, by which corporations try to teach employees on the way up methods for success in business. 'But again and again, we find women hesitate – to the point of stupidity – to put what they know into play. They aren't stupid, so you have to ask why. They think their superior strategic and political planning is somehow cheating. When they enter the office, they park this kind of skill at the door. In Powerplay, they tend to want to give back all their winnings when the game is over. Many are afraid to beat out the other girls. They don't want to destroy relationships.'

I know a travel agency staffed by women that has

'eliminated' competition by doing away with titles. 'When a senior position is open,' one of the partners says proudly, 'we don't make a big deal of it. Competitive feelings don't get stirred up. Someone gets the position and that's that.' The story makes my heart sink.

Who is fooling whom? When there is no open power relationship, it does not mean there is no power relationship at all. Everybody knows who decides that the office will open a branch in Florida, who decides Mary Anne will get that lush assignment to Paris while Sally will type up the reports. Some people want to run organizations, some do not. Unless the rules of competition are spelled out, nobody is comfortable. The dominant personalities rule the roost by their own rules, and usually for their own comfort, while paternalistically (!) telling the subordinates they are one big happy family with the good of all as the common goal. Nor do the people at the top win totally: because their place in the hierarchy is unacknowledged and thus nonlegitimate, they suffer from anxiety too.

To deny women their right to feel competitive reinforces old stereotypes of passivity. Power is being exercised, but everyone pretends it is not. Only we are nasty enough, competitive enough to feel angry. Better shut up, pretend not to be competitive at all. To do anything else is to risk being labeled unwomanly. Even as we pass laws to force corporations to put more women into management positions, there are few women who will step up and say with self-confidence, 'I am a competitive person.' Back in the boardroom, it is decided not to give a female executive that big job in Chicago. 'Women just aren't tough enough to hack it at the top. We'd better go with Harry.'

We think we will be rewarded for being good girls, for not making waves. The other guy gets the promotion.

In *African Genesis*, Robert Ardrey says that the most neurotic, unhappy animal in the world is the American woman: she is trying to do something 'nature' did not adapt her to do.⁸ I totally disagree – beginning with the fact that while we are animals, we are something more too. Nature did not adapt us for playing the piano or flying airplanes. We taught ourselves. If we take this idea of *training* and substitute it for Ardrey's quasi-religious notion of *nature*, I could agree with him.

'Why has there never been a woman who has been the bridge or chess champion of the world?' asks Dr Robertiello. 'The way this question is usually put by male chauvinists is, "Why haven't there been more great women artists, scientists, etc?" The answer is a function of the culture in which women are brought up. After all, in comparative IQs, women come out brighter than men.'

Working for yourself, getting ahead, usually means beating out another person, *breaking a bond*. Says Dr Peabody: 'Women have been trained to be somebody's "other", not to have an independent sense of identity. When you get to be Number One, you can't be somebody's other. If your lifelong habit is to think of your identity only in terms of being somebody's wife, somebody's secretary or assistant, it is scary not to be in that position. It means you have no identity. But as soon as you can tell women that it's not cheating, not naughty, to go after what they want, that they can do it and still be feminine – that assertiveness does not mean putting other people down – then women can give themselves permission to use their great skills and they move marvelously. It is almost a shock to them to find people don't fall apart when they say No.'

We have been trained not to initiate, but to respond – not to choose but to be chosen. 'My job,' Dr Peabody continues, 'is to help women over the fear of clear self-definition and self-responsibility; it's the only way to move into top management. Sometimes it takes six to eight months to get even the best women through that knothole. But they can learn!'

In most women's lives, the rewards for seeing ourselves as capable and valuable on our own come late, after our deepest beliefs have been formed. It is like trying to learn to be a ballet dancer in your twenties. Our psyche has already been conditioned to respond only to certain kinds of praise; it is difficult to adjust to a whole new range of stimuli, attractive as they may be.

'You're terrific!' says the boss. 'What a job you did!'

We blush. He really didn't mean it. It was a fluke; we'll never be able to pull it off again.

This is the split in which we live. We may hear praise when it is given. We just can't believe it. We see recognition of our accomplishments as a kind of flattery, mistaken or insincere. But if you cannot take in praise and recognition during the uphill battle to get a hold on who you are, how long are you going to stick with it? We have been trained to gain confidence not through efforts for ourselves but through meeting the needs of others. 'Women,' says Jessie Bernard, 'are the ones who keep families together. All the studies show that women are the mediators in kinship relations.' We are good at compromise. Men take the extreme positions that, right or wrong, define identity. They let people know 'where they stand.' 'A lady,' the old proverb used to run, 'gets her name in the newspapers only twice in her life. When she marries and when she dies.'

A successful woman tells me, 'I work so hard. I know I do my job well, but when people praise me, I think, "Oh, they're just being nice." Why can't I just smile, say, "thanks a lot," and maybe buy everyone a drink the way men do to nail the good feeling in? But no, I just slink away after the compliment, as if I've done something shameful.' She has – she has separated herself from the other women. Not only is she slightly ashamed of the competitive glow she felt for being praised, but she is frightened too. We are overwhelmed with the fear of growing too big. We are losing our right to the feminine option: becoming so self-sufficient no man will want to take care of us.

I do not believe that 'making it' is an absolute good, and that anyone who does not try is infantile. I might even say the opposite. But it is one thing to decide you don't want power, to make a conscious decision that the rat race isn't worth it, that you don't want to become unfeeling and domination-hungry 'like a man'. All this is reasonable, even admirable. But it is something else to pretend you aren't trying for success because you don't want to become masculinized, when the real reason is that you are surrendering to your baby fears that success and autonomy will separate you. Choice cannot be truly made unless it is conscious.

The notion of choice is beset with philosophical difficulties, but in our own lives it is usually possible to distinguish between genuinely deciding we don't want something, and merely crying 'Sour grapes.' A woman who has just come out of a devastating love affair says, 'To hell with men, now I'm going to concentrate on my career.' To the outward eye, she may then seem purposive and self-contained, but unless she finds someone to provide the closeness and intimacy we all need, she may simply be practicing denial when she says, 'I can take care of myself. I don't need a man.'

Another woman 'chooses' not to see men because 'they don't give me the support I want, either emotionally or financially.' Hearing a woman speak out is still such a rarity that we often take her loud declarations as strength of character. It is important to ask, Is her choice that of an adult or the demands of a disappointed child?

Says psychoanalyst and sex therapist Helen Kaplan: 'We are in a transitional period. Women want to be successful on our own, but we still look for superdaddy, who will be more successful still. In terms of numbers, there are more men available to the career-oriented woman. She is more likely to be sexually active than the home-oriented person. But the great number of work-oriented women are thrown by the notion that most men they meet are less successful than they are. For women like these, a man who is less powerful than they may not be attractive.'

Women marry up, men marry down. Says sociologist Cynthia Fuchs Epstein: 'For all the talk about the women's revolution, there are no figures to indicate this is changing.' And yet if women could get over our learned need to attach ourselves to someone more powerful than we – and accept the more democratic notion of a relationship between peers – new numbers of men would become available to us. 'I won't even go out to dinner with a man who makes less money than I do,' says a divorced woman who is an advertising copy chief. She eats dinner, night after night, alone.

It is not our success but leftover, childish symbiotic needs that push so many men out of our lives. In cool and sophisticated disguise, these needs surface in our grown-up years. Jackie Onassis went from President Kennedy to Aristotle Onassis. How many men can there be left for her if she continues on that trajectory? As it is, popular speculation is that she will never marry again.

Says Dr Kaplan: 'I think many men are happy to accept women of superior accomplishment. *We* aren't able to accept ourselves yet. We keep on thinking we have to look for men superior to us. Women have to learn that their self-esteem cannot depend on "superior" males. We shouldn't need daddy.'

A man who is tight with money destroys our illusion that we have found the powerful, overabundant father who will give us everything we feel we cannot earn for ourselves. 'When a woman marries,' says Sonya Friedman, 'and finds out her husband is cheap, or she buys a dress and he has a fit, it's tremendously jarring. Stinginess is the one thing women resent more than anything else. They can even tolerate impotence, sadism, and infidelity. Cheapness rules him out.'

Symbolically, nothing says you are big and strong as forcibly as money. The last thing I want to do here is set up money as the kind of value for which men have thought it worth killing themselves – but it is vital that women understand their choices regarding money, how often unconscious separation anxieties get played out in our attitudes toward the dreamy stuff.

From the time we are children, we begin to learn not how to earn money but how to manipulate for it. Half the fights between mother and father are about money. We sense her feeling that if he loved her more, there would be more money available for him to give her. Money is proof he wants to take care of her. (It is a truism of psychoanalysis that when a child steals money from her mother's purse, she is stealing love.) If mother had to earn money for herself, that would mean she was not so dependent on daddy, not nearly so loved by him. What we must do is turn the whole game around. Instead of making money ourselves, which means we are separate, unloved, and independent, we want to have our husband put us on an allowance, as mother did. This uses money not to threaten the symbiotic connection but to establish it more firmly.

The man thinks setting up a reward system of giving the woman something extra to buy a new dress is his idea; the woman is at least complicit in this maneuver from the start. When we are grown and have a 'big daddy' of our own, we still like to get that nice little extra something for being 'a good girl'. In this way, money becomes involved with closeness, rather than separation. 'Nevertheless,' says Professor Jeanne McFarland, 'while the wife is proud of how she can cajole money out of him, she knows the real money power is with him. When the man threatens to leave her, instead of quickly thinking of ways to support herself, she feels the old paralysis. By the time you're a wife, you don't really have economic options because you've bought the model that says you're dependent.'

When the American Council of Life Insurance asks in its annual national sample, 'What does masculinity mean to you?' – each year at least 80 percent of the population answers, 'A good provider.' (Sexuality is so far down the list it doesn't get a mention.) For the single working woman trying to find her elusive identity, this means one thing: in becoming too good a provider, she becomes unfeminine. She is depriving a man of his role in life, emasculating her own man – should she have one. At AT&T, women can get a college education on company pay while going up the corporate ladder. 'If the gulf between what she makes and her husband's salary is not too wide,' says Personnel Director Amy Hanan, 'she takes advantage of the offer. But when it is too wide, the marriage is often jeopardized. It is too much of a threat.'

Traditionally, when women had money of their own, a bank, a husband, or father took care of it. This socially sanctioned ignorance masks an immense concern with money, along with a feeling of powerlessness. Says Jeanne McFarland: 'Women profess a stupidity about money, they are willing to take on this foolish caricature in order to buy the socially accepted role of womanhood. I don't know any woman, however, who actually lives out this stereotype.'

Women, who made up 33 percent of the national labor force in 1960, now account for 40.7 percent, a proportion that was not expected to be reached until 1985.⁹ Economist Eli Ginzburg calls the flood of women into the work force 'the single most outstanding phenomenon of our century.'¹⁰ And yet most women like to give the impression that 'the man of the house' runs the money, while they not only contribute to it but make most of the consumer decisions.

All of which leads to dreadful arguments because of the double message women send out: Little me, I know nothing about money, take care of me. At the same time we broadcast: Money is very important, I can't make it, so you've got to make enough for both of us, and if I do make it, then goddamn it, I'm going to make a lot of the big decisions about it. (To say nothing of the third message: Despite all I've just said, I want to feel you're making the decisions anyway.)

'The issue of what money does for a woman and what it doesn't is a puzzle,' says Emily Jane Goodman, lawyer and co-author of *Money, Women and Power*. 'If she doesn't have a man to turn it over to, she is in a dilemma. A shorthand way of saying it is, What woman goes out and buys herself a Porsche? It boils down to a sexual thing. For men, financial success is a very sexual experience. For women, it is not. If we make money, we don't really know how to enjoy it in the same way as a man. We do not accumulate men, we do not accumulate wealth. We don't see them as interchangeable. Men are not sexually attracted to us by our wealth and power. If money is indeed an aphrodisiac when obtained by men, it is a turn-off when obtained by women.'

Even if we can come to terms with the role reversal inherent in the idea of earning more than our husband, we have to live with the disapproval in other people's voices: 'I don't like the way people looked askance that I made more money than Jack,' says a divorced woman executive. 'I tried not to let it bother me. In the end, it got to him. I know money, my money, was the reason we split.'

One way to solve our childish need to have a man more powerful than we is to 'choose' to make less money ourselves. Very rarely have I heard a woman say she wanted to make a million. I can't count the number who've told me, 'I want to marry a millionaire.' By deliberately deciding to leave the issue of making money to someone else, by marrying *up* so we feel we have someone powerful to lean on, we have not strengthened the grown woman within, but reinforced the baby.

As undeniably and simply as rain makes you wet, a paycheck is proof we can make it on our own. Once we have succeeded in a job, once we have the feel of money, it loses much of its awe. We know how much it costs to earn; how to spend it, save it, what it can do for us. It no longer is some mystery that only men can understand. Money in your pocket gives you firm ground on which to stand. Until we have an economic alternative to marriage, we have no alternative at all. We will try to make it perform a function it is not meant to do. Love does not easily survive a power relationship in which one partner can economically blackmail the other.

When we were little, if mother had a job or career, we may have resented her for not being there when we got home from school. In the same way, if she did not subvert her sexuality in the service of motherhood, we resented that she wasn't comfy, and homey, like all the other moms. When we are grown, we may realize she gave us something better: the image of sexuality, of independence, of a woman earning money, spending it, enjoying the freedom from anxiety that comes with knowing you can support yourself if anything happens. 'The girls who are being best taught that autonomy presupposes economic independence,' says Jeanne McFarland, 'are those who have career mothers.'

Sometimes, even as we pursue career and sexuality, we continue to be angry she wasn't the way we, as children, would have liked. Anger is a way of maintaining some form of tie. As long as we remain fixed on resentment of what she didn't do, we don't have to think of what we must do for ourselves. 'Children,' says Jessie Bernard, 'have always had the option to call on mother for help and support until they were fifty. Mother must have the right to say, "OK, I've done my share. I'm finished." '

'The money I would ordinarily have given my daughter, I spent on a trip to Paris,' a woman tells me. 'The day I got on the plane, I said to myself, "This is my declaration of independence!"'

CHAPTER ELEVEN

Marriage: The Return to Symbiosis

Bill and I decided to get married our first hour alone together. He had never touched me. I had known him two years and during that time I had not expected he should. I had always been with another man, he had been with someone too. One morning I phoned and said, 'It's my birthday.' 'I'll get my shoes shined and take you to lunch,' he said as casually as if we had been meeting for years. We went to the Drake and sat in the darkness at the far end of the bar. 'When you and I begin,' he said with our first martinis, 'it's not going to be like all the other times.'

Nothing in me argued. 'You get out of your thing with Tom,' he said, 'and I'll get out of mine. I'll be waiting.' We never had lunch. When we left the bar, we paused on the corner of Fifth Avenue and 55th Street and looked at one another. We had decided to spend the rest of our lives together and we had never kissed.

My call to him had said I was a very separate person. It was what drew him from the very start. 'I love it that I'm not your life,' he said. The only advice my mother ever gave me about men was 'Marry a man who loves you more than you love him.' She didn't hand it to me like a bulletin. I can't even remember the context in which it was said. I thought I'd dismissed it as yet one more of my mother's well-intentioned, but mostly irrelevant bits of advice. The eerie way that sentence has remained isolated in my mind says how profound an effect it had on me. I wasn't ready to marry; my life as a single woman was at its zenith. But I never doubted this was the man for me.

Because he loved me more than I loved him? Other men

371

had loved me for different reasons. When they asked me to marry, when they spoke of their love, I did not respond – I could not match the emotions they were talking about. Bill saw the part of me I wanted to become.

Bill wasn't ready to get married either. He had written several books on the pleasures of bachelorhood. I loved what he saw in me that had made him change his mind; as I grew to love him more, I became more the person he admired. And yet I have always felt I defrauded him. He had seen me on a good day. The woman who called him, the woman who left men easily and flew around the world on her own, was only independent until she was in love. I was only secure as long as he loved me more than I loved him. The way he loves me binds me to him. 'Don't ever leave me,' I whisper to him at night. It puzzles him. He thinks of me as the woman self-determined enough to write books like this. I am, but I am that frightened person too.

I have always liked it that my mother is so attracted to Bill. She responds to him physically. When she's on the dance floor with him she never wants the night to end. She never criticizes him as she does my sister's husband. The first time I took Bill home, my mother gave a cocktail party. A local banker offered Bill a job. 'We're sailing to Europe,' Bill announced. Mother looked from him to me. 'On the same ship?' she asked, and then quickly rose above that first clutch of anxiety. 'How romantic!' she said. Because I was with a man she respected, she acted like a woman instead of a mother.

Before we sailed, she and my stepfather came to New York. Bill was taking part in a literary symposium. Very quickly it changed from polite conversation to a heated argument about 'What has happened to fucking in literature?' During the intermission, Bill looked uneasily at my mother. 'Shall we leave?' My mother was crushed, 'Oh, no!' she said, 'Let's stay.' Afterward we went to a bar in the Village. 'Once,' my mother said, 'when I was twenty-eight, I met a man at a railroad station. He was an army captain. There was a line in front of the telephone booth, and he gave me his place. That night he took me to dinner. When I got to daddy's the next day there were roses from the captain. He wanted to see me again, but I couldn't . . .' Her voice trailed off. She was smiling, flushed. My stepfather had gotten up from the table and was sitting a few feet away at the bar, staring at my mother. He had never heard this story. 'Why didn't you see him?' I asked, fascinated by something I had never seen in her before.'Because,' she said, 'daddy wouldn't let me.' 'I'll tell you what, Jane,' Bill said to my mother. 'We'll make up for the adventure you missed. There's a taxi outside. Let's the four of us get in and go to Kennedy and take the first plane to Puerto Rico. We'll buy the toothbrushes there.' When we dropped mother and Scotty off at their hotel that night, she was still pleading, 'Oh, Scotty, forget your business appointments tomorrow. *Let's go!*'

Seeing me with Bill changed our relationship. It opened up something in her she hadn't dared expose before. Had I become the mother, giving her permission to give in for once to the antic side of her nature? Was it competition? Had she just slipped into my skin? Probably a bit of all these reasons, but mostly I think it was exhilaration that I had gotten past a barrier and in so doing had made the way safe for her. I felt comfortable with Bill and me in the lead because I believe more in us than in them. 'Marry a man your mother is half in love with,' is the advice I give my single women friends.

Four months later when we cabled her from Rome that we were getting married, she swallowed her fear of flying and came to Europe for the first time. We had planned a beautiful wedding at Michelangelo's Campidoglio – Rome's city hall. Afterward, there was a wedding lunch at the Casina Valadier – it had been Napoleon's son's villa, overlooking the fountains of the Piazza di Popolo. As I planned the details of the menu, the flowers, the ceremony, and the parties surrounding those days, I think I had her pleasure in mind as much as Bill's and my own. It was our wedding, taking place on ground we had chosen, but for the first time in my life when a judgment of taste had to be made, I did it her way. The night before the wedding, I asked Bill to move out, not just to another room but to a different hotel. While my mother was speeding forward to meet her adventurous daughter, I was retreating back to her.

I argued with Bill all the way to the altar. Terrible fights up until the moment I swore to the man in the red, white, and green sash of Italian civil law that I would live in Bill's 'stanza' (room) forever. Much as I wanted to be married to Bill, I didn't want everything to stop – the men, the travel, the possibilities for change. Did half of me hope Bill would call it all off? I'll never know. The moment I married, I was triple married. Overnight I became a wife. I wrote home to mother for recipes. I bought a series of prim little double-seamed dresses. I banished even the remotest thoughts of infidelity by never looking at another man. I gave all the money to Bill; no, I didn't even want my name on the checks. I would just ask him for cash when I needed it.

I loved the picture of my mother with her man and me with mine, as two jolly couples. When they came to New York we would take them dancing. When they came to Italy, we would abandon our work and drive them to Florence or Positano. I was meticulous about the arrangements and would call ahead to be sure they got the best room, the one with the cantilevered bathroom so my mother could lie in her tub surrounded by the Mediterranean. 'Nancy, you're planning too many things,' Bill would say as I scheduled activities to please them from dawn to midnight. 'No, no,' I would say, and call the restaurant to be sure the fiddler remembered my mother's favorite tune was 'Fascination'. Now that I was married, I wanted to be a good daughter; now that I was married, I was able.

When men approached me I felt the old excitement, but it frightened me. One night at a bar, a man said, 'You are too much together, you and your husband.' Five minutes earlier, when I had rejected him, I had felt a twinge of regret. Now I took his criticism as a compliment.

When we moved to London we found a beautiful house for sale. Being writers, we had no credit rating. 'I'll write mother,' I said. 'Don't,' Bill said. 'Don't ask your mother for money.' 'It's not asking for money,' I pointed out. 'We're just asking her to countersign a loan.' I reminded him of how often my mother helped out my sister and brother-in-law. I had never asked her for anything, not in my whole life. How could she possibly say no? I smiled at Bill's resistance. He didn't have a close family like mine. 'One for all and all for one!' was my grandfather's toast at family dinners. I smiled now when I said it, but had grown up believing in those words. I wrote mother. I remember the day her letter arrived, a fat envelope on the hall table containing five pages explaining why she couldn't countersign the loan. Bill put his arms around me. He didn't say a word.

I didn't answer my mother's letter. My silence was nothing as simple as a desire to get back at her. I needed desperately to understand. When I can't sleep, Bill's joke is that 'Even in her dreams, Nancy is always asking "What does it all mean?" ' The pain I felt questioned my whole relationship with my mother, a lifetime was balanced in the air. If family was so important, if being a good daughter was superior to being good at anything else – then why was this refusal my reward?

My mother's letters over the subsequent months never mentioned the issue of the loan. 'I'm sorry you're so busy, darling,' she would write. 'I wish you'd find time to send just a note.' When I did write at last, I did not mention the house, but the subject roiled in me like a storm.

Six months later we found another, less expensive house which we bought on our own. It is the only place I have ever lived that I felt was *my* home, Bill's and mine. Was it because we bought it without assistance? Only partially. Unlike other places we had lived, I had no hesitation decorating that house. I knew exactly what I wanted. One sunny afternoon as I was lying on an antique British Officer's campaign bed in a sitting room that fit me like a second skin, I picked up a book on women's sexuality. The author's theory was that the basis for a woman's orgasmic potential lay primarily in her trust of men, first developed in her relationship to her father. 'But what about mother?' was my immediate response. The idea for this book was born in that house.

Eventually my mother and stepfather came to visit us. Content in my new home, past angers forgotten, I went into my old good-daughter gear and staged a lavish cocktail party so they could meet our English friends.

Bill and I took time off from work and flew to France to show them the Paris we loved. Late one night, when I was seated beside my mother in a restaurant, she edged toward me on the banquette, almost cuddling up to me. I wanted to shove her away. Instead I leaned far away from her toward Bill – half furious, half repentant and guilty that I could not give her the affection she wanted from me. Sometimes the anger would rise in the middle of a tour of Notre Dame, or a walk through a department store. Once I got up and left her sitting alone in the Café de Paris. We never talked about these scenes, she never ceased to show me a smile the next time we met. My anger seemed to belong to another person, another time. It did.

Oh, perhaps she should have countersigned that loan. Perhaps it was wrong of me to ask. These are questions that have no answer. Who was right, who was wrong can never be fixed. The anger that came out of the collision between my expectations of my mother and her own estimate of what she could or could not do for me – that was real. It was the beginning of my responsibility to be me.

So sweet is the first feel of marriage that we give up everything. We abandon our names, say good-bye to old lovers and friends, and close our savings and checking accounts, putting everything in our (his) name. We are losing our credit rating for life – should this man ever die or leave us – but we don't want to hear those arguments. We have come full cycle. We are home. Nothing has ever felt so right as putting ourselves in his hands.

The uncertain rewards of autonomy now seem like so much rebellion, merely a childish phase we had to go through to get here. 'When I was single,' a divorced woman of thirty-two says, 'I had this crazy life. A terrific apartment, work that sent me all over the world, lovers . . . Oh, the men I used to fall in love with! Then I got married. I stopped seeing my single friends. Even though I had argued with my mother for years about how provincial she had become by living in the suburbs, my husband and I moved out of the city ourselves. Mother and I became great friends. When I married, I started re-enacting my mother's life, like a sleep-walker. I used to refer to my single years as "my rebellion". Now I refer to my marriage as "my regression".'

When we marry, we don't know how to be. We intend to 'make up' our marriage with this man we love, just as we planned to make ourselves up when we were single. We will incorporate only those warm and loving aspects of mother's marriage, and throw out the rest. One day our husband says angrily, 'You are just like your mother.' Nothing cuts so deep.

Everything reminds us of her. When we decorate our house, when we stand at our kitchen stove, or buy clothes to fit our new married persona, who comes to mind? When he pays the bills, when he tells us how to cope with the world and holds us in his arms, promising love forever, what we feel is what we once had with her. Or grieve that we did not. In our union with him we are reunited with her.

'What makes symbiosis hard to break through,' says Dr Robertiello, 'is that it is so endorsed by society. This sticky, gooey closeness between mother and daughter is seen as some idyllic, wonderful thing. In fact past age one and one half or two, it's an absolutely terrible thing. When you have this symbiotic dependency between a mother and daughter who is eight or eighteen, it's nothing to cheer about. If the woman is twenty-five and married and still telephoning mommy every day, it means there's something wrong. Society always prefers to endorse people's insecurities rather than their health, independence, and tradition-breaking possibilities.' An almost superhuman conscious effort is demanded if we are to maintain our individuality in marriage.

'Lean on me,' our husband says. Little does he realize the profundity of the invitation. 'How was I to know,' says a divorced man, 'what she meant by asking me to take care of her? Of course I said yes. It made me feel proud of myself, and competent.'

'I need a lot of sleep,' his wife would say.

'Fine,' was his reply. 'Just tell me when you're tired, and we'll leave the party.'

'No, you don't understand. You must tell me when to go to bed. If you leave it to me, I'll stay up all night and be wretched tomorrow.'

'I was too dumb to recognize what a dirty bargain was being struck,' the man says. 'From then on, she could be as irresponsible as she liked and if anything went wrong, it was because I hadn't taken care of her. Who was I supposed to be? Her mother?'

Not for independence, not for an apartment of our own, not for experimenting with jobs, careers, work, sex, men, but for this – *this* is what mother raised us to be good at: to live for, through, and protected by, others. It makes us feel more at peace than anything we ever did for and by ourselves.

When we were single our independence may have reminded us how much like our father we were – he too had a life away from home and mother. Many married women still say father was the determining person in their character, the one who shaped their attitudes. It is understandable. Mother stands for worry, anxiety, fear. She is connected with the baby embarrassments of dependency, feeding tantrums, etc. All that is long behind us. We are like father now – women of the world. But who was our sexual model? The act of marriage makes us feel more womanly. Is that identification with father? We have taken mother's model into ourselves; an added strength runs through our veins. With the circle of gold on our finger, we wake like sleeping giants. Lying on his breast, we feel omnipotent, as once we must have done lying on hers.

Our marriage puts mother's heart at rest too. It is proof that she has been a good mother. Accomplishments prior to marriage may have made her proud, but they also put distance between us. Marriage builds a bridge back. She helps us decorate the house, sends us *The Joy of Cooking*, lends us money. *She is available.* We think the change is in her. It is we who have changed, taking a step back in time to meet her again. So complete is the reunion it doesn't matter if our husband is richer or more powerful than her own: she lives in our triumph as if it were hers. Marriage is the great equalizer.

'All my life I wanted my mother's approval,' a woman says. 'For her to say, "Well done!" Nothing I accomplished in my single years did it for me like finding a husband. Now she wants my approval.' We think our reunion with mother is self-chosen, that it is a step forward in our relationship, growth toward maturity. Because she treats us as an equal now, phones for advice, and even depends on us in a way she never did before, the assumption is we are bigger people. The truth is that in marriage we become the little girl who once took down the cookie sheet and imitated mommy. We also become mommy.

Very often the new mother-daughter friendship comes at the expense of what should be our prime union – with our husband. We do not mean to ally with her, but whose standards are we living up to when we give up our identity? Did he ask it of us? When a husband is unfaithful but the wife does not take the same freedom for herself, to whom is she remaining true? If sex once divided mother and daughter, The Rules in marriage make us friends again. Monogamy is the vow made for our husband but even more to placate the introjected mother within. The Rules make a prison, but they give us rest; they inhibit each woman equally.

'After we'd been married six months,' a thirty-year-old woman recalls, 'my husband said he didn't want me to talk to my mother on the phone so much. "I don't want you to see her," he said, "until you understand a new habit you've gotten into. If I want to put a chair here, the table there, the two of you get together and decide they would look better in a third place. She's done it for years to your father. I won't have you lining up against me with your mother. You and I will decide and then we'll tell her how we want things done, if we tell her at all." He was right. I wasn't even aware of slipping into this thing with mother – which, in a way, was against him.'

Hence, the terrible mother-in-law jokes that men tell.

For some people, the blissful 'in love' stage of the honeymoon may go on for years. We idealize the other person – and through him, ourselves. 'It is a very heightened symbiosis,' says Dr Robertiello, 'a merger with the fantasized ideal. The other person is seen not as he is, but as the glorious person we want him to be.' The unspoken self-flattery here is that we must be pretty special too, to have been chosen by this incredible being. For others, reality presents its harsh face when the two weeks in Bermuda end and he calmly goes back to his job or golf foursomes. He walks out the door alone, and doesn't think of it as betrayal at all. When he leaves home for work in the morning, his feeling of doing the right thing is unmistakable. Much as we love our new house, our new name, they have not brought us what we expected of marriage. The rational self knows the mortgage must be paid, but somewhere within we feel his 9 to 5 life – *anything separate from us* – is a rival. We want love, more love, love without end. Doesn't he want it too?

We are told we are womanly to need love so badly but the issue is not love. It is the longing to be merged. If we take a job for a salary our new family needs just as much as it does his, why don't we feel as wholeheartedly right about working as he does? 'Everything is OK,' he says reassuringly. We don't believe him. The independence of a job, life in the office with other people, do not seem to compliment what we have at home, but carry jeopardy. New friends and adventures when we were little, sex itself, were all the more exciting because they were *away* from mother, but that was why they were tinged with anxiety too. We didn't tell her about these experiences because we believed they would frighten her; the truth is we were frightened that if she knew, she would get angry. Our tie to her would be weakened. This way of thinking was confirmed when we found out later that more men, more success and accomplishment often lost us the love of other girls. They experienced our gains as somehow leaving less of the pie for them. How can our husband be any different? How can he not fear the added life we get from work as a betrayal too? Won't he love us less, even leave us?

A successful career woman tells me she feels no conflict at all between marriage and career. 'It was my husband who encouraged me to continue my job,' she tells me proudly. But when we part, she calls me back; 'I've been thinking,' she says. 'Sometimes I do feel guilty that I'm not there with a hot meal when Jim comes home from work. It's irrational, but there it is. There's this niggling fear that maybe I'm disenfranchising myself from my femininity. He's never said anything, but I feel it.'

The anxiety here is not between husband and wife but within the woman herself. On TV, she sees commercials of families moving ever together in tight, compact groups. She has her own history of closeness within her childhood family. She and her husband may have worked out more economic divisions of time; she may be getting rewards more real and appropriate from her marriage – but it is not what she was raised to look for. The majority of American divorces – higher than ever last year – come in the second year of marriage. The third year is almost as bad. More women than ever are working outside the home, but our culture has taught us so successfully that a woman's place is tied to a man as securely as once we were tied to mother that we are guilty about our efforts to be free. Men too have been raised to think of women in this way. Though they may give our work separate from them verbal encouragement, the other half of the unspoken double message is often there too; why aren't you the way my mother was with my father?

It is important to emphasize that wanting to be taken care of is not always negative. Men and women are drawn together because we all need a close, intimate relationship. In a good one we can satisfy each other's needs with pleasure, or at least at low psychic cost. To be held in someone's arms, to be able to say, 'I'm scared, lonely, tell me everything will be all right. Comfort me and I'll do the same for you when you feel this way' — that is not asking to be guaranteed against all the vicissitudes of life. The woman who says this is merely asking for a resting place, a fueling station in which to gather her strength to go on again. It is not quitting the job of adulthood, nor submitting to a superior-inferior relationship. It is the pause that refreshes.

When 'take care of me' means asking someone to permanently interpose himself between us and reality, the wish is destructive to the self, and therefore to the marriage. In the 1936 movie *Dodsworth* there is a scene I once would have dismissed as cute movie dialog. Walter Huston's wife has a shipboard flirtation with suave David Niven and quickly finds herself beyond her depth. Humiliated, she says to her husband, 'Sam, you've got to take care of me. I frighten myself. And if I'm bad, promise you'll beat me.' Walter Huston dismisses this as foolish woman talk, but the need to be nurtured, disciplined, and protected by a man as if he were our mother speaks of unformed identity: take care of me, tell me how to be, who to be, let me be your child.

This behavior is often found in women whose total orientation toward life is a kind of reliving out of the dissatisfactions they experienced from a cold, nongiving mother. Even in sex, such a woman expects to be passively gratified at all times, with little concern for the man's needs or satisfactions. If her primary aim is to be nurtured, to be petted, soothed, *suckled* (in any of its unconscious disguises including the sexual), it is not orgasmic satisfaction she is looking for; I've heard men say sex with women like these makes them feel, not refreshed, renewed and satisfied, but exhausted.

A psychiatrist describes a sexual problem she often sees in women: 'She won't do anything during sex because that means giving. All she wants is to receive. She speaks of sex as "letting him make love to me". The idea that she might make love to him is inconceivable. She just wants to lie there. The typical mother of a woman like this simply hadn't been there, emotionally or physically, when the woman was little. Therefore, the daughter's orientation toward life was that she had to be constantly reassured, told how good she was, to be nurtured and done for. She can't give, partly because she was afraid she would be smacked down if she did, but mostly because she has very little to give.' You can't learn to give without having been initially given to.

I don't think most women question the rightness of expecting a man to take care of them. We have been raised to think that handing men our will is as precious a gift as our virginity. A friend of my husband's speaks about a woman he met after fifteen years of marriage. 'I didn't realize it was an affair, at first,' he said. 'I had always thought of women – especially a wife – as some kind of burden, some heavy weight you had a duty to carry around on your back. This new woman is such fun, she pulls her own weight at all times. So I didn't realize I was entering something serious with her. Now that I realize it is serious, I don't want the feeling of lightness I get from her to stop.'

No wonder so many couples who have lived together worry that marriage may ruin what they have. 'We're as much as married now,' one of them may say, 'what would be different if we went through a legal ceremony?' But marriage does change us; it brings a formal element into our lives, the rigidity of the model of our parents. The friend of my husband's mentioned above, who began an affair after fifteen years of marriage, had been as symbiosed as his wife. It wasn't just his wife who fell into old patterns, he did too.

Women too can find breaking symbiosis exhilarating. A woman who had been faithfully married to an increasingly indifferent husband for the past ten years tells me about her affair: 'I began to think there must be something wrong with me because I never wanted to confess to my husband. I just frankly enjoyed the relationship very much. It's hard to explain, but it had been a very close friendship for many years, before it turned into an affair. We had worked together for six years. My job has been responsible for a lot of growth on my part.'

Without putting any value judgment on adultery, let's try to understand what this woman is saying about symbiosis and freedom of choice. What surprised her is how little guilt she felt – as opposed to how much she had always assumed she would. Once she'd experienced the security and self-esteem that came from having a job and life apart from her husband, she could reassess her marriage, decide it was not fulfilling her needs – and do something about the decision. Symbiotic dependence upon her husband had been broken – as evidenced by the fact that she feels no need to 'guiltily' inform him. What she is doing is separate from him, her own affair. No wonder she enjoys it so much.

Having a life of our own outside marriage does not necessarily mean we will go in for adultery. Instead, when he goes off for a business trip, we don't simply wait for him to return but take an art class. If he wants to go to a Chinese restaurant but we want to go to a movie, we meet again after each has done his/her thing and it doesn't feel like an unhappy, lonely compromise. The evening leaves us feeling refreshed, each pleased for a little time on her/his own, glad to see each other again. Symbiotic union puts a premium not on doing what the individual wants but on finding something with a low enough common denominator so both can do it together. It is a low-intensity relationship.

It isn't even safe – you never know when, without even looking for it, one partner is suddenly going to be swept off his/her feet by some new person who comes along as a reminder of all the electricity life once offered.

'Before I was married, I functioned very independently,' says psychologist Liz Hauser. 'I had a job that took me all over the country. I was months on the road on and off an airplane almost every day. But when I married at twenty-seven, I went directly back into a symbiotic thing. It's really where I'd been all along. When I was growing up my mother used to say, "Now when you get married, you won't move away. You'll have a little house nearby." I would not say a word but I had my plans. I wanted out of all that smothering and overprotecting. But if someone hung on to you too long when you were little, or you didn't get enough mothering, you tend to go through life not knowing how to relate except symbiotically. When I got married it was simple transference. There is tremendous regression in symbiosis with the mate, if you haven't settled it earlier. It's important to stress this because women may be able to recognize their regressive behavior in their marriage easier than they can with their child. Marriage is less sacred than motherhood. Our child is where we want to face separation last.

'I was self-supporting before marriage, but after – I began waiting for him to come home and bring me news of the outside world. I was upset that he wasn't there all the time. I began to think of myself only as his wife – no other identity. And so I only felt really alive when he was around the house, when we were together. When he was home, I wanted him to talk to *me*, to be with *me*. I didn't want to travel anywhere without him.

'The moment wasn't real, time wasn't whole when he was absent. *That* is the symbiotic bind. After about six months, he said to me, "For God's sake, get yourself something to do and go do it." I knew he was right. I was whining and whimpering like a baby because he was busy with his work, not with me. So I went back to work, thank God.'

Symbiosis is not a dirty word. When we are grown, fleeting, temporary symbiosis and merging can play as lovely a role as it did in infancy. There are times when we don't want to be separate, when it is indeed exhilarating within a loving relationship to feel merged – a satisfying sense of closeness, almost a transcendent oneness with the other person. For instance, if we would let ourselves feel this kind of depth of union with our husbands or lovers tonight, it would be a marvelous experience. During sex, when we suspend our adult lives and get back into those almost primitive feelings of symbiosis that we once had as trusting infants, the joining with the other person is going to give the sexual experience all kinds of different dimensions than it would have had we stayed on an adult level.

The feeling of life that comes from symbiosis isn't exclusive to sex; you can feel it in other moments of deep intimacy with a person. Creative people experience it when they suspend their day-by-day adult consciousnesses and dip back into buried emotions, their earliest, unconscious experiences, to dredge up raw, powerful feelings and ideas to be sublimated into art. *What distinguishes bad symbiosis from good is the loss of choice.*

When the need for symbiosis is so desperate that you cannot turn it on or off at will, you lose your sense of self. The other person, the outside world, loses its urgency and excitement, sex becomes tame, autonomy is gone. Pleasurable, positive symbiosis is entered into at will, enhancing moments of union with the other so that both feel a larger identity than ever before; and yet it is easily broken or interrupted when it is time to separate, to be people with your own ego, autonomy, and jobs to do in the world. The conventional name for the feeling is 'being in love'. In destructive symbiosis the two people meet, feel the initial enlargement of the self due to merging of identities – but can't seem to part. They stay glued to one another. Absence from the partner is tinged with anxiety, peace comes only when they are together. But with so little stimulation and energy coming in to the situation, they use each other up. They go stale, but still can't let go.

Women have an important confusion about being taken care of emotionally, and being taken care of financially. It compounds the problems of symbiosis, and so will be discussed here at some length. The difficulty begins with the fact that men and women see money's role in their lives in different ways. This causes almost hopeless frictions compounded by the fact that all of us have been trained to think there is something intrinsically not nice in talking about money at all.

Psychoanalysts speak of stubborn aspects of behavior in the same way they speak of misers or stingy people: they say these are 'anal retentive' character formations. It surprises no one to learn that stingy people are often constipated. Whether you believe in psychoanalysis or not, ideas like these resonate on a deep, intuitive level of everyday wisdom; they help explain a great deal about people's furtiveness about money. Most of us have noted how someone would rather tell you his most intimate bedroom secrets than reveal his yearly income. Therefore, it is easy to see that money discussions between husbands and wives begin with a great handicap. Money is symbolic of too many aspects of emotional life to be dealt with on a simple, factual level; too many angry repressions – equations of money, filthy lucre and shit, for instance – are boiling just beneath the surface.

By the time a man is old enough to think of marriage, he is usually on his way to having solved the material side of living. Socialized masculinity tells him that as long as he is a good provider, women will tend to his emotions for him. 'Take care of me,' he says when he comes home from the office. He means he is exhausted by the battles of the day, and wants his wife to help him feel better. He is asking for emotional support.

The wife too is exhausted by battling it out with the carpool, the repairman, the PTA, and her loneliness. 'Take care of me,' she says. Her emotional request is as legitimate as his, but she wants more from him. You might say there is a hidden clause in her request. In defense of women, it must be added that this usually operates outside our conscious knowledge: mixed in with any request to be emotionally taken care of is the expectation that this includes being taken care of financially as well – an assumption men do not fully understand. From here, it is easy to fuse and confuse emotional and material needs: we expect that meeting one need implies the man is ready, willing, and able to meet the other too. That is what love 'means'. If he buys us expensive gifts, a house on the lake, or takes us for a trip to Paris, the economic half of the gift becomes suffused with a romantic, emotional glow: he has 'proved' he loves us.

'I will marry for love,' a woman says, but the unspoken half of her definition is that love will make her feel free of material anxieties. It is only after marriage that many women become aware that what they love is not just the man but the material security he is supposed to bring. Married couples fight over money more than any other single cause.

On the other hand, a marriage in which all bills are paid promptly is not necessarily a happy one. It is only a negative event, an anxiety subtracted. The cliché is old and tired, but that is because it is so often true: a man often works so hard and long to make the money for the marriage that he has little time or energy left for emotions. After the house in the suburbs, two pretty children and charge accounts at five expensive stores, a wife in a marriage like this may realize she is emotionally starving to death, right in the midst of material plenty. 'Why did she leave good old reliable Charley, with his solid job as vice-president at the bank, to run off with a guitar player?' people ask. 'She must be crazy.' She is hungry. Her confusion and merging of two different needs – financial and emotional – into one, led her to a dead end.

Not every wife in this situation runs off, of course. She may look for the emotional support she needs elsewhere. Charity work, children, adultery, women's consciousness-raising groups, alcohol, divorce itself. Some of these options may work, some may not; questions of value are not the point here. I want only to show that while a woman may turn to various outlets in her search, perhaps a wiser start would be to look at her assumptions. Mother's love and milk gave her both emotional and material well-being; in fact, they were indistinguishable one from the other. When she met a man who could materially take care of her, did she assume – as it had been with mother – she would automatically feel emotionally taken care of too?

Money is the rub, and when marriage fails, often enough it is money that women use to 'get back at him'. How much of the unrealistic amounts asked for in divorce settlements is meant for support, how much for revenge? When they were in love, she told him money didn't matter, love was all. Now that the unrealistic promise of symbiotic live has failed, money matters very much. But, says lawyer Emily Jane Goodman: 'When I tell women that if they do not own and control their own money, they do not control their lives, I always meet resistance. "Oh, no," they say. "I'm the one who keeps the checkbook, pays the telephone bills on time, we have a joint account," etc. They never want to face that when he stops putting money into the joint account, everything stops.'

A cliché says that women control the wealth of the United States. It supports women's refusal to understand our powerlessness over money. If women own the major share of stocks on the New York Stock Exchange, it somehow is supposed to mean we don't have to get angry about impotence over money in our individual lives. 'If you are convinced you are part of the ruling class that controls the nation's wealth,' says Emily Jane Goodman, 'it's hard to get angry over the fact that in your family, you have no say about the money at all.'

The day all this changes is when the wife goes to an attorney to seek a divorce. Up to now, she's 'chosen' not to know her husband's income, she doesn't know whose name the house is in, what are their total assets in stocks, bonds, or whatever. 'Who me? My husband handles all that.' When her lawyer asks for figures, income tax statements, bank balances, etc., in order to make a case for alimony and/or child support, the soon-to-be-ex-wife can only weep.

'Women come into my office in divorce cases,' says Ms Goodman. 'They've been beaten by their husbands. "Do you know what assets your husband has?" I say. Their reply is, "No, but all I have to do is ask him. I know he'll never try to trick me." It is almost impossible to make her see that this is the man who broke her nose. Why does she think he's going to be level with her about money? Her attitude is, "If I don't trust him, everything has been in vain."' If a child cannot trust her mother, what is the purpose of living?

I have heard many an otherwise articulate single woman stammer in her efforts to express her confusion when, the morning after the night of love at his place, there is the matter of the long, expensive taxi ride back to her apartment. Should she pay it herself when he makes four times her salary – merely because she is sufficiently liberated to see herself home? She wants to be equal, but she is broke. Isn't there an easy way for him to slip her $10? Even if he does it gracefully, why does she still feel angry, humiliated, like a greedy child who has just wheedled an extra $10 allowance? No one wants to talk about money, she doesn't know how, but it is her reality.

A common defense wives adopt against economic powerlessness is to live by a kind of unspoken formula. 'Your money is our money, but my money is mine.' When the husband wants to know how she can justify not pooling all her money, she cannot tell him. Feeling sneaky and sly, she squirrels away part of the housekeeping money in a cookie jar or secret account. She has some unconscious feeling that money – keeping money, hiding money, *her* money – is not nice. On a more conscious level, she has been trained never to mention it. Saddest of all, the amount being withheld is not going to give her autonomy anyway.

My own feeling is that far from behaving childishly, women who defend the unspoken formula 'Yours is ours and mine is mine' may be showing a certain amount of common sense. Says psychologist Sonya Friedman: 'I don't think it's unrealistic for a woman with no income to put money away as a margin of safety. In marriage counseling, I often see men who are getting ready to leave their wives. He sells the home, then puts her in a new $80,000 house with a $70,000 mortgage and departs, keeping most of the cash realized on the sale of the old house for himself. A woman must always ask herself, "Am I being financially wise to depend on him totally?"'

Millions of women do contribute to the family income. More than 30 million women work outside the home today – over one-third the labor force.[1] When children must be fed or clothed, there is no question of whose money is whose. A recent University of Michigan survey shows that a third of working women are the sole wage earners of the family.[2] Some women have been raised by their mothers to think of themselves as providers and take pride in it. Other women find feelings of deeply satisfied symbiosis with the husband

and children when they hand over their paycheck for the good of the family. 'It is when the money in the family rises above the baseline of survival,' says Dr Friedman, 'that the trouble starts. It's up to him, the wife thinks, always to provide the economic baseline on which they live. If she earns anything, it is on top. He is not supposed to count on it. She thinks she is entitled to do whatever she wants with her money.' She has been raised to think she needn't earn any money at all, so if she does, it is extra, hers alone. And if a money need should arise that she considers to lie within his province of day-to-day family expenses – like a repair bill for the car – and he asks her to help pay for it, she may stubbornly resist.

She usually gives in to him on everything else. Why does she balk here?

Ever since we can remember, mother has held out marriage as the grand payoff for all our sacrifices and restraints. It is put as a kind of reality principle: deferring satisfaction today will lead to a greater reward tomorrow. If we curb our temper, deny ourselves sex, give up assertiveness – all will bring a better man, a safer marriage, one in which it is the man's job to support us. For the wife to contribute money to her own support is to break the symbiotic illusion that the husband will always take care of her.

Money is power, the woman without money is a victim. Most wives realize this means they are living on the edge of a financial precipice. But to say it might make it come true. 'When my wife told me she was putting her salary into a savings account in her name,' a highly successful surgeon tells me, 'I was mildly surprised. But I didn't mind. She makes only a fraction of what I do. She has a good reason to want a nest egg of her own. I've been married four times. I hope this is the last, but if it isn't, her standard of living could go from upper class to welfare overnight.' Seen this way, the wife who insists on keeping whatever little money she can earn in her own name is trying to right an unequal power balance – a balance that our society still rigs in favor of men and their greater earning ability. She is also responding to fear: if he breaks the symbiotic promise to take care of her by asking her to pool her money, how can she know he will not break the rest of it and leave her?

It is difficult to tell a husband: 'I'm not getting enough emotion from you.' It sounds neurotic and childish. It is easier to say, 'Why don't you ask for a raise? Why can't we take a trip to South America? The people next door have a new car. Can't we?' Asking for pleasures that money can buy when what we really feel is emotionally poor makes money arguments family-killers. Trapped in role-playing postures, talking about one thing when they mean another, and unable to understand the difference between emotional and material 'taking care of', both husband and wife are doomed to endless Rashomon arguments. Each is defending unnamed positions the other doesn't suspect.

'Ask a housewife if she's happy,' says Jessie Bernard, 'and she'll say, "Oh, yes, I'm just as happy as can be." And yet she's taking all these tranquilizers . . .' In northwest Washington, DC, Dr Bernard goes on to report, 'The suicide rate among women is higher than almost anywhere else – even though it is a very prosperous area.' In fact, since 1950, the number of female suicides in this country has practically doubled.[3]

A woman may resist the new tide of feminism and reject all its tenets, but she cannot forget she has alternatives her mother did not. Grandmother may have gotten enough narcissistic gratification through identification with her husband, his achievements and her status as his wife. Today, television makes it impossible not to know many women out there are getting a lot more out of life. This is not to say being a housewife and mother is not enough for millions of women. It obviously is. But if you are the sort of person who wants more than being *Mrs* Harry Brown, living through him may not be enough. He is not taking in enough air, life, success, and/or achievements for two.

'But the insufficiency,' says Dr Shaefer, 'is not seen by the woman as her problem. She thinks it is his. She may feel like a nobody, but the way she puts it is: "Oh, I'm very happy, but I wish George were better organized so he could get a better job." Her implication is, If I were George, I could do it better. Another wife will say to her husband, "If you just tried harder, with all your brilliance you could be making a lot more money." To the superficial observer, this sounds like the wife has unbounded confidence in her husband. *He* knows this is criticism.'

Dr Schaefer continues: 'A woman like this is afraid to take the risks her husband does. She would like a more interesting, stimulating life, but she sees it as something only he can get for her. It never occurs to her the problem is hers. She is so meshed, so dependent on him, she can't see where he begins and she leaves off. She fears that separating out a problem as her own will divide them – that it will force her to act on her own. "Why not get a job?" I suggest to a woman like this. "You're terrific with clothes, you could sell dresses in a boutique." But she is terrified. "Oh, no, I could never fill out one of those sales slips!" she says. She clings to him and complains instead.'

To people like this, the contemporary message that women have a responsibility for their own gratification in life seems like so much theoretical hooey. A woman who is as talented as her husband will put him through law or medical school because she has been trained to feel the life she will get from his success far surpasses what she could get on her own.

In those marriages where roles are shared – where women help carry the financial load and men help in the housework and raising the children, studies show, says sociologist Jessie Bernard, 'that women end up working at least 25 percent more than the men.'

'Wives have too much at stake to admit unhappiness,' says sociologist Cynthia Fuchs Epstein. 'You really can't interview people about how happy they are. I did a survey on women lawyers married to male lawyers, and in practice with them. Though these women told me they were living in husband-and-wife partnerships of utter equality, when I observed the actual behavior of a good proportion of them, I found the women were doing the "housekeeping" of the law firm – the hiring, firing, and administration – while the husband went out, met the clients and did the interesting cases in court. By outside standards, these were very assertive, commanding women. By their own standards, they were "happy", but when they said theirs was an equal partnership with their husbands, they were deluding themselves. When you were around them for a while you saw how the woman deferred to their husbands. They made the meals, they asked, "More coffee, dear?" They took the back seat.'

There has been a recent backlash among certain male writers who warn that unless women return to traditional roles and get out of the male marketplace, a whole new generation of frustrated and angry males will be unleashed upon the world.

I would like to talk about the rage of women.

We bear a burden of anger all our lives. Just like men, some of us are more angry than others. Although some authorities would like to convince us that men's greater potential for anger is sex-linked (hormones, testosterones, etc.), I remain unconvinced. The difference between the angers of the sexes is that women's are the more repressed.

If I choose to discuss anger within the context of marriage, it is not because I believe there are no happy marriages. I know many. And yet any institution sold to women as a reward for lifelong inhibition must cause anger and disappointment. But how many women can name marriage itself as a source of our turbulence? More often than not, we were the ones who most wanted to get married. Besides, if not marriage, what *do* we want? Divorce? That is too fearsome. 'The more I talk to a woman,' says Sonya Friedman, 'the more anger I uncover. All the depression, the going to sleep early, not having energy, the fact that it's three in the afternoon and she is still sitting around in her housecoat – all these are various forms of anger. "I'm bored," she says, "I went through all this schooling, I used to have dreams but now I know they aren't going to be met. I'm even afraid to go back to school, to get out there and compete." Most of the anger has to do with the way she was raised.

Marriage, she was told, would be the answer to all problems. The typical American housewife has no identity apart from her husband, so can't let the anger out. Her only way to deal with it is to turn it upon herself. That is why so many women are depressed.'

I was very moved by the following interview. The woman is thirty-five years old. At first I thought her gentleness of speech was part of her early, learned passivity. What she said made me realize it is the calm that comes after the battle of facing one's own raging emotions.

'My mother died five years ago, of emphysema. She was submissive and my father was very dominant. All my life, I watched her swallow her anger. Mother was such a gentle, loving person. She wouldn't want me to bottle up the turbulent emotions I've been going through but she never showed me how to get them out. I thought my parents had a perfect marriage because I never heard them fight. It was a difficult experience for me, working out my anger toward mother after she died. But it was a freeing experience too, to be able to admit the anger, the hate, as well as the love. Part of my anger is having held back getting my postgraduate degree until my husband had his. From my mother, I got the feeling that, as a woman, I had to let him go first. I had learned that kind of deference to men from her, and I was angry at her for teaching me this. I married someone totally different from my father and have had trouble accepting his regard for me. I have only recently stopped thinking of him as weak for what is in essence his high opinion and tender feelings for me. I couldn't appreciate this because I was looking for what mother had settled on. I have deep respect for my mother and for my father. I am not angry at my father. I am angry at her because I am like her, because she taught me to be like her. Because she loved me, she taught me to swallow my anger.'

Speech is the least harmful outlet for anger. The easiest way to dissipate it or to change the environment in a beneficial way is with words. But one of the first things girls are deprived of is the direct translation of thought into speech. While we are little, the clever, articulate child is mother's darling. It is the commonplace experience of pediatricians that little girls learn to speak earlier and more fluently than boys. As we become young women, this changes. The subtle training in silence begins.

We learn that spontaneity in speech can lose you people. We learn to edit our thoughts, to reduce strong emotions to bland euphemisms. 'When I go places with my husband,' says a thirty-year-old woman, 'I'd like to participate more in the discussions. But by the time I've formed a sentence in my head, the talk has already gone on to a new subject.'

We are not practiced in spontaneity. What fluency in speech this woman picked up in college has been lost in the ten years she has spent at home raising children. She does not regret the choice of motherhood; she just can't understand her uneasiness about joining in dinner-party conversation. 'Many men aren't necessarily bright, but that doesn't stop them from going nonstop. Why can't I let myself get in a word?'

Like any other facility, the conduit between brain and tongue requires use if it is not to go rusty. Without practice, the prospect of humiliation, fear of saying the wrong thing and finding ourselves stranded midsentence, keeps us silent.

We also have the social disadvantage of a woman's voice. I've often sat in my own living room and heard my opinion ignored as if I were invisible; the same idea spoken five minutes later in a sonorous male voice is applauded. These experiences do not equip us to handle differences of opinion about a movie or even teasing about a tennis game. How can they equip us for the sudden and violent emotions of anger?

How many women have you ever heard express hostility intelligently? Our voices become charged, not with anger's force and determination, but with an anxious quality that makes listeners turn away. They are afraid we will lose control; they are 'bored' by our overemotional delivery. 'That's how women are. They can't argue logically.' What drives us to fury is not the illogic of our argument, but inexperience in speaking aggressively. We ourselves fear hysteria. I have watched socially organized groups of intelligent women disintegrate into anxious little knots of dismay when faced with someone's inability to speak her anger at another woman who is present. It is easier to show anger to a man: it was a woman who taught us to suppress our rage. Tears and weeping are the only sound of anger we are allowed.

Without female models able to show us how to vent anger in socially acceptable ways, we fear the emotion, deny it. 'When I was in college,' a woman tells me, 'I took fencing lessons. Part of the rules are that you are required to stomp aggressively on the floor to start a match. You don't have to say a thing, just *stomp!* That was the part I loved best.'

In her book on rape, *Against Our Will*, Susan Brownmiller describes a self-defense karate class in which the male instructor ordered the women students to hit him as hard as they could. He assured them they could not hurt his professionally hardened muscles and gave them permission to be as aggressive as they liked. Ms Brownmiller reports that at first not a single woman could allow herself to hit the instructor with all her force, and many could not strike a blow at all.[4] Learning how to protect ourselves begins as an emotional problem.

Because society would rather we always wore a pretty face, women have been trained to cut off anger, much as surgeons in the nineteenth century, for similar reasons of keeping 'the sex' tame, popularized the clitorectomy. 'Help me,' we cry, running to psychiatrists, surgeons, doctors, priests, or even back to mother. We say we are 'nervous' and take tranquilizers, aspirin, gin, and courses in Total Womanhood. We say we are 'happy' but find ourselves unaccountably suffering from headaches, ulcers, or chronic fatigue. We say we are bored and gamble, take lovers or spend too much money in the department store. We say we are not in the mood and deny our husband sex. We say we are menopausal and live in states of chronic physical and/or mental anguish for a decade. There is a respectable body of medical opinion which believes that our buried, long-smoldering anger can even lead to the silent explosion of the body against itself: cancer. Our anger against the false idealization of marriage is so unacceptable that we have turned it against ourselves in the profoundest sense of the word.

A forty-five-year-old woman speaks: 'I was married at high noon at St Patrick's Cathedral. You can't do better than that. I did so many things right. I suppose I was acting out my mother's desires. When she was growing up, she didn't have the opportunities so she made them for me. She was a career woman, worked all her life, and she expected me to be an achiever too. She got a lot of vicarious pleasure out of whatever my sister and I did, but she never gave us praise directly. We'd hear it from her friends. So there was this ambivalence we got from her: "You should do better than I did . . ." but a feeling of jealousy too.

'Along with making my mark in the world, I was brought up to marry and raise a family. My mother used to pray for me to St Anne . . . you know, "St Anne, get my daughter a man." When I was twenty-eight and still not married, she switched to St Jude, the patron saint of hopeless cases. This set up a kind of split in me. Especially on the job. It is hard to work alongside a man, and even compete with him for the same promotion – but nevertheless need his approval as a woman at the same time.

'Marriage made it easier for me to be nice to my mother. When I married, I stopped working. I was going to be the typical Irish Catholic East Side New York young matron. But my husband died and I had to go back to work. That was fifteen years ago, and I've made a professional success of my life. But I am left with this anger. If I had been raised to be even normally aggressive, I would not have had to always assume the soft position in career situations; I always needed male approval of me as a woman before I could think about getting it as a professional and a peer. All those years of smiling at men who were less capable than I . . .

'Nowadays, my mother depends on me. I am not angry at her any more for withholding her approval when I was a kid. That's how she was. She called me at the office today and asked if she should wear a pants suit on an airplane. A few years ago, I would have been angry at her for bothering me with such a stupid question at work. Today, I have my anger under control. Perhaps I have mellowed. I made time for her call, even though it meant I had to delay a meeting. At this point, I guess I view her very much as I do my children. It's a responsibility, part of my dues-paying. It leaves me with a good feeling. The latent hostilities, the things that bugged me when I was younger, are still there, but I avoid them.'

The woman in this interview died of cancer a year after I spoke to her. Her two daughters are being raised by her sister, who asked if she could read the interview. 'It made me sad to see how emphatically my sister denied being angry about certain things,' she wrote me. 'She said that because she understood, she didn't have to get mad . . . How I wish she had been angry at some things, some people. She wasn't even angry about life's final assault on her.'

Says Dr Schaefer: 'I see so many women whose lives are dominated by the idea, "He won't let me." The whole women's movement is based on personal responsibility, but many people think as soon as they've liberated themselves, all the goodies will drop in their lap. They think, Now that I've dumped the old man who was holding me back, now the boss will give me, the world is going to give me, the sisterhood is going to give me. Because women were never raised to be autonomous, they don't understand the personal responsibility needed to make the liberation slogans mean something.' We want to be 'free' but taken care of anyway.

The bottled-up fury resulting from overidealizing marriage as the solution to all our problems makes for a kind of agoraphobia. 'You might even call it "housewife phobia",' says Sonya Friedman. 'It is not uncommon, and describes the great number of women who don't like, or are afraid, to leave the house alone. It has to do with the fear that once she gets out there in the wide-open spaces, she'll get this irresistible urge to run away.'

A private detective who works for a large agency in New York gives me a description of the average runaway housewife. It reads like someone in a TV soap opera: she got married at nineteen, had children shortly thereafter, and has had little or no work experience. She's thirty-four when she differs from her more conventional sisters and disappears to find a new life.

In a symbiotic marriage, you feel protected, close – in fact, so close that no separation can be tolerated. Any emphasis put on individual choice, any anger expressed, is betrayal. I've heard this kind of marriage called 'the long quiet walk, hand in hand, to the grave.' A psychiatrist I know calls it the 'tit-lined coffin'. Men have long run away from it. Women are beginning to.

'I was a lot more passionately in love with other men than the man I married,' a woman tells her marriage counselor. 'There was an actor I was crazy about. He was extremely emotional, and it gave our affair that extra zing. But the idea of marrying him? It frightened me. So I married someone I thought was stable as a rock, like my father. By the time I saw that behind Larry's surface calm he was selfish and unreliable, it was too late. I was already emotionally dependent on him. He would stay out late. He wouldn't telephone. I blamed myself. I was going slowly, desperately mad. But the next morning, I wouldn't want to muddy the waters. There were so many things to do that I would forget my desperation. I made breakfast, got the children off to school and always tried to put a good face on things.'

Our culture rewards women for swallowing their anger and/ or directing it away from its source. The compulsive housekeeper, the lioness of the Anti-Porn Society, the nonstop charity-worker, the overprotective and critical mother who does it all for someone else's good – who can fault these people out loud? We don't know where they get their energy, we don't know what they get out of it. We may avoid them and their company; but we can't call them bad women/wives/mothers.

Very often, these women are obsessive/compulsives – suffering from forms of behavior that seem to have nothing to do with anger. Unlike depressed people who turn their anger within, against themselves, the obsessive/compulsives express theirs outwardly – but in such an indirect way they never face their furies at all.

While usually discussed together, compulsions and obsessions differ slightly. Compulsions are repeated acts of behavior, like constantly emptying ashtrays while the smoker is using them, or fluffing up the sofa pillows the minute somebody gets up. If you've ever been around compulsive people and seen how they fray the nerves of anyone they come into contact with, you will recognize that a great deal of hostility is being loosed nonspecifically into the environment. On the other hand, obsessions are not actions, but thoughts. Obsessional people have their minds constantly flooded with repetitive ideas – like the woman who is ever worried that something terrible has happened to the children, that her husband will leave. Once again, anger has taken on a disguise, a constant conjuring-up of pain, loss, and death. Nobody has happy obsessive thoughts. Both obsessions and compulsions are repetitive because underground anger must be defeated against, over and over.

'What I remember most about my mother,' says a twenty-eight-year-old wife, 'is the incredible amount of anger she brought to little things, like tracking dirt across the kitchen floor. She would get as hot about a button missing as she would at a sin like lying. I've decided her anger was because she was afraid. Each thing I did wrong was a clue that I was so careless I would do something far worse. I see her anger in myself nowadays toward my little girl, and it frightens me.'

Says Sonya Friedman: 'Women have problems with anger because they don't have a sense of security within. Women go from being an extension of their families to being an extension of their husbands. Most marry before they complete growing. The man usually has more power, so whatever sense of identity she has can easily be snuffed out. Men don't *do* this *to* women, they do it *with* women's compliance. Women have been so conditioned for marriage that they buy the contract, the trade-off of autonomy for dependence. Later they cry: "What can I

do to save my marriage?" You have to tell these women there
are no ready-made answers. Maybe in time they get in touch
with their anger, but that means going back to the beginning to
when they first learned the double-edged reward they got from
mother was paid for by playing down their self-confidence and
independence.'

Dr Friedman continues: 'Anger is positive. When a woman
is unhappy about her marriage, but apathetic, I know it's going
to be a tough job to help her. If she's angry, I know I've got a
good shot. If I can get a woman to see that she's bought a
shoddy bill of goods, she doesn't go into anger. She goes into
rage.'

Says Dr Sidney Q. Cohlan: 'Just as no child ever meets the
mother's fantasy, so does no mother ever live up to the
daughter's fantasy of what a mother should be.' To continue
the fiction that we have some ideal relationship with mother
behind the superficial, day-by-day frictions, we often invent a
pat phrase to sum up what we have with her. Like sentences in
code, they disguise the real situation. 'Mother and I get along
fine these days, as long as we don't live too near one another.'
Or, 'I don't blame my mother for the way she raised me, she did
the best she could.' Indeed, unless mother was one of the rare
malevolents, she *did* do the best she could. Nevertheless, what
she did or did not do, hurt us. The child within is furious still. If
you will go back and reread those two sentences quoted just
above, you will see there is anger in each one.

'The job of the grown-up part of you is not to deny that
angry child within,' says Dr Robertiello. 'If you do, that child is
going to get out and displace the anger onto other people, like
your husband, or take it out in psychosomatics, depression, or
compulsions.'

Here is an example of how a twenty-five-year-old woman
both knows and doesn't know that she is angry at her mother:
'My mother had this idea that if you didn't talk about sex it
wouldn't happen. Even when my sister became pregnant and
had to have an abortion, the matter was never discussed. I went
into marriage a virgin because I believed what my mother said.

That if you were a good girl everything would turn out all right. But all my life I've wondered how important that was. I know it wasn't my mother's fault, but I feel cheated that I was never able to talk about feelings, emotions when I was growing up. I have this anger toward men, and I don't want my daughter to see it. But she can't help but see my resentment toward my husband. He's a good man. I married him because I loved him and because he was accepted by my family. I wanted my mother to approve of my marriage.'

This woman is angry at her husband because he didn't make the dream come true. She says she doesn't blame her mother; that is supposed to mean that she's not angry with her – which is not the case at all. Side by side with the love she has for her mother is another emotion: fury. We have trouble understanding that we can be angry and forgiving at the same time. The two are not mutually exclusive. We think if we hate someone we hate them all the way through. This is to misunderstand the split between the conscious and the unconscious, between the adult self and the child.

The solution is not to call up mother and give her hell for what happened twenty years ago. *It is not today's mother we are in a rage with*. She probably wouldn't understand what we are talking about. Or mother may be dead – which does not mean we are not still angry at her. 'It is only when you understand the source of your anger,' says Dr Robertiello, 'that you may be able to stop displacing it onto your husband or yourself.'

There is a big difference between being angry at someone and 'blaming' them. If a psychotic comes up and socks you in the nose because he thinks you are his boss's wife, you may be angry, but you don't blame him. You can understand that he is not a responsible person. You might even be sympathetic. But still you got the slap in the face, it hurt, and you're angry. In a similar manner, perhaps what mother did or didn't do came from the best intentions. That doesn't lessen the sting. You were hurt. You were angry. 'So it behoves you,' says Dr Robertiello, 'to acknowledge your anger and not hide from it by saying, "Poor mom, she did the best she could." Just knowing that your anger is inappropriate to the present situation, that it is childish, helps put things in perspective. It frees you from having to relive the past situation in the present.'

Part of the problem is even when we are grown, the little girl within is still fixed, *vis-à-vis* mother, at some period of life so primitive, so imbued with leftover ideas of infantile omnipotence, that there is no distinction between anger and annihilation. Our unconscious won't allow us to feel, let alone express, our rage at mother. To do so brings with it the guilt and fear of killing her. 'Thoughts of rage against our mothers are just not acceptable,' says psychiatrist Dr Lilly Engler. 'The only thing more difficult to face is a mother's rage against the child. That is almost impossible. There's too much guilt.'

Besides headaches, depression, ulcers, and other illnesses, repressed anger can also take the form of sexual masochism – an abhorrent idea which is often gratuitously applied to all women. Freud found it in so many of his female patients he thought it was biological, that it came with our genes. He was wrong, of course. It is cultural and can be changed.

As an example of the roots of a particular kind of psychosexual masochism, take the mother who says to her child: 'You've been naughty. Wait till your father get home.' Says a young mother: 'In our house, discipline was always handled by my father. I'd be sent to my room to wait until he got home, and I'd sit there quivering. I was terrified of my father, and I would say that my fear of rejection from men stems from him. But even more than I feared him, I needed my mother's approval. It seemed she was the only bulwark I had against him. She dominated the household, including him. And so having established him as the fake authority figure, the bad guy, she would then use him. We would conspire together. If I were going out she'd say, "Be in by twelve, but if you're really having a good time, call me and I'll tell him it's not as late as he thinks."'

In time, this woman came to regard her mother as a victim of this terrifying male creature who had to be cajoled, lied to, and above all, controlled – or his savage temper would be loosed. She goes on:

'It was only when I got far enough away from home in distance and time that I began to see what a raw deal my father had. I used to think he was such an ogre, but my mother *ran him*. There is a parallel in my own marriage, in that I accepted the face-value aspect of my parents' marriage. When my husband would storm and rage at me – for ten years he told me I was frigid, castrating, and sexually nothing at all! – I accepted it. That's how men were supposed to be – perpetually storming and angry. I never could get mad back at him because my mother had shown me that a *real woman* handles a man with the soft answer and the cunning trick. If I stormed back at him, it would be acting like a man!'

When mother sets up the father as the daughter's disciplinarian, the unspoken message is: 'I'm mad at you, but I'm not going to express it because women don't. The bad guys, the sadists of the world, are men. That's what daddy is – he's going to hurt you.' Later, when the daughter is married, she does what she had been taught is woman's role: she looks to the man to put her down, to hurt her psychologically or even physically. She may hate it, but it feels right to her. It's what she's been taught to expect. She's a woman, isn't she?

Most important of all, and with dire consequences for women's sexuality, when she does feel angry she maneuvers the man to express it for her, as mother did. She projects her anger onto him. She tricks, goads, or taunts him into expressing his rage – for instance, by letting him somehow find out that the $20 dress really cost $75. Then she has the melancholy satisfaction of having made herself the victim of the man's anger. He is vile, but male. She is submissive, but female. The psychosexual pattern, established as a child, is lived out by the woman.

On the other hand, if our needs are to be as symbiotic and unseparate from our husband as possible, we will not do anything that might arouse his anger. Instead of using him to express our anger, we turn it inward. We feel we are failures, become insomniacs, compulsive housekeepers, victims of obsessive ideas of aging, death. One very frequent face this inner fear and anger wears is that of the controlling woman. The nagging, critical, hen-pecking little woman.

Says Dr Friedman: 'We think the controlling wife is so sure of herself. The opposite is true. Very often there is such a terror of *being* controlled or abandoned that she assumes control. A woman who had a very controlling mother often becomes inflexible herself because she has this fear of·becoming the helpless child again, on the bottom. She controls the man before he can control her or leave her. But the more she nags and controls him, the more she fears his retaliation – the more she becomes terrified he is going to get fed up and leave her. Any spontaneous impulse on his part must be checked because the next one might be the impulse to leave her.'

In human relations, fear is almost always counter-productive. The more a wife fears the husband will leave her, the more she nags, the more she will try to run him like a child. He gets fed up with all the tears, the going through his pockets for evidence, the anxiety. He goes.

As the girl watches her mother play martyr rather than express her anger directly, she learns techniques of masochistic manipulation. 'Oh, that's all right,' mother tells father, 'don't worry about me if you have to work tonight. I'll just have dinner alone.' This kind of nonexpressive, nonassertive behavior once again tells the girl she must bow to men's evil ways. The message is: 'Any resentment or anger that women might show is nothing compared to men with their tempers, ruthless business ethics, their delight in wars and the mayhem of Sunday pro-football games.' Techniques of passive-aggression are being taught – a method of letting the man know you are angry at him, all the while denying you are, giving him no handhold with which to grasp the problem. Passive-aggressive actions may be very subtle, not conscious or even verbal: withholding an appropriate response, for example. A classic case is the man who becomes aware that he has said or done 'something'. 'What's wrong?' he says to his wife, who has gone dead and silent on him. 'Oh, nothing,' she replies. She says it without feeling although everything about her – her face, body, her attitude and posture – is screaming that everything is wrong.

These methods of avoiding expression of anger create an alliance between the women in the family; often it is a method of avoiding sexual competition. Setting daddy up as the bogey man warns the daughter off from wanting to be close to such a stormy, hurtful creature. Only mother is unfailingly kind and nice. It is a way for mother to win the almost universal competition between the parents as to whom the child loves most.

After marriage, in any quarrel, the man is set up as the aggressor, we are the victim. We knew it would come to this. Men only bring pain. Men can't love. A basic insecurity is being expressed: it all depends on this other. His anger, loss, disappearance, or death wipe us out. We would be unnatural if we did not at times resent needing someone so much. But our very dependency forces us to smother any hostility. If the marriage breaks up, we have more to lose than he. Says Dr Sonya Friedman: 'Mothers tell their daughters. "It's up to you to make the marriage work. It takes 80 percent from you, only 20 percent from him." No wonder all the studies show that women tend to blame themselves for whatever goes wrong in a relationship.'

Except for sex. That is the man's job, 100 percent. If this is so, how is the wife to cope when sex doesn't run smooth? 'Sam couldn't keep his hands off me before we were married,' a young wife sadly says. 'Now he couldn't be less interested.' The only advice she gets from popular wisdom is to experiment on the safe margins: try a new perfume, go off for 'a second honeymoon' to Hawaii. Says Dr Schaefer: 'The wife is not conditioned to realize that she's just as responsible for their sexuality as he is. She can't imagine initiating sex in totally different ways, to vary the usual active/passive roles.' 'You're cold and frigid!' cries the man, his anger at peak because he knows he is at least half at fault. But he is the sexual expert. If he labels us a sexual dud, we believe him. It is *all* our fault.

It is only in some buried, central core of being that we know better. It is here where the residual anger lives.

There is little we can do about it. The power relation has been set since adolescence: We are the malleable clay, he is the master sculptor. Do with me as you will. The tyranny of the orgasm begins: true sex, real sex, orgasmically fulfilled sex with your husband will make a different woman of you, a real woman, a prettier woman, one more relaxed, more energetic, happy to be alive. In our secular society, a kind of sexual mysticism is one of our last faiths, and the 'right' orgasm comes to be its tangible sign.

It is a medical fact that many women report having wonderful feelings about sex without orgasm, just as it is true that many women have orgasms without sexual pleasure, or happiness. Freud's heavy legacy is the notion that 'vaginal orgasm' is in some mysterious manner the measure of womanliness or psychic health. 'A very dependent and neurotic woman can be very orgasmic,' says Dr Robertiello. 'In my clinical experience I have found women in the back wards of psychiatric hospitals who are multiorgasmic. There are other women who are well-functioning, who enjoy sex, but who have never had an orgasm in their lives. When we say there is a diminution of sexuality with the loss of the self in symbiosis, we must not confuse sex with orgasm. We don't know what makes some people have orgasms and others not. There are no exact correlations between sexual pleasure and orgasm.'

'The reason a woman chooses sex to demonstrate her rage,' says Sonya Friedman, 'is that it is the only weapon she has. On the surface her tendency is to accept the blame, but underneath, because she can't be assertive in any other way, she withholds sex. In almost every marital problem I see, there is sexual incompatibility. Men don't understand that sex doesn't begin in the bedroom. He thinks he can criticize her, yell that she's a lousy mother or housekeeper, and then take her into the bedroom where she'll receive him gladly. He has been able to separate love and sex, but most women cannot. For him, marriage is not the central core of his life. For the full-time wife and mother, *it is*.'

A significant number of women do not hold out on their husbands totally but use sex as a form of barter – candy for getting something she wants from him, when she feels guilty or afraid he might leave her. The penalty of turning sex into a commodity in this manner is that it – and she – are reduced to a cheap bribe, and the man who takes that foolish bribe is a chump. Respect is gone from marriage. So is romance and genuine excitement.

Withholding sex is not always a coldly conscious maneuver. The wife may get sudden headaches; she is tired, fatigued, she says the children may hear them, etc. It doesn't matter that by denying the man she is denying herself. She is gaining something preferable to sex in her state of dependency: the poisoned joys of control.

Says Dr Friedman: 'When a woman turns her anger upon herself and becomes nonsexual or nonorgasmic, she is doing several things. On an unconscious level, she refuses to give him the deepest part of herself, perhaps the only area in which she feels full control. Many women simply don't want to share sex with the man they are married to. I see a lot of women who are selectively orgasmic – just as some men are selectively impotent. It has nothing to do with technique. She is angry, bitter. She doesn't want to give this pleasure to him, to let him see her abandon herself. She doesn't want him to see he has this kind of power over her. She doesn't want to enhance his pleasure. If a woman goes into marriage thinking he must take care of her, which includes making her sexual, fully orgasmic and fulfilled, she's too frightened to tell him what she wants.'

Dr Friedman continues: 'To change this way of thinking in which the man is responsible not only for her sex but also for her orgasm is simply not possible for many women. Making herself understand that sex is for her own pleasure, something she actively does for herself, demands rethinking her entire sexual training.' We would rather be silent, angry, and asexual.

It is a common enough idea that orgasm correlates very strongly with the trust a woman feels for her sexual partner. 'If you are angry, wary, or suspicious,' says Dr Engler, 'then you feel you must control yourself. You have to control him too. If you are constantly trying to control, you can't let go and be spontaneous in sex or anything else.'

Some men are trustworthy and good as gold – and still their wives are unable to let their suspicions go. I do not think that ease in sex is merely a matter of faith in the man, or his knowledge of erotic tricks. Along with Erik Erikson, I believe 'basic trust' is first learned in the relationship to mother. Father is immensely important, of course, but unless he genuinely shared in our early mothering, it is years before he enters our life with any degree of significance. One of the fundamentals of our attitude toward our body is the attitude toward it of the person who held, bathed, and toilet-trained us. Was that father? Trust is the issue in sex. It may be altered, affected, augmented, or diminished by what goes on with men. It begins with mother.

Leah Schaefer once told me that when her mother refused to lend her the money that would help finance her training to become a therapist, the resulting anger gave her courage enough to write her book *Women and Sex*. 'But from the time I began my research,' says Dr Schaefer, 'my relationship with my mother improved. It may have taken anger to get there, but increased anger was not the result of facing it. The opposite was true. My relationship to my mother improved to the day she died because I was released from my old rages against her.'

The child is afraid to sexually defy mother. The woman carries her inhibitions with her into experiences with men, but now he is the one at fault: he did not 'give' her an orgasm. And yet, simple logic tells us that either partner can only be 50 percent responsible. It is easier to blame our husbands than to rearouse our buried furies at mother.

Nevertheless, if the rages of childhood are faced and

expressed – if only to ourselves – they do not kill any real love between mother and daughter. I am beginning to see that there is nothing I can ever do that will destroy my mother. I can be as sexual, as free, as different from her in my work and life as I choose, but can have a relationship with her too. It will be far more real than the mythic All-Loving Mommy I had been unconsciously holding out for.

I had always resented feeling that to keep my mother's love and approval I had to be perfect. I had to show her what she wanted to see, and not the me who had grown up in the years away from her. What I know now is that this pact I had set up killed any chance of being myself whether I was with her or not. And wasn't I doing the same to her?

We make our own ghosts.

CHAPTER TWELVE

A Mother Dies. A Daughter is Born.
The Cycle Repeats

During our honeymoon I began to menstruate two weeks early. It had never happened before. I took it as a sign: the mystery of marriage was full upon me. Ten months later, I had a pregnancy scare.

The words are apt because I was as terrified as a sixteen-year-old. Marriage had once loomed like The End of adventure. Now pregnancy threatened like the finish of life itself. With the fervor of a nun, I prayed I was mistaken.

I went to a young American doctor on one of those pretty, shady streets just off the Via Veneto, who confounded me still more with his disdain for a married woman who did not want to be a mother. Afterward I met Bill at the Café de Paris. We sat at one of the cramped tables indoors instead of our usual place on the sidewalk with a view of the afternoon *passagiata*. Bill ordered me a brandy. I was shaking. What was so terrible? Why were we acting like two conspirators hiding from the consequences of a dubious act? We thought it had to do with not being able to afford a family yet. We wanted more time for ourselves. Or so we said. The idea that we simply did not want to be parents was something neither could voice.

I don't think I was really married until two or three years after we'd gone through the ceremony. 'Playing at marriage' was how I'd describe that first year in our pretty apartment in Rome. Play-acting in a foreign country. How can the mere signing of a document change a life? Young girls imagine being married so long; when reality comes, it seems a dream. It took me time to become a wife, to give up my fantasies of what marriage would be. I did not love Bill that first year or two, not as I would grow to. I was right to be worried that day. Children, Bill and I had decided, would come later. We were both still absorbed in our marriage. Bill was beginning a new career, as a writer. We were young. We never doubted that one day we would be parents. Not now.

Several years later my mother and I were going through a revolving door in Bergdorf Goodman's when I caught the tail end of a sentence: '. . . and the magazine said that birth defects are more frequent among couples who do not have sex frequently . . .' *What?*

Had my mother said that? By the time I caught up to her, she was deep into discussions about the palest shade of lipstick with the saleswoman at the Estée Lauder counter. My mother's medicine cabinet is filled with barely used tubes and vials of cosmetics. They are the softest colors available but she still can't bear to use them. I wasn't sure whether I wanted to pick up on her comment. She settled the issue by buying us each a lipstick brush and heading for the shoe department. She had always avoided any discussion of sex.

'Can't you two write about anything else?' she would ask. 'Don't you know there are other things in life?' It was never really criticism – these half-embarrassed, half-titillated remarks over martinis. She was playing her part. We had ours: to be 'different', not like her neighbors' children, not like my sister, who'd had three children in the first four years of marriage.

I have always wondered if I blew it that day at Bergdorf's. Was it a mother-daughter talk on babies she was after? I think not. She had all the grandmother role she could handle: my sister spoke to her daily about the children, relied on her for advice and financial support, and suffered her constant criticism; which my mother took as her right. My sister might be a mother herself but in my mother's eyes she is still thirteen, wears too much make-up, talks too fast, overdresses, and shouldn't smoke.

No, to this day I do not think my mother was urging me to get on with beginning a family. Out of her own dark history of being left with two babies to raise on her own when she was twenty, I feel she was obscurely trying to warn me that there are unpredictable hazards in marriage, that all the lovely fantasies of motherhood do not automatically come true at the end of nine months, and that there is sometimes a stiff price to pay. More than being put off by Bill's and my 'preoccupation' with sex, she was warming her hands at our fire, trying to tell me that if I became a mother, this quality in us that she enjoys might be lost. To this day, I don't think she regrets that Bill and I decided not to have children.

Four years ago I went off the pill. We were living in England and a close friend was having a baby. My London doctor – like gynecologists in every country we'd lived – kept pointing at the clock and making doomsday noises: I was not getting younger. What is frightening is that I don't remember Bill and me sitting down to have a discussion about parenthood. We seemed to have come to this crossroad of our lives by an almost negative route: since we had always assumed one day we would have children, when the time struck me as right – a friend of my own age having her first baby – he just went along with it.

'We drifted into that decision-without-making-a-decision,' Bill recently said. 'Neither one of us was expressing his own wishes. We had not gone along with conventional ideas about jobs, career, money, where and how to live, or what we wanted out of marriage. But this one was too big, too deeply implanted in us. In our own defense, we have to remember this was before the whole nonparenthood movement came to consciousness. Still, backing into that decision to have a child meant we'd lost confidence in ourselves. We were surrendering to unconscious assumptions about what the world seemed to be asking of us. *They were right*. Never to have a child was too large a decision to question by our own values. As for me, I was undercut in my reluctance by feeling I must be strange, inhuman, not to want to be a father. Alienation from my true feelings made me indecisive and passive. I didn't feel I had the right to make you live by my strangeness.'

The whole exercise wasn't an idea I entered into passionately either, merely one I assented to, and with less weighing of the pro and con than the decision to move to another country. Nevertheless, since my friend had had trouble conceiving, I too began taking my temperature every morning and keeping charts. I even went into the hospital for a day to have everything checked, to be sure I was in tip-top shape for the trip. (In the back of my mind were ten years of gynecologists' queries: 'What, never been pregnant, never had an abortion?' they would say, giving no points at all for carefulness.) I was going to be as responsible about having a baby as I'd been about not having one. Once pronounced in perfect running order, I set about getting pregnant.

The dispassionate nonquestioning of the decision still puzzles me. Like Bill, perhaps I too thought I didn't have the right to keep fatherhood from him. It is frightening to think that we, who always discussed every aspect of our lives together, were so passive and silent about this. Being married, living together, moving around the world as we willed – *that* was natural for us. To have a child – *that* was the really radical thing for us to do, not our style, not born of our own imagination. And yet we accepted it, even though we knew that if I did conceive, our lives would be totally and dramatically changed. With no guarantee at all that the change would be for the better.

I was passionate about one aspect of motherhood: it must be a boy. The idea of a little Bill with dark hair and big brown eyes was a wonderful fantasy. Growing up without a father, I told myself that I'd had enough of living with women. Nothing but a boy would do, I said to Bill, as we were driving to Mexico on a shaky assignment that might enable us to live there a year. Infrequent as our talks were about children, joke as I might about my insistence on a boy, I was deadly serious about not wanting a daughter. Something in me knew I would never, for instance, let her take journeys like this into the unknown. I would be a mother more afraid for her daughter than for herself.

*   *   *

Two months after I went off the pill I was back on it. Once again it was not really a conscious decision about motherhood. Work demanded we return to New York; starting a family was being postponed as haphazardly as it had been entertained. A year later I switched from the pill to a diaphragm, and about two years ago Bill and I decided not to have children. No, to put it correctly, the decision went like this: One day he said, 'Isn't it a good thing that we didn't have children?'

Today I look over my history of contraceptions, pregnancy scares, temperature charts, and I wonder what the hell two intelligent people were doing, never consciously making a decision about one of the most important steps in their lives. I said that I wasn't really married until the second or third year; today, the way I am married makes the first six years look like an acquaintance. I sometimes tell Bill I don't even mind growing old so long as we're together. The life we have made, the kind of marriage we have applied talent and imagination to create, would change if there were a child. No matter how much we loved that child, no matter how good parents we were, Bill and I would be different, I do not know that it would be better. I know the kind of wife I am, and I have an idea of the kind of mother I would have been.

Those things I like best in myself are never far from the things I like least: anxiety, which I hope brings a creative tension to my work, fear that makes me want to be close to someone. To the degree that on any given day that I can believe in what my husband feels for me, and in my work, that is the degree to which I have surmounted that day's residual anxiety of being my mother's daughter. I can handle the anonymous telephone call in the night, my fears of failure and success, the neighbors' opinions. They no longer run me because I acknowledge the space between the me I am today and the me I used to be. I can pull it off for myself. But if I had a daughter, I could never trust that she could be as lucky. That space between autonomy and fear would narrow and I would make her anxious with my own anxiety. To protect her I would limit her world, and thereby my own. It would put what I have with

Bill and my work into question. I would be my mother's daughter all over again.

When I was interviewing Helene Deutsch for this book, she spoke of the maternal instinct. 'Are you telling me, Dr Deutsch,' I asked with some incredulity, 'that one day I'm going to wish I'd been a mother?' 'Yes,' she said without hesitation, 'You will always regret never having had a child.' Even now words like this fill me with anxiety. They seem to speak the wisdom of the ages. A moment later I have my certainty back. Today, should a person talk about these regrets, my reply would be that I will never try sky diving, or be the President of the United States. These must be very fulfilling too. I have learned to live without them.

I don't expect my story is exactly like any other woman's but I suspect most of us have had ideas like these. I will always have a fantasy of a son. I imagine Bill talking to him about the books he read when he was a boy, Norse mythology, and *The Water Babies*. Because I have decided not to have a child doesn't mean I never dream of what might have been.

Let's begin with a story of classical mother-daughter role-modeling:

Peggy is cooking her first big meal for her parents since her marriage – a glorious Virginia ham. Standing up to carve, her new husband asks Peggy why she sliced off three or four inches from the shank end before baking. Peggy looks surprised. 'Mother always does it that way.'

Everyone at the table looks at Peggy's mother. 'That's how my mother did it too,' she says, a bit puzzled. 'Doesn't everyone?'

Peggy phones her grandmother the next day, and asks why, in their family, has the shank end always been cut off before baking. 'I've always done it that way,' grandmother says, 'because that is how my mother did it.'

It happens that four generations of women are still alive in this family. A call is put in to great-grandmother, and the mystery is solved. Once when her daughter – Peggy's grandmother – was a little girl and learning to cook, they were baking a large ham. The family roasting pan was small, and so the shank end had been cut off to make it fit.

Four generations of women, each one ignoring present reality, each one conforming, unquestioningly, to a circumstance that was no longer relevant; each one certain in her mind 'that's how you do it' because she had seen her mother do it that way. An amusing story, an illustration of how we incorporate those parts of mother we choose to imitate – like her skill in cooking – but right along with them we also take in less rational and unexamined aspects all unaware.

It is here that one of the great feminine mysteries begins. Everyone else can see we've taken in many of mother's most negative character traits; we cannot. We deny it, treat the imputation as an accusation, get angry and deny it again. And yet one day we realize that we are acting to our daughter exactly in the same repressive way mother once acted to us. How did it happen? We swore it never would. We would show our child only the wonderful warmth and love we got from mother. As for the rest – mother's nagging, anxiety, sexual timidity and general lack of adventurousness – why, we would just leave them out. And yet, generation after generation of daughters become women still carrying the inheritance of mother's sad luggage, passing it on to daughters of their own.

Why does the cycle repeat?

Says Dr Schaefer: 'There are times when I catch a glimpse of myself in the mirror, and I hate the way I look. It is when I most look like my mother. It's a kind of driven expression she used to have when she was busy with one of her projects. When I was a child, I was very close to my mother. I adored her, but when I saw that purposeful, nothing-will-get-in-my-way look on her face, I hated it. Lately, I've realized it wasn't the driven trait I hated in my mother. It was how she *behaved toward me* when she was this way. It meant she was so busy with her charity work that she would ignore me.

'I couldn't admit to myself that I hated her. I had to think it was the driven *quality* that I disliked. In other words, I was saying that this characteristic was not my mother. My real mother – she was this other good, kind person who always had time for me. This driven, purposeful side of her was a foreign aspect, someone else. *I had split the good mother off from the bad one.* I refused to recognize the bad side. Then, when I had a daughter of my own, I came to realize that Katie hated me for having this same quality. When I was finishing my thesis I was locked away in my office for weeks. One night Katie said to me, "I hate you, I don't like you anymore. Stay in your office forever." I felt awful. I had ignored her in the same way my mother had me. I had repeated exactly what I hated most about my mother.'

The pathos of the parental double bind is in this story. Mother didn't nag or restrict us because she was cruel. Dr Schaefer didn't lock herself away from her daughter because she was selfish. There was a lot of reality in Leah Schaefer's need to write her thesis, get her degree, complete her training; she had to support herself and her daughter. Remembering her own unhappiness as a child when her mother was unavailable to her, one might think she would have *made* more time for her daughter. That is not how the unconscious works. Since she was acting as her mother had, *it felt right*. To maintain her tie to her own mother, to avoid anger at that mother of childhood, Leah Schaefer *became* her mother.

Why do daughters repeat in their lives many aspects of mother, including those they hated? Says Dr Robertiello: 'Two mechanisms are at work. *Role-modeling* is largely conscious, and has a lot to do with those parts of the "good" mother we liked. For this reason, it is usually the work of a moment's introspection to see that mother's ease with strangers, and our skill at entertaining, are connected. At some point, role-modeling shades into *introjection*. This process is harder to understand because it is mostly un-conscious, and is marked by a lot of repressed anger directed against the "bad" mother. We take in her negative aspects in order not to see them in her. If they are in us, we don't have to hate her – and run the risk of her retaliatory anger. We are the bad ones. The evil, split half of mother has been introjected.'

Even a child who has been deserted or sent away cannot think, 'Mother doesn't want me.' She has to rationalize. 'Mother loves me, but is punishing me because I've done this or that bad thing. The fault is not in mother. She is trying to correct me. She is sending me away out of love, so I'll learn to be better. She is good. The badness is in me.'

A more everyday example might be when mother refuses to let us go to the movies with friends. We hate her, splitting her off from the good mother who bought us a pretty dress yesterday. However, should one of our friends say, 'That's mean, your mother is too strict,' we rush to mom's defense. 'Oh, no, I probably deserve it,' we say. 'I've been a real pain around the house lately.' We don't like to hear our parents, especially mother, criticized by others. It externalizes the bad mother, threatening release of our pent-up rage, which would destroy the relationship. It is easier, safer to feel we are bad, not she.

This process is automatic, unthinking, unconscious and inevitable. The child cannot take the fearful loneliness that hating mother brings. Introjection is an almost mindless union in the depths of being, a merger at the level of the baby who could not hear – and indeed could not survive – being separated from mother.

In ideal developmental circumstances, by the end of the first year the child will have fused the image of the good and bad mother into one person – she will have come to the realistic conclusion that mother is a mixture of both. This is a highly sophisticated idea, a judgment of such difficult and mature perception that even adults have difficulty with it. We get stuck with a kind of dichotomous view of the people with whom we are intimately involved, repeating with them the split we never resolved with mother. If we get mad at our husband, he becomes the biggest bastard in the world, and our entire marriage to date has been a mistake; the next day, when he brings us flowers, we realize that he's really the sweetest guy of all time. It is a child's way of seeing the world – the way we liked to see movies when we were little. The white hats were all good. The black hats were all bad. Any effort on the screenwriter's part to show us that there was shades of gray in the good guys, some redeeming features in the bad, ended by confusing us. It is only when we are able to achieve a higher level of psychic integration that we can accept others as a mix of good and bad and not swing to extremes when they disappoint or hurt us.

In his book *The Uses of Enchantment,* Dr Bruno Bettelheim examines why so many fairy tales of witches and deadly dragons survive – even though they were passed down through the centuries unwritten – while most published contemporary and supposedly 'creatively healthy' children's stories are soon forgotten. As each generation verbally passes on the version of what it heard from the generation before, all unnecessary, contingent, or purely personal elements are dropped. The dross is burned away. Only those elements with golden meaning for every succeeding age survive. In the end, says Dr Bettelheim, fairy tales become universal stories, 'communicating in a manner which reaches the uneducated mind of the child . . . [they speak to the child's] budding ego and encourage its development, while at the same time relieving preconscious and unconscious pressures.'

One of the elements that gives the old fairy tales their power is the frequency with which they deal in images of the mother, split into good and bad. Cinderella is treated miserably by the cruel stepmother, but the kind fairy godmother makes her into a princess. In story after story, there is this opposition between a wicked stepmother, or evil old fairy, and a protective, magical figure who is on the child's side. In writing about how Little Red Riding Hood's grandmother suddenly turns into a wolf wearing the benevolent old lady's clothes, Dr Bettelheim says, 'How silly a transformation when viewed objectively, and how frightening . . . But when viewed in terms of a child's ways of experiencing, is it really any more scary than the sudden transformation of his own kindly grandma into a figure who threatens his very sense of self when she humiliates him for a pants-wetting accident? To the child, grandma is no longer the same person she was just a moment before; she has become an ogre.'[2]

As we grow up, we repress the attachment the needy child within still has to the powerful mother of infancy, and come to the seemingly mature conclusion, 'Oh, well, there are some parts of mother I don't like, but I understand why she was that way. They are not important.' The 'bad' parent is being ignored. We both know and don't know there are parts of mother we dislike.

While we are young enough to live at home, there is even a degree of tolerance for those aspects of mother that irritate. We can afford to see them because separation anxiety is not too great: we are both living under the same roof. We may hate or rage at mother, but there she is, waiting. An hour later, a kiss and a few tears, and symbiosis is back, strong as ever. Even if we are not affectionate, she is physically near, available.

As we get older and the tie to mother is weakened by physical or psychological separation, introjection gathers momentum. When we move into an apartment of our own, when we find a job, take a lover, get married and have a child of our own – in all these important rites of passage away from her, as we take one step forward, we take another one back, and find ourselves doing things her way. *Becoming like her overcomes our separation anxieties*.

It is a kind of symbolic rapprochement. Just as the infant who crawls away from mama into the next room gets frightened and rushes back for confirmation that she is still there, so, emotionally, as we edge away from mother in our adult lives, do we incorporate parts of her. Having her with us – *in* us – makes the journey less fearsome.

We are offered a promotion at the office. It is deserved, we can do the work. But mother's entire life warned us, a long time ago, that people don't like aggressive women. We decide to stay with the job we've been doing. 'I'm not all that competitive,' we say, 'not career mad.' We have lovers but are never free of mother's anxiety that men will trick and desert us. It is unsettling. We can almost see ourselves, split into a double image: the woman who goes to bed with men and enjoys sex, the woman who wakes up the next morning already wondering, Will he telephone tonight? These are mother's fears. Which woman are we? We are both.

The process of introjection continues even if we never see mother any more, even if she is dead or living in Paris. It is not the present mother who is being introjected, but that bad one of long ago, whom we could not afford to 'know' was making us so unhappy we hated her. When we have an outburst of fury at someone, how often is it because what that person is doing makes us aware of something we dislike in ourselves?

When we were little and saw mama running her house, we admired how firm she was with the repairman who did a bad job, the department store that sent the wrong bill. She spoke her mind, got the job done. We're as good at these things as she. But we also remember her panic when father was driving and took a wrong turn, how angry she got over spilled milk, her fear of noises in the house when alone. Above all, we have introjected her anxiety about sex.

Marriage is our chance at last to become as sexually daring as we would like. Instead, we are preoccupied with furniture, neatness, entertaining. The clothes we wore when we were single had plunging necklines. Now we run to suburban styles that don't raise an eyebrow. The reason sex was easier when we were single was that we had never seen mother unmarried and without a child. This was a role we could create on our own. She was far away – emotionally, at least – and we felt the zip of at least temporary separation. Marriage reunites us with her. To openly declare our sexuality now would make us too different from the picture of how she was as a wife. We would have to face our anger at last at that frustrating mother who hated the sexual pleasure we wanted from the time we were infants, who made us renounce it to keep her love.

When we become mothers ourselves, introjection speeds up even more. When we hold our little girl in our arms, we are reminded of mother, feel at one with her, as never before. Since sex was always a powerful force toward individuation, it is hardly surprising that sex is one of the first things to go.

To please mother, we gave up the right to our bodies and erotic gratification when we were little. Now when baby touches her genitals, we don't just frown. As mother did to us, we take her hand away. We become child-centered caretakers, madonnas, 'not always thinking about sex'. Mother used to be the enemy of sex. We are tired of the war. For our daughter's sake, and our own, we join her. Continuity is preserved.

When we were single, the joys of sexuality were their own reward and reinforcement. Allowing the same autonomy to our daughter is too risky. We have no models of a mother who encourages her daughter's sexuality. To ensure our little girl does not get any funny ideas, we present her with the right one: a nonsexual image of ourselves. Nothing must excite forbidden thoughts in our daughter. Soon, nothing excites them in us either.

Most women I interview are aware they became less sexual after motherhood, but cannot say why. They were too tired, they had to listen for the baby's cries, etc. Good reasons, but not convincing. If you want something badly enough, you establish priorities so you get it. Child psychologist Helen Prentiss looks at the issue subjectively and objectively:

'Before my daughter was born, I had been very proud of my sexual union with my husband. More than anything, I felt this distinguished me from the kind of woman my mother was. But when I became pregnant, I began to lose this contact with him, with the feeling I'd always had opposite him. I knew Jack loved my body, but that was my old slim body. How could he be turned on by this fat lady? He would put his arms around me, start kissing me, but I would make excuses. It felt wrong, sex, and me almost a mother. I was into this whole other picture of myself – one of those warm clean, dedicated mothers you see in women's magazines. Those pretty women don't have sex! They're good mothers, and I was going to be one too.

'My own mother being around a great deal speeded this

idea. She was always dropping by with clothes for the baby, helping me fix the nursery. It was very reassuring to have her around because I was a little scared. Even though I was teaching courses in child psychology, being responsible for a baby loomed up as a frightening responsibility. Just as my mother had always steered away from "knowing" about the strong sexuality Jack and I had between us, so did she steer right into knowing all about my pregnancy. Suddenly she seemed to have all the answers, just as she hadn't had any before I was pregnant. She told me about her pregnancies. She even admitted having doubts about being a good mother!

'As she and I became closer, my physical thing with Jack diminished. It was as though I couldn't have both – my closeness with her and with Jack. Sex became something silly or frivolous, perhaps a bit shameful, that you did before you became a mother. Now that I was pregnant, well, this was serious business, and those long hours in bed, those nights and mornings Jack and I used to spend exploring one another, closed away from the world – they seemed like selfish devilishness, kid stuff. So, you see, because I entered into motherhood without any clear assessment of myself, of my priorities in my own life and with my husband, I just automatically slipped into this picture of my own mother. Unwittingly and without any hesitation in the world, I gave up one of the most important things in my life and with my husband – our sexual tie.

'It was as though I'd been programmed from birth like some female Manchurian Candidate. I just allied with my mother in this feminine mystery she and I shared, and Jack was left out – some Dagwood Bumstead who perhaps had been necessary to get the whole thing started, but now it was time for him to get out and let us women handle the realities of life. It was almost as though what I was setting up with my mother was against him!'

Dr Prentiss went on to say that while she knew – theoretically, intellectually, from everything she had read and lectured on herself – that it is necessary for a mother to be as symbiotic as possible with her baby during the first months of life, this union should not be allowed to interfere with what goes on between husband and wife. 'There's a six-week prohibition against sex after the baby is born. Well, in my case six grew into ten, and what with me listening for the baby every time Jack touched me and feeling like this Super Mother, I would say, *"Jack, please!"* in this tone of indignation, as though he'd touched the Holy Grail.

'In my mind, I knew that without a connection to your adult identity, you stay symbiotically tied to your baby long beyond the period when you should let your child start to separate. Sex is the call of the adult world, reminding you of who you are. Reminding you that you may be a mother, but you are a woman too, a wife. But deeply as this knowledge was planted in me, something deeper, more unconscious, was working too. Sex had always been one of the strongest forces working on me to get out in the world, to leave home and become my own person. I loved my mom but I wanted a bigger life, and when I met Jack, sex with him became the final definition that divided me, in my mind's eye, from the picture of my mom. I was a different kind of woman, or so I thought. Holding this baby in my arms changed all that. It never occurred to me that Jack might like to be included in taking care of Sally during those first months. And since I seemed to have no confidence in him, he lost whatever confidence he might have had in himself. He stopped volunteering. So there I was – a case out of one of my own textbooks. Symbiotically tied to my baby, reunited with my mother, and excluding my husband from "our" (me, my baby, and my mother's) life!

'I got an enormous amount of emotion from this thing with my baby. And my libido, if you want to use those kinds of terms, was very much directed toward the baby. All my libidinal energy went there. My body was still not the beautiful body it used to be, my narcissistic view of myself was diminished. I just didn't feel like a sexual woman. I can see now that all my old notions – all my mother's old notions – had come back: that sex was dirty, or selfish. *It was unmotherly.*

A Mother Dies. A Daughter is Born. The Cycle Repeats

'If you don't think about sex during those first months when you are so meshed with your baby, you wake up six years later not a woman, but a mom. Being sexual and being a person with a strong sense of who she is are ideas that are very tied together. Women cannot focus on this enough. It is hard enough to be sexual people before we become mothers. The outside world may see us as sexual women, but inside we are not at home with that idea ourselves. It's so easy – and dangerous – to lapse back into being a "nice lady", a mother. Giving yourself to union with your child at the beginning of your baby's life is healthy and necessary. After that, it is resignation from the problems, joys, and pleasures of an adult life of your own.'

Resignation or not, it is what most women do. 'Not in front of the children,' sounds like a musical-comedy joke, but it is a fact of marital life. We gladly make the sacrifice because it is 'for our child's good'. The idea is debatable. Frustration and anger lie just behind the curtain we have pulled down between ourselves and our sexuality.

If we have to sacrifice so much for her good, well – she'd better be damned good. We are determined not to be as inhibiting as our own mothers, but much stricter codes of conduct are enforced on our daughters than our sons. After the latest outburst at the girl, we sit down and get hold of ourselves. Never again! How frightening it used to be when we were little to have mother furious. And so we start out once more with the best intentions: to be calm, cool, kind, to let her do things her way. But even as we act out this part, an inner anger comes up to sabotage all good intents. It is not possible to be this 'perfect' mother without comparing the ideal way we are trying to act, with the restrictive way mother used to be. To see this comparison too clearly would be to become furious at the old 'bad' mother hidden in the unconscious. This rage would separate us from her. That is intolerable. The anger gets diverted, back onto ourselves, onto our husband, the unfairness of the world in general. Part of it inevitably spills out onto the daughter.

Why should she get this perfect treatment when we had such

a hard time? One part of our anger becomes subverted, and is experienced as a kind of forgiveness. 'When women have children of their own,' says Dr Mio Fredland, 'they begin to feel much more empathetic with their mothers. They make up old quarrels. They realize what their mother's life was like. They forgive whatever obscure angers have plagued them in the past, and they become loving and close. Especially if they have a daughter. There's a strange kind of direct line between mother, daughter, and granddaughter. My own mother told me that while she loves my brother's children, she doesn't have this same feeling about them as she does about my little girl. They didn't come out of the uterus of the child she carried in her own uterus. My mother looks ahead to the child my daughter will bear in time, and sees her own immortality. She is transformed by the idea, rejuvenated.'

'A major reason,' says Dr Sirgay Sanger, 'why women's anger at the mother often diminishes when they have a child is that the good mother image can now be acted out in real life. The negative, internalized image can be repressed, and there is the existence now of a new capacity – to love the new baby with a pure, unfettered giving of one's self. This is the mother one wished to have and to be. There often exists a euphoria after birth that women radiate. It casts a glow of warmth over her family, her husband, and friends. It is also biologically necessary for the early growth and development of the infant. Post-partum depression in some ways is not a depression of the usual variety. It is a limiting of the euphoria. The woman's feeling that here is her chance to heal and solidify her sense of being a worthwhile and productive person has been punctured. The desire – "I want to be a good mother to my infant" – explains why some women who never asserted themselves before can say no now in the name of that infant. The wish for a perfect mother has been transformed into becoming that perfection.'

You hear it again and again: 'When I became a mother, I began to understand what my mother went through. I'm not so mad at her anymore.' Fine – unless this forgiveness goes beyond healthy recognition of the real problems of motherhood and becomes the strengthening of the original symbiosis. Does this 'understanding' mean identification with everything in mother we once hated? Does rapprochement give us permission to act as she did, to overprotect our daughter and so limit her separation? Is the green light on once again for bringing all mother's old anxiety, nagging, sexual repression and inhibition to bear upon another generation?

When we have a child, we think we will be able to give up the old symbiotic need of mother (call it by what name you will), and find new security with our baby. Instead of needing someone to take care of us, we will be happily fulfilled by taking care of someone else. This is a kind of distorted notion of separation: because I will be most tied to my infant daughter, I will be less dependent on my mother for union and strength.

To nobody's surprise, the new mother finds the need for her own mother increasing. By this I don't mean the need for physical help and practical advice so much as the longing for an emotional reconciliation, a bonding with her. Now, more than any other time in our lives, when we hold our helpless baby in our arms, we cannot afford the old angers at mother. Ironically, mom herself is mellowing, becoming more like the mother we always hoped she would be. But not to us – to our little girl.

Says psychologist Liz Hauser: 'My mother was loving and patient with my daughter Liza and would play cards with her for hours. When I was little, I got the idea that you should always be doing something productive. So I don't have the patience for cards. She didn't smother Liza as she did me because there was enough separation. That's why it is so much easier to be a grandmother. The sticky symbiosis never began, so you don't bring all that anxiety and fear to the relationship, the need to hold on. As for me – no sooner do I get through listening to a patient tell me how much she hated it when her mother nagged her, than I'll go home and begin on Liza. "Look at your room!" It's so hard to remember to do things differently with your daughter than your mother did with you.'

Before motherhood, we tried to find with men and other women what we missed with mother. Our husbands may have failed us in that search for a perfect, blissful union. (How could he not?) Becoming a mother ends the search. We will never be alone again. We will find in the bond with our baby's need for us an identity we can recognize, all the emotion we want.

Says the poet Anne Sexton in 'The Double Image':

> I, who was never quite sure
> about being a girl, needed another
> life, another image to remind me.
> And this was my worst guilt; you
>   could not cure
> nor soothe it. I made you find me.[3]

'As a new mother,' says Liz Hauser, 'part of what you're looking for in this heavenly blurring of dependency and closeness between you and your child is the desire to be taken care of yourself. If you didn't get enough mothering when you were a baby, this is your chance to do the mothering. It is as if you can make up to the baby for what you didn't get yourself. So in your befuddled, symbiotic way, you get the feeling of tight attachment and unending love. *But you are not the one being taken care of.* The child is getting it all. There is an immense satisfaction in being a mother but not the kind of satisfaction you wanted. You are not the child in this relationship. You are the mother. This is the problem of symbiosis: undefined boundaries. You don't know where you leave off and the child begins. Eventually you become angry because your child is not satisfying your needs.'

Dr Hauser may be speaking in terms of psychological theory, but she is speaking from the inside too. She is a mother with a daughter of her own. All the women quoted in this chapter are both mothers and professionals trained to handle symbiotic problems. And yet they could not avoid nonseparation themselves when they had children. The almost hypnotic way symbiosis took them over is a warning of how delusory may be the boast, 'I'm raising my daughter in a totally different way than my mother raised me.'

Dr Hauser continues: 'To think your daughter is somehow going to make up for what you missed yourself as a baby is like hanging around a bakery when you're hungry and just smelling the brownies. It isn't satisfying, but it's irresistible: at least you are *around* mothering. Eventually, of course, out of this unsatisfied hunger are born the terrible angers that mothers feel. Their children are "selfish" and "ungrateful" – angers that are all the worse because they are so defended against and unadmitted. But if you stop to think about it, you can see that the mother who is raging against her child because the child isn't giving her enough, isn't grateful enough – she has turned the tables around. It is as if the mother is the baby, screaming at *her* mother for love. She's twenty, thirty, forty years old, and she's still raging for that tight, all-encompassing love infants need.

'One of the first things I heard when I was studying psychology,' she continues, 'was the remark, "Of course she's hostile. She's dependent, and dependent people have to be hostile." That idea stuck with me. It's simple, but it is the whole dynamic. If you're utterly dependent, then you're always waiting for someone to give you a handout – even if it is a small baby. You expect that baby to *give* to you, and in that sense you are dependent on your child.

'I've made these mistakes, felt these angers myself. I love Liza and I get a tremendous feeling when I make her happy. But sometimes it's like there's an endless request going on. This is natural to a child, but to the mother, it can seem like the little girl is a bottomless pit. You can't satisfy her. You want her to stop and be happy at what she's got. Your anger boils up. I can remember so vividly being on the other end and hearing the words I say to Liza from my own mother: "Now, you've already had this, we've done that together, you should be grateful you have so much and not keep asking for more and more . . ." This is why women should be aware of separation before they decide to become mothers. They should run checks on themselves after the baby is born. For instance, when you get terribly angry at a child that's been crying and won't stop, ask yourself if the intensity of your anger at that moment isn't derived from your own frustrations that the baby is making you miserable when you want *her* to make *you* happy. All those feelings of closeness and security and mother love you've been dreaming about – where's your payoff?'

There is a story ascribed to Freud about an eagle who had to bring her three children to safety when a flood covered the earth and they were too young to fly the great distance. She picked up the first child in her talons and began to fly. 'I will always be grateful to you, Mother,' said the baby eagle. 'Liar', said the mother, and dropped him into the flood. The same thing happened with the second child. When the mother picked up the third little eagle and began flying him to safety, this eaglet said, 'I hope I will be as good a parent to my children as you are to me.' The mother saved that child.

The debt of gratitude we owe our mother and father goes forward, not backward. What we owe our parents is the bill presented to us by our children. Having a daughter is one of life's fulfillments, but to expect her to reward us in a time, place or manner of our choosing is to distort the nature of the parent-child relationship.

Over vast periods of time, the process of evolution weeds out any trait that is not fundamental to the survival of the race. Conversely, anything on which the race depends cannot be left to whim, fashion, or accident: it must be carried forward in the gene. I believe the rewards of motherhood are biologically imbued, but the degree of satisfaction can vary with circumstances. The new mother who feels her baby nursing at her breast does not have to be told she is happy. A slum mother with nine children who finds she is again pregnant may feel differently. Biology and anatomy go on whether we like it or not. The unmarried mother may decide she will have her baby put out for adoption. When the baby is born she is suddenly caught up in a rush of emotion. She wants to keep the baby. She is certain her decision is right. Is she? There is no 'correct' answer. What I wish to discuss here is individual choice. Motherhood furnishes great feelings of worth and value, function and pleasure. The question some women are beginning to ask is, Is there something else I would rather do with my life that would be more satisfying still? In a recent public-opinion poll, three out of four people – men and women alike – thought it OK for women not to have children.[4] My own feeling is that this reflects our changing attitudes – not necessarily our deepest feelings: *It's OK for other people, not me*. But if most women don't think of marriage without children as a permissible option, can it be said that they *chose* to be mothers.

Says Dr Prentiss: 'My own story sounds like I made a conscious decision about motherhood, but it was only an illusion. As a child I always felt I was getting only my mother's "official" emotions – what she thought would be good for me. Not her real emotions. And so I learned to show her only what she wanted to see, the daughter in me – not the full person. The result was that while we were loving, it was not very honest. This is what I wanted to make up for in children of my own. Especially a little girl, because I could understand a girl's feelings. But don't let me mislead you. It sounds like I was deciding to have a baby for this reason or that. The fact is that I never decided at all I would or would not have a baby. I never consciously felt I had a choice. I always assumed I would get married and have a child. It was part of the sequence that was already set up for me. I just knew I would be a mother. Every woman was. This kind of automatic falling into a role has caused me and my daughter a lot of trouble.'

Having a child is still so expected of us, so programmed into our development, that we drift into what is perhaps the most important act of our lives. Our reason for becoming mothers – difficult as they may be to get at – are the first clue as to whether we will maintain our own identity, and let our child grow into a person – individual and separate from us.

The manner in which a woman relates to her child is one of the marks of her development – or arrested development. If she related symbiotically to her mother, and does the same with her husband, it cannot be said she has grown. Only the cast of characters has changed. In time, the wife may become a bit more independent of her husband, but when their daughter is born, the symbiotic switch is made to the girl. 'It goes from mother to husband to daughter,' says Dr Robertiello, 'but the woman's emotional age, her stage of development, remains fixed. She has not grown up one single day. The husband has just been a kind of intermediate stage between the old symbiosis with mother and the new one with the daughter. The woman, as an independent individual in her own right, never fully emerged.'

Everyone – man or woman – has a stake in preserving the idea of unique identity. *'I'm me!'* Few things threaten this notion of autonomy so much as being told we are like our mother.

Last night at dinner I was asked what I was working on. 'A book about the mother-daughter relationship.' Instantly, the four women present turned to listen, ignoring the men. 'What aspect are you writing about now?' one asked. 'How we become like our mothers,' I said. The light faded from four pairs of mascaraed eyes. 'Oh, no, I'm not at all like my mother. It was my father – my grandmother – who influenced me most.'

Denial. Flat denial that the woman with whom we once lived so intimately – who taught us how to speak, to eat, to walk, to dress ourselves, and on whose smile we lived – had any determining influence. Two of the four said they loved their mothers, but still repeated that their greatest influences were other people. I felt as though I had just heard it denied that two and two are four.

Of course other people – father, Aunt Sal, or an older sister – may be crucially important, but why deny so vehemently that mother was too? Why hold our attachment to these other figures as evidence of our uniqueness? Says Dr Robertiello: 'It

434

sounds much more adult and self-affirming to say you are like your aunt or grandmother, with whom you don't have that sticky closeness and half-remembered dependencies. To say you are like your father is best of all. It implies decision. After all, he is a man. It says you are sexual, while to be like mom is practically to label yourself nonsexual. To declare you are like dad brings in choice. Being like mother sounds automatic and passive. Being like father shows a certain strength of character. You've crossed the sexual line, you're big enough to move easily in a man's world. You are one hell of a woman and you did it all yourself!'

Cutting the symbiotic tie between mother and daughter can be aided by identification with father or an aunt, but it is best begun through an effort of absolute honesty, introspection, and memory. We have to see who mother was, and who we are. What was mother really like when we were little? Was she withholding, not quite attentive enough? Or did she overprotect, intrude, and make us fearful of life without her? Have we been able to face both the good mother and the bad, to know what we love and what we hate, and begun to fuse them all at last without sentimental gloss?

If the reason for having a child is to give yourself an identity, to replay childhood over again the way it should have been, to preserve the marriage, to have someone to live through, or a half dozen other crippling reasons, separation will be very difficult. The daughter cannot be let go because *she is doing something for you.* If she leaves and becomes her own person, you lose your identity, function, the chance to live life all over again.

Making a conscious decision about motherhood is one of the most liberating things that can be done both for ourselves and the unconceived child. Even if we want to become a mother for unrealistic reasons, *just knowing it,* says we are more separate than someone who doesn't make a decision at all, who passively slides from growing up into getting married and then automatically has a child. That kind of sequential thinking – or nonthinking – says we have no real feeling of self.

The woman who says, 'I want a child because I want to hang on to my husband,' has been proved again and again to be acting for wrong and self-defeating reasons, but even she is ahead of the wife who gives birth because that's what you do if you're a woman. Right or wrong, the first woman had decided, she has been active, and taken the responsibility for becoming pregnant.

Deciding that we want a child, knowing why, helps us escape the feeling 'they' made us do it. If motherhood is disappointing, if the work of having a baby is more than we reckoned, remembering it was our own idea helps put a damper on making the child feel responsible for being alive.

If the inexorable pattern of repetition between mother and daughter is to be changed, all the denied aspects of our mothers and ourselves must be faced. We have the right to acknowledge at last the fury felt when we were five and she neglected us. But she has the right, now that we are twenty-five, to be allowed to be less than perfect. Seeing mother plain, seeing her whole, a mixture of good and bad, is in itself an enormous step toward separation. Even better, it helps us from cutting ourselves off from her so totally that we throw away all our good inheritance from her, as well as the parts we don't like.

There are two times in women's lives when the unconscious drive to become the mother we dislike speeds up. The first is when we become mothers ourselves. The second is when our mother dies.

Even beyond the grave, mother continues to be split. The person who died was good. The bad person lives on in us, vile daughters who did not appreciate mother enough while she was still alive. It is a complex business, this eerie monument we make to our mothers within ourselves.

'My mother died six years ago,' says Leah Schaefer, 'and I'd had problems of separation from her all my life. I think I took my biggest step toward autonomy when my daughter Katie was born. In my years of psychoanalytic study and practice, I'd come to an intellectual grasp on the symbiotic problem between my mother and me, but I'd never been able to resolve it, when Katie was born, I was forty-two. Only then was I ready to take this giant step in separation from my mother. If I say I did it for the sake of my daugher, I know now it was I who benefited from it most. I had always thought it was my mother who insisted on keeping this symbiotic hold on me. Typical wishful thinking, the sheerest projection. I learned I was the major contributor to keeping alive this suffocating attachment between my mother and me.

'All my life I had never denied my mother anything. If I wanted to do something she might not like, I did it secretly. I always believed something terrible would happen if she knew of this other me, my secret self. She would die or reject me if I defeated or denied her. When Katie was born, she wanted to come live with us. I realized that if she did, it would be the end of me. If I gave in to her, as I always had in the past, she would just take over my life and my child. I understood the symbiosis between my mother and me, I could handle that. But now I was a mother and I wanted to raise my daughter to be the individual I was still trying to become. Telling my mother No, that she could not move in with us, was one of the major turning points in my life – a lifelong dependency on her broken.

'It didn't kill her, she didn't reject me. In fact, it was the best thing I ever did for both of us. We think we cannot be straight with our mothers, that they can't take the honesty of who we really are. But it is we who are the cowards, the babies; we are afraid that if we stand up to them, they will abandon us.

'It was a terrible confrontation when I told my mother No. We both cried. I felt miserable, as though I'd put a knife in her heart. Then several days later, she announced she was returning home to California. "I think married people need to live alone," she said to me, as though she had come to this decision herself. She was perfectly content with the explanation. She was basically a very independent person, but she had this terrific tie to me, her only daughter. When we said good-bye she was as light-hearted as I'd ever seen her. I felt miserable. You know what my biggest emotion was after she'd left? One word kept running through my mind: *rooked!*

'All my life had been one big compromise because I'd believed that if I ever denied my mother anything, it would mean a withdrawal of her love. I'd had my secret life where I did those things she wouldn't approve of anyway, but it had been paid for by all this guilt. The revelation that I could be myself in front of my mother, tell her No, and that she didn't die and I didn't die, that nothing terrible happened – was incredible. I was married and the mother of a daughter of my own, but emotionally I was still acting like a child who had to have her mother's approval. It was the purest symbiosis. All those years I had spent being less of the person I wanted to be because I also felt I had to be her kind of person. Now, here she was tolerating my separation from her very happily.'

Dr Schaefer continues:

'Before my mother died, I was with her in the hospital. She was confused, her loss of memory troubled her. My mother had never been able to accept my profession, she believed in *physical* medicine, not mental therapy. But now I was able to give her back some of the rewards of the work I'd been able to pursue because of the habits of professionalism she taught me. For the first time in my life, I could help her, talk to her about her past, about her husband and our family, remind her who she was. I was able to give her what she wanted most in those last weeks: her sense of self. When I said good-bye to her that last time, she turned away and began to talk to my brother. She never could stand separation.

'The break with my mother that began when my daughter was born allowed me to begin to see in myself, before she died, the good things I had inherited from her. My mother's dedication to her work made her effective and admirable. I had hated it as a kid because it left me out. Now that I had gained some distance from her, I could see this wasn't "compulsive" but rather, it was professionalism. Without this dedication to my work, I would not have been able to support myself, to make her last days in the hospital easier, or to pay her final bills. Unless I had separated from my mother, I would never have allowed myself to see the value of how I am like her in the best ways.'

The idea of *melancholia* – in connection with the death of someone toward whom we have ambivalent feelings of love and hate – was developed by Freud and one of his disciples, Dr Karl Abraham.[5] It is very different from genuine mourning. To mourn a mother who has died is a healthy process, the acceptance of loss, a gradual letting go. It is a sign she was 'a good enough' mother, and that our feelings about her were relatively unambivalent – much more love than anger or hate. 'Even if she was not a good enough mother,' says Dr Robertiello, 'if you have come to terms with that idea before she dies, you may be able to avoid melancholia. If you can recognize her for what she was, that is a mature evaluation. You have at least begun separation.'

In the melancholic, grief is not whole-hearted because the ambivalent rage at the bad mother of infancy has not been resolved. Sorrow cannot be fully expressed and so gotten out. Old feelings of infantile omnipotence come to plague the daughter: her unconscious conscience accuses her of murder.

It is too terrible an idea. We must deny our hatred for the bad mother more strongly than ever. This repression seems to solve the problem. We begin to walk like mother, talk like her; *we become her*. We take in all those parts that once we hated. In this way, we can answer the self-accusation that we are glad she is dead: we are keeping her alive!

By turning our aggression inward, hating those aspects of her we have introjected, we do not have to see it is really directed at her. We hate ourselves instead. The result is a sadness and self-hate that goes on and on, feelings of futility and bewilderment, flashes of seemingly pointless rage amid a general air of depression. Melancholia. The introjection of the bad mother after she dies is a mystery. It has been too universally remarked to doubt.

Dr Robertiello: 'My father had his first heart attack six

months ago. It gave me time to face what was coming. I never got on well with my father. All my life I had denied I was like him at all. And yet, during these last six months, I became aware that I was taking in the aspects of my father I'd always hated: his imperious nature, his hypochondria, and all the rest. This was introjection and I realized that if I didn't face my father squarely, the kind of man he was – good and bad – the guilt when he died would be too great. The melancholia would have gone on for years. I knew only a more complete separation could stop the process. Otherwise, I would have continued to hate my father totally. I would never have seen the many good things I took over from him. As it was, I felt: The king is dead, Long live the king!'

Four years ago I told my mother's sister that I was going to write a book on the mother-daughter relationship. She said, 'Nancy, some day your mother is going to die. How can you do this to her?' I was startled, guilty, hurt that my aunt would think that I was setting out to injure my mother. Why did she automatically assume any unblinking examination of the mother-daughter relationship must be hurtful? Simple projection, forbidden images of the repressed 'bad mother' surround notions like these. If we daughters feel enormous guilt at the thought of our mother's mortality, mothers too mirror our anxiety about taking a hard look at the relationship with eyes rendered unsentimental by the importance of death. Why is honesty so fearful? What can there be between us that is so bad that two lives must be spent, each showing the other only what they feel the other can tolerate – while simultaneously seeing in the other only what we want to see?

Says Dr Robertiello: 'If people say it is cold and calculating to analyze who you are, and who your mother is – to acknowledge what you hate and love in her – they are still trying to hold on to her as children. They are afraid to think these things because at some deep level they still fear she can be hurt by their thoughts. They are also demanding that she be immortal, postponing their separation.'

'If only I had been able to tell my mother how much I loved

her while she was still alive!' a woman tells me. 'She had her faults but they were just reflexes. She couldn't help nagging and criticizing any more than you can help sneezing when your nose itches. It was just something built into her nervous system. Now, I'll never be able to tell her what I really felt for her. It's too late.'

It is a conversation I find chilling, sad, and bewildering. If anything, this woman is even more nagging and critical than her mother. It has led to her divorce from her husband and alienated her daughter. Even when we have a destructive relationship with our mothers, why do we turn it all around when she dies, and only talk about our love for her?

When I began this book, I too would have told you that I loved my mother and all my angers at her were unimportant. 'She didn't mean to hurt me. That's just the way she was, a bad habit.' In the service of maintaining a fantasy that beneath her 'bad habits' was all-encompassing love, I'd refused to recognize the 'bad mother' of childhood. I once would have said that ignoring my petty angers was my adult way of keeping the relationship to my mother affectionate and easy. I know now this 'forgetting' only ensures the angers beneath are kept alive and boiling.

The usual way to avoid the fear of seeing there are parts of mother we hate is to sentimentalize her. Literature tells us very little about what really goes on between children and their mothers. The saccharine sweetness of Mother's Day poetry protests too much.

Says Dr Robertiello: 'These forms of sentimentality are a defense against anger. Rather than feel like a murderer, we doubly repress our hostility with a smile. Whatever it is we didn't like – her nagging, the controls she tried to put on us, her sexual repressiveness – we say they weren't important. We "understand" them. Which means we forgive them, and try to focus instead on the "loving" parts of her, and how much we loved her. To talk like this is not proof that you loved your mother, but that you are sentimentalizing. The word "love" is used to cover so many destructive emotions, like possessiveness, anxiety, et cetera. You tell yourself soft remorseful lies that protect her – which means you are blurring your own perception that you are repeating her. You are stuck with your rage, and the only way you can keep that alive is by incorporating into yourself the parts of her that you hated. It's all in the service of continuing the symbiosis, even though mother may be far away or dead.' In the unconscious where the first connection was forged, the mother of our infancy never dies.

When we are not sentimentalizing her, we go to the other extreme. If the telephone call home didn't go well, if she said the wrong thing during our visit, all the old angers rise up again. We were right to decide to be as different from her as possible. She becomes the measure of everything we dislike – which means we will denigrate or hate every echo of her we find in ourselves. Everything in the 'bad mother' is bad, and so if we have her straightforwardness and honesty, we will say it is unkindness and hostility. Leah Schaefer took in her mother's professionalism and called it being a compulsive worker. If we have mother's powers of organization, we will dislike ourselves for being bossy and controlling.

No matter if the world or our husbands love us for these qualities. That only means we are temporarily fooling them. If they don't find us out, they are dumb. If they do, they will leave us. Our choice is to be loved by a fool or not to be loved at all.

'It was denial of what really went on between my mother and me,' said Helen Prentiss, 'that made me hide out and symbiose with my daughter. To deny your sexuality is a way of avoiding competition with your daughter. I hope to break the chain women pass on from one generation to another – that paralyzing nonaggression, noncompetitive pact. I know you can be a good mother and sexual too – even if it took me a long time to find it out. It's so simple. I can explain it to my six-year-old but I could never get it through to my mother.'

At this stage in our lives, mother probably needs us more than the other way around – but we are still afraid to ask her those difficult but clarifying questions about childhood. Her

442

involvement in our introspective process of separation can help, but is not necessary. The question is, If our questions should lead her into a rage so violent that she throws us out of the house – to name the worst fantasy – what has been lost? Only the illusion of symbiotic love.

Most of us need to get over the fear that separation is going to kill her. Being a good mother to a thirty-five-year-old (dependent) daughter is just as confining and anachronistic as playing the good daughter when we are grown with a daughter of our own. Mother is stronger than we wish to give her credit for. Part of this fear of hurting her is puffing up our own importance. Another part is just wishful thinking, maintaining the symbiosis. Both ideas may be summed up by the thought, 'She cannot live without me.' Another part is, 'My anger is so terrible, that if I show it to her, it'll kill her.'

The Greeks had a word for all this: *hubris*. It meant a kind of overweening self-importance, pride, and arrogance. It always led to destruction. Now that we are grown, to decide that mother must be protected as if she were the child – isn't that hubris too?

Guilt is the name we give anxiety at the fear of losing symbiosis with mother. Guilt is what we feel when we leave her ourselves. All our lives, whenever we say good-bye, there is this feeling we have not been able to give her something she wanted. What does she want from us that we can't seem to provide? Next time we meet, we promise ourselves, we will try harder, we will be 'a good daughter', we will give her this magic something that will make her happy. But the next time we fail again, and after she dies we know we have failed forever.

I have heard ideas like these from many women, and in a recent talk with Dr Robertiello mentioned how often I'd felt them myself. We'd been talking about introjection, and about his father's death; it had occurred while I was writing this chapter. I went on to say that I hoped what I'd learned from my research would 'help me avoid all that old sadness and guilt the next time I go home and it comes time to say good-bye.' Richard shook his head in mock despair. 'Ah, Nancy, Nancy,' he said. 'You still haven't integrated what you know intellectually with what you feel down deep. It is not guilt you feel, that you cannot make your mother happy. You feel *anxious* that you do not say the right thing, open the magic door, through which all the love you once wanted from her would come flooding through. You still cannot let go of your infantile need of that magic mother of long ago. Your mother is still vigorous and alive, but if you don't come to understand what you are doing, you will continue to blame yourself after she dies. The forsaken feeling will not be that you didn't make her happy, but that you did not do or say the magic thing that would force her – in the sense of infantile omnipotence – to love you as you have waited for all your life.'

How many times have I said in this book that my mother and I are totally different women? Oh, I have acknowledged certain minor virtues I got from her – housekeeping, an easy hostess, etc. But compared to those qualities of hers I have always disliked but taken over anyway – her anxiety and the fear which lies beneath my surface independence – how paltry appeared my 'good' inheritance. I have always thought I had to leave home to reinforce the qualities in myself I wanted because I felt by nature my mother is a very timid person.

For every step I have taken away from her – my sexuality, my work, the whole dramatic design of my life which overshadows her conservative one – I have been aware of her tugging at my heels, pulling me back. Maybe I 'made myself up', but there is not a daring thing I have ever done that has not been accompanied by anxiety. At the beginning of this chapter I had said that one of my strongest reasons for not becoming a mother was I did not want to turn into the kind of nervous, frightened mother she had been to me. Alone, I can control the helpless mother who lives inside me. A mother myself, I would become just like her.

Helpless? Why do I automatically associate that word with her? A woman who raised two daughters on her own, who ran her house smoothly, paid her bills on time, and never set a table or planned a trip where anything was left out? Is she indeed so timid and afraid, so unlike me – the adventurous daughter? To turn that around: am I so unlike her?

I have mentioned the silver cups she won in cross-country steeplechasing. She demeans this courage as if it were girlish stupidity, and stored the cups in the basement until I retrieved them. They are now in my home, polished – a tribute to something I too am reluctant to acknowledge. Whenever Bill tells people how responsible and well organized I am, it rankles me. Why have I always seen these qualities in myself as something I must hide, not to be proud of? So long as I could not recognize and appreciate them in my mother, and was determined to see her 'helplessness' as the mark of being a woman, being capable and organized made me sound masculine.

It has taken me the entire writing of this book to acknowledge in my heart that the qualities I am proudest of in myself I learned from her. It is unbelievable to me now to think I did not know them last week. 'Why, you look just like your mother!' a woman said to me recently. I thought she meant I was wearing my mother's tight, anxious look. But she was thinking of something else. 'The last time I saw her,' this woman went on, 'your mother bid a grand slam. It was four o'clock in the morning, and she made it!'

Stories of my mother's courage have always excited me. The photos of her I love so much hang over my desk – jumping a horse over a high brick wall, wearing a daring two-piece bathing suit twenty-five years ago when she was my age. Why have I refused to credit her for the abilities and emotions I have tried to incorporate in myself?

At one time I would have told you that more than anything else, my sexuality differentiated me from my mother. But she likes men tremendously, and they her. When we are together, I am usually the one who calls the evening to an end; she'd

445

prefer to dance all night. More important, why have I always discounted that when my mother was seventeen she ran away with the handsomest man in Pittsburgh, and married him against her father's wishes? I used to make her elopement sound like some out-of-character phenomenon, as if the idea had been totally my father's and she had only passively gone along. The fact is, my 'asexual' and 'timid' mother was into sex *four years younger than I, who didn't give up her virginity until twenty-one!*

In my absolutism about having made myself up out of no cloth taken from her, I have disinherited myself from my grandmother too. Didn't she leave her dominating husband and their oldest children when she could no longer stand the tyranny – and that in the 1920s, long before liberation, long before the time when a decision like this could be thought anything but mad and irredeemably unfeminine?

There is a strong current in the women in my family that I am bound and determined not to recognize. I come from three generations of sexual, adventurous, self-sufficient women. Is this not more exciting, more profound, than the shallow notion of making myself up? Aren't these the qualities I want most to reinforce in myself? In the service of maintaining a childish tie to a mother who never existed, I have turned my back on the best of my inheritance.

I am suddenly afraid that the mother I have depicted throughout this book is false.

Does this mean that everything I have written so far is false?

'No!' says Dr Robertiello. 'Like everyone else you keep changing your idea of your mother. One day she's good, kind, and loving. The next day, she's frightened, timid, and asexual. One day all you can see is your anger. Right now you want to go into a period of seeing her as all good. Either way, it means you are still avoiding the job of seeing her realistically. You are determined to invest your mother with magic importance – to see her, not as a human being, but in some childlike, monolithic, total way. *That is the way the baby sees her mother.* You are still lost in that first attachment to her, as you were when she was the Giantess of the Nursery.'

Seeing mother divested of the symbiotic glamour she once held for us means she becomes another person, someone else, outside of us. Which means we have separated at last. As long as we remained symbiotically linked, there was always hope that it was not too late to get from her the perfect love we always wanted. Now we are grown, and know we never will. We must give up the fantasy and look elsewhere. The idea is sobering. It is maturing too. Most important of all, it is the truth.

I can see now that while I liked my sexuality and wanted to give my mother no credit for it at all, that part of me rested on an uneasy base: if my mother, my image of femininity, was 'asexual', then my own sexuality must be 'masculine'. I was proud of it, but didn't trust it. In this way, until we learn to fuse our mother into one person, we will be at war with ourselves. The cries and slogans of liberation from outside can serve at best to cheer us on. There is no changed history for women until each faces her own.

I said in the first chapter of this book that I'd often wished my mother had had my life. Hubris again, snidely competitive, and damned impertinent too. I don't think she'd want it. The more I grow away from her and define myself, the more I see in her this other person she was before she became Nancy Friday's mother. That is the magic: not that we can ever recreate that nirvana of love that may or may not have existed between us as mother-and-child, but that once we have separated we can give each other life, extra life, each out of the abundance of her own.

Recognizing the woman who can bid a grand slam at four in the morning when the rest of the world is asleep, I sleep better myself. Now that I have granted her the right to have run off with my father at seventeen because she was a sexual adventuress at heart – and not because it was some atypical bit of foolishness which had nothing to do with her true character at all – I can be proud of that part of myself that is a sexual woman too.

Notes

CHAPTER TWO

1. Will McBride and Helga Fleischauer-Hardt, *Show Me* (New York: St Martin's Press, 1975).
2. See D. W. Winnicott, *Playing and Reality*, pp. 47–52.
3. Adrienne Rich, *Of Woman Born*, p. 259.
4. Edward Shorter, *The Making of the Modern Family*, pp. 168–9.
5. Helene Deutsch, *The Psychology of Women*, vol. I, *Girlhood*, p. 151.

CHAPTER TWO

1. D. W. Winnicott, *The Maturational Processes and the Facilitating Environment*.
2. Erik H. Erikson. The theory of basic trust runs throughout Erikson's work. See *Childhood and Society*, 1950. Also *Psychological Issues* (1959), pp. 55–6: 'For the first component of a healthy personality, I nominate a sense of basic trust.'
3. Margaret Mahler is a pioneer in ego psychology and child development. Her theory of the nature of the child's attachment to the mother (symbiosis) and the gradual breaking of this attachment (separation-individuation) has been one of the major contributions to psychoanalytic theory in recent decades. This theory was set forth in *On Human Symbiosis and the Vicissitudes of Individuation, vol. 1, Infantile Psychosis*, 1968. She has recently written *The Psychological Development of the Human Infant*, 1976, which is a continuation and elaboration of her theories.
4. Erik H. Erikson, *Childhood and Society*, p. 247.
5. *Ibid.*
6. Heinz Kohut, MD, a practicing psychoanalyst in Chicago, is one of the most important psychoanalytic theorists on the subject of narcissism. His book *The Analysis of the Self* affirms the development of narcissism as a healthy drive that is necessary for the formation of a positive self-image.

CHAPTER THREE

1. Leah Schaefer's doctoral study was completed in 1964, at Teachers College, Columbia University. It is titled 'Sexual Experiences and Reactions of a group of 30 Women as Told to a Female Psychotherapist.' This study grew into her book *Women and Sex*, published by Pantheon in 1973.
2. John Bowlby is an English psychoanalyst whose books on attachment and separation are considered classics in the field. His work has focused on the effects of the child's separation from its parents, his argument being that an early closeness to mother is the bedrock of later emotional stability and that anxiety is caused by fear of loss of this attachment. See *Attachment and Loss*, vol. I, *Attachment*; and *Attachment and Loss*, vol. II, *Separation*.
3. Margaret Mahler, *On Human Symbiosis and the Vicissitudes of Individuation*, vol. I.
4. Quote from the poem 'Effort at Speech Between Two People,' from the book *Waterlily Fire, Poems 1935–1962* by Muriel Rukeyser, p. 3.
5. See Seymour Fisher, *The Female Orgasm*.

CHAPTER FOUR

1. Germaine Greer, *The Female Eunuch*, p. 142.
2. Clara Thompson, 'Penis Envy in Women'. *Psychiatry*, vol. VI, 1943, pp. 123–5.
3. Quoted from a review by Anatole Broyard of *The Curse: A Cultural History of Menstruation*, by Janice Delaney, Mary Jane Lupton, and Emily Toth. Review appeared in *The New York Times*, September 21, 1976.
4. Karen Page's studies were conducted in 1971 and 1973. Her findings appeared in an article, 'Women Learn to Sing the Menstrual Blues.' *Psychology Today*, September 1973, pp. 41–6. Karen Page is a psychologist at the University of California at Davis, where she continues to do work on this subject.

CHAPTER FIVE

1. *American College Dictionary*. New York: Harper, 1950, p. 246.
2. See Reuben Fine, *The Psychology of the Chess Player*.
3. Jessie Bernard tells me she has seen informal studies in recent years that show girls are beginning to remain on the honor roll right through high school. In the *Journal of Counseling Psychology* (January 1975, pp. 35–8), Rosalind C. Barnett statistically demonstrates in a study of 988 females and 1,531 males from ages 9 to 17 that boys tend to prefer high-prestige occupations, the more they enter adolescence. The article is titled 'Sex Differences and Age Trends in Occupational Preferences and Occupational Prestige.' 'What do these differing studies say to us?' asks Jessie Bernard. 'That we're still very much betwixt and between.'
4. Aurealia Schober Plath, *Letters Home by Sylvia Plath*, p. 38.

Notes

1. 'The age of the menarche [onset of menstruation],' says Seymour Reichlin, MD, chief of the endocrine division at the New England Medical Center Hospital in Boston, 'has changed from 17.5 years in about 1860 to 11.7 years in 1976. We are talking about Western societies. The relevant factor is size; a girl can't conceive and bear a live child until her body has the fat content to carry her through a pregnancy. A certain height and weight is necessary for the onset of puberty. And with the better nutrition and freedom from infections today, young girls are reaching this height and weight earlier.'

2. Lillian Hellman, Pentimento: A Book of Portraits, p. 119.

CHAPTER EIGHT

1. Sigmund Freud, 'A Case of Paranoia Running Counter to the Psycho-Analytic Theory of the Disease,' Standard Edition of Complete Psychological Works of Sigmund Freud, p. 261.

2. Quote appeared in an interview with Elizabeth Ashley by Ila Stanger. The article was titled 'Extraordinary Women Talk About the Single Life,' Harper's Bazaar, March 1975.

3. This study was titled 'The Effects of Mass Media on the Sexual Behavior of Adolescent Females' and was distributed by The American Association of Sex Counselors and Therapists, of which Dr Schiller is executive director.

4. Margaret Hennig's doctoral dissertation was done in 1970 for the Graduate School of Business Administration at Harvard University. It is titled 'Career Development for Women Executives.' Her work was further developed in the book written with Anne Jardim. The Managerial Woman.

CHAPTER NINE

1. A. C. Kinsey et al., Sexual Behavior in the Human Female, p. 170.

2. Leah Schaefer, Women and Sex, pp. 88–106.

3. Robert Sorensen, Adolescent Sexuality in Contemporary America, pp. 129–145.

4. This study was done on 300 undergraduates at the University of Iowa in 1963. The study is contained in a book by Ira Reiss, The Social Context of Premarital Sexual Permissiveness, pp. 105–125.

5. This is an ongoing study being conducted by Ira Reiss.

6. These findings were in the same study quoted above, Note 4.

7. Mirra Komarovsky, Dilemmas of Masculinity: A Study of College Youth, pp. 78–81.

8. SIECUS Study Guide No. 5, 'Premarital Sexual Standards', p. 14.

9. Zelnik and Kantner's figures were published in 1972 by the US Commission on Population Growth and The American Future. This study was only on

15- to 19-year-olds. 'But recent national samples,' says Ira Reiss, 'conducted by the US Department of Health, Education and Welfare, back up both Kinsey and Zelnik and Kantner.'

10. I heard of this study from Ira Reiss. The study was done by Robert Walsh and was his PhD dissertation, 1970, titled 'Survey of Parents and Their Own Children's Sexual Attitudes.' The study began in 1967 and is ongoing. Walsh did his research at Illinois State University, got his degree at the University of Iowa. He is teaching now at Illinois State University.

11. This survey was conducted on 500 coeds at the University of Minnesota between the years 1970 and 1972. It was titled 'Premarital Contraceptive Usage: A Study and Some Theoretical Explorations,' and was published in the *Journal of Marriage and Family*, August 1975, pp. 619–30.

CHAPTER TEN

1. See Jessie Bernard's paper 'Homosociality and Female Depression,' *Journal of Social Issues*, to be published in 1977. In this paper, Dr Bernard states that 'never married women fared better in terms of mental health than never married men.' She cites the studies done by psychologist Lenore Radloff which show that 'The never married [women who were] heads of households in which the household income was $16,000 and over − presumably successful career women − fared spectacularly well [in terms of mental health]. As well, in fact, as married men, usually the best off in all studies. It is interesting that the category of never-married was the only one in which women showed up better than men.'

2. Quote from an article, 'I Weep for the Party of Lincoln and My Father,' by Richard Reeves, *New York Magazine*, August 30, 1976, p. 8.

3. Komarovsky, p. 31.

4. Figures are for 1975, from the US Department of Commerce, Bureau of the Census.

5. M. Elizabeth Tidball is a professor of physiology at George Washington Medical Center in Washington, DC. An account of her study on achieving women appeared in *The Executive Woman*, vol. 2, no. 6, February 1975, pp. 1–2.

6. Margaret Hennig's doctoral dissertation was done in 1970, at the Graduate School of Business Administration at Harvard University. It is titled 'Career Development for Women Executives.'

7. Psychologist Matina Horner was a doctoral student at the University of Michigan. Her dissertation is titled 'Sex Differences in Achievement Motivation and Performance in Competitive and Non-Competitive Situations.'

8. Robert Ardrey, *African Genesis*, p. 165.

9. Figures quoted from the US Labor Department, as they appeared in the article 'Women Entering Job Market at An "Extraordinary Pace",' by Robert Lindsey, *New York Times*, September 12, 1976.

Notes

10. Eli Ginzburg is a Columbia University economist and chairman of the National Commission for Manpower Policy. This quote appeared in the *New York Times* article cited above.

CHAPTER ELEVEN

1. Figures from the US Labor Department. Almost 48 percent of American women over 16 years of age now work or want a job. Some economists think that within two or three years it is possible that half of American women over 16 will be in the work force.
2. Dr Joyce Brothers, 'How to Be Unafraid of Success,' *Harper's Bazaar*, January 1976, p. 96.
3. In 1950, 3,848 women committed suicide. In 1974, 7,088 women committed suicide. These figures were obtained from US Department of Commerce, Bureau of the Census, Statistical Abstract of the US, 1976.
4. Susan Brownmiller, *Against Our Will*, p. 403.

CHAPTER TWELVE

1. Bruno Bettelheim, *The Uses of Enchantment*, pp. 5–6.
2. *Ibid.*, p. 66.
3. Anne Sexton, 'The Double Image', *To Bedlam and Part Way Back*, p. 61.
4. In a national sample, the American Council of Life Insurance asks: 'Is it perfectly all right to be married and to choose not to have children.' In 1973 and 1974, three out of four adults, age 18 and over, agreed with that statement. In 1976, it went up to 83 percent in agreement, which is four out of five people.
5. Sigmund Freud, 'Mourning and Melancholia', written in 1917. *Standard Edition*, vol. XIV., pp. 243–58. See also Karl Abraham, 'The Process of Introjection in Melancholia', *Selected Papers*, pp. 442–53.

Bibliography

Abraham, Karl. *Selected Papers*. London: Hogarth Press, 1927.
Ardrey, Robert. *African Genesis*. New York: Atheneum, 1961.

Bardwick, Judith. 'The Dynamics of Successful People.' *New Research on Women*. Ann Arbor: University of Michigan.
Barker-Benfield, G. J. *The Horrors of the Half-Known Life: Male Attitudes Toward Women and Sexuality in Nineteenth Century America*. New York: Harper & Row, 1976.
Barnett, Rosalind C. 'Sex Differences and Age Trends in Occupational Preference and Occupational Prestige.' *Journal of Counseling Psychology*. Jan. 1975, Vol. 22 (1), pp. 35–8.
Bernard, Jessie. *The Future of Marriage*. New York: World, 1972.
———. *The Future of Motherhood*. New York: Dial Press, 1975.
———. *Women, Wives, Mothers: Values and Options*. Chicago: Aldine Press, 1975.
Bettelheim, Bruno. *The Uses of Enchantment*. New York: Knopf, 1976.
Blos, Peter. *On Adolescence: A Psychoanalytic Interpretation*. New York: The Free Press, 1962.
Bowlby, John. *Attachment and Loss*. Vol. I, *Attachment*. New York: Basic Books, 1969.
———. *Attachment and Loss*. Vol. II, *Separation – Anxiety and Anger*. New York: Basic Books, 1973.
Brothers, Joyce. 'How to Be Unafraid of Success.' *Harper's Bazaar*, Jan. 1976, p. 96.
Brownmiller, Susan. *Against Our Will: Men, Women and Rape*. New York: Simon and Schuster, 1975.

Delaney, Janice and Mary Jane Lupton. *The Curse: A Cultural History of Menstruation*. New York: Dutton, 1976.
Deutsch, Helene. *The Psychology of Women*. Vol. 1, *Girlhood*. New York: Bantam Edition, 1973.
———. *The Psychology of Women*, Vol. 2, *Motherhood*. New York: Bantam Edition, 1973.

Erikson, Erik H. *Childhood and Society*. New York: Norton, 1950.
———. *Identity, Youth and Crisis*. New York: Norton, 1968.

Fine, Reuben. *The Psychology of the Chess Player*. New York: Dover Publications, 1967.

Fisher, Seymour. *The Female Orgasm*. New York: Basic Books, 1973.

Freud, Sigmund. *Standard Edition of Complete Psychological Works of Sigmund Freud*. London: Hogarth Press, 1957–64.

Friday, Nancy. *My Secret Garden*. New York: Trident, 1973.

Goodman, Emily Jane and Phyllis Chesler. *Women, Money and Power*. New York: Morrow, 1976.

Greer, Germaine. *The Female Eunuch*. London: MacGibbon and Kee, 1970.

Haskell, Molly. *From Reverence to Rape: The Treatment of Women in the Movies*. New York: Holt, Rinehart and Winston, 1974.

Hellman, Lillian. *Pentimento: A Book of Portraits*. Boston: Little, Brown, 1973.

Hennig, Margaret. 'Career Development for Women Executives.' Doctoral dissertation for the Graduate School of Business Administration at Harvard University, 1970. Developed into a book, *The Managerial Woman*, co-authored with Anne Jardim. New York: Doubleday, 1977.

Horner, Matina. 'Sex Differences in Achievement Motivation and Performance in Competitive and Non-Competitive Situations.' Unpublished doctoral dissertation for the University of Minnesota, 1968.

Hunt, Morton. *Sexual Behavior in the 1970s*. Chicago: Playboy Press, 1974.

Janeway, Elizabeth. *Man's World, Woman's Place*. New York: Delta, 1971.

Kaplan, Helen. *The New Sex Therapy*. New York: Brunner/Mazel, 1974.

Kinsey, A. C. et al. *Sexual Behavior in the Human Female*. Philadelphia: W. B. Saunders, 1953.

Kohut, H. *The Analysis of the Self*. New York: International University Press, 1971.

Komarovsky, Mirra. *Dilemmas of Masculinity: A Study of College Youth*. New York: Norton, 1976.

Maddux, Hilary C. *Menstruation*. New Canaan: Tobey Publishing, 1975.

Mahler, M. S. *On Human Symbiosis and the Vicissitudes of Individuation*. Vol. I, *Infantile Psychosis*. New York: International University Press, 1968.

———. *The Psychological Development of the Human Infant*. New York: Basic Books, 1976.

Masters, William H. and Virginia E. Johnson. *Human Sexual Response*. Boston: Little, Brown, 1969.

Mitchell, Juliet. *Psychoanalysis and Feminism*. New York: Vintage, 1974.

Money, John. *Sexual Signatures*. Boston: Little, Brown, 1975.

Page, Karen. 'Women Learn to Sing the Menstrual Blues.' *Psychology Today*. September 1973.

Bibliography

Plath, Aurelia Schober. *Letters Home by Sylvia Plath*. New York: Harper and Row, 1975.

Pomeroy, Wardell B. *Girls and Sex*. New York: Delacorte Press, 1969.

Reiss, Ira L. *The Social Context of Premarital Sexual Permissiveness*. New York: Holt, Rinehart and Winston, 1967.

———. 'Premarital Contraceptive Usage: A Study and Some Theoretical Explorations.' *Journal of Marriage and Family*. August 1975.

Rich, Adrienne. *Of Woman Born: Motherhood as Experience and Institution*. New York: Norton, 1976.

Robertiello, Richard C. *Hold Them Very Close, Then Let Them Go*. New York: Dial, 1975.

———. and Grace Elish Kirsten. *Big You, Little You*. New York: Dial, 1977.

———. and Rena M. Shadmi. 'Dynamics in Female Sexual Problems.' *Journal of Contemporary Psychotherapy*. Vol. 1, No. 1. Fall 1968.

———. 'Masochism and the Female Sexual Role.' *Journal of Sex Research*. Vol. 6, No. 1, Feb. 1970, pp. 56–8.

———. 'Penis Envy.' *Psychotherapy: Theory, Research and Practice*. Vol. 7, No. 4. Winter 1970.

Rukeyser, Muriel. *Waterlily Fire, Poems 1935–1962*. New York: Macmillan, 1962.

Schaefer, Leah Cahan. *Woman and Sex*. New York: Pantheon, 1973.

———. 'Female Adolescent Sexuality.' An unpublished paper given at International Forum on Adolescence, Jerusalem, Israel. July 1976.

Schiller, Patricia. 'The Effects of Mass Media on the Sexual Behavior of Adolescent Females.' Study distributed by the American Association of Sex Educators and Counselors.

Sheehy, Gail. *Passages: Predictable Crises of Adult Life*. New York: Dutton, 1976.

Sex Information and Education Council of the US. *SIECUS Study Guide* No. 5 (revised edition), 'Premarital Sexual Standards.' New York: SIECUS, 1967.

Sexton, Anne. *To Bedlam and Part Way Back*. Boston: Houghton Mifflin, 1960.

Shorter, Edward. *The Making of the Modern Family*. New York: Basic Books, 1975.

Sorenson, Robert. *Adolescent Sexuality in Contemporary America*. New York: World Publishing, 1972.

Stanger, Ila. 'Extraordinary Women Talk About the Single Life.' *Harper's Bazaar*, March 1975.

Sullivan, H. S. *The Interpersonal Theory of Psychiatry*. New York: Norton, 1953.

Thompson, Clara. 'Penis Envy in Women.' *Psychiatry*. Vol. VI, 1943.

Tiger, Lionel, and Robin Fox. *The Imperial Animal*. New York: Holt, Rinehart and Winston, 1971.

Weideger, Paula. *Menstruation and Menopause*. New York: Knopf, 1976.

Winnicott, D. W. *The Maturational Processes and the Facilitating Environment*. New York: International University Press, 1965.

————. *Playing and Reality*. New York: Basic Books, 1971.

Zelnik, Melvin, and John Kantner. 'Sexuality, Contraception and Pregnancy Among Young Unwed Females in the United States.' In US Commission on Population Growth and the American Future. *Demographic and Social Aspects of Population Growth*, Vol. 1 of Commission Research Reports. Government Printing Office, 1972.

Wanting Everything
The Art of Happiness

Dorothy Rowe

'I would like to see it on every bookshelf in the country. We would be the happier for it' FAY WELDON

To be human is to suffer. We enter this world expecting that we can have everything, but we learn very quickly that we can't always get what we want. The accompanying and constant feelings of loss, frustration, anger, aggression, resentment and sadness can dominate us for the rest of our lives.

The strategies we evolve to cope with these feelings – greed for possessions or power, a propensity for assuming responsibility for everything, saddling ourself with guilt for the world, martyr-dom, envy or utter selfishness – do not lead to happiness. But Dorothy Rowe shows us how, once we understand the nature of our longing and the conditions that prevent its fulfilment, we can arrive at a state of wanting which does hold the possibility of fulfilment, and which does lead to happiness.

'Dorothy Rowe is essentially a chronicler of emotional pain, a suggester of solutions. Her perspective on existence acknowledges sadness, pain, anger, but it instantly makes things seem meaningful' *Guardian*

ISBN 0 00 637430 1

The Silent Passage
Menopause

Gail Sheehy

Gail Sheehy has broken the last taboo.

All women face menopause, but, as Gail Sheehy compellingly reveals in interviews with women from a broad spectrum of different backgrounds, the passage is seldom easy. Distracting symptoms, confusing medical advice, unsympathetic reactions from loved ones, and scornful attitudes of society often make menopause a lonely and distressing experience.

Sheehy brings together the latest information and assesses women's options and risks. She writes frankly about her own experiences, and more importantly she plays back the words of numerous women who have talked to her about how they have coped and what they think of the treatments they have tried.

Myth-shattering, funny and vibrant, this is a book of candour and hope that places menopause in the cycle of life as the gateway to a second adulthood and post-menopausal zest.

Includes interviews with:
Fay Weldon · Kate O'Mara · Edwina Currie ·
Barbara Taylor Bradford · Eve Pollard · Antonia Fraser

ISBN 0 00 637967 2

Dorothy Rowe's Guide to Life

'Dorothy Rowe is full of robust good sense, rare intuitive wisdom and unhurried sensitivity ... she is a giver of courage'
NIGELLA LAWSON, *The Times*

The central theme of all Dorothy Rowe's work is that, while the world and ourselves might *seem* to be solid and real, the way in which we are constituted means that we can never know reality directly, only the meanings we have created about reality.

It is when we don't understand this, when we mistakenly think that we, our life and the world are fixed, unalterable parts of reality which we have to put up with and cope with as best we can, that we find we can't handle life's problems – we make mistakes, feel trapped, and often despair.

When we do understand it, we realize that we are free to change.

Dorothy Rowe has helped tens of thousands of people reach this understanding through her books on fear, depression and unhappiness. She has shown how, by understanding our nature, we can end our suffering. Her *Guide to Life* is a summation of this wisdom but with more besides, for there is no end to self-understanding. Like all her books, it is clear and compassionate, witty and wise.

ISBN 0 00 638422 6

The Women's History of the World

Rosalind Miles

Men dominate history because they write it. Women's vital part
in the shaping of the world has been consistently undervalued or
ignored. Rosalind Miles now offers a fundamental reappraisal
that sets the record straight – history is also her story!

This brilliant and absorbing book turns the spotlight on the
hidden side of history to present a fascinating new view of the
world, overturning our preconceptions to restore women to their
rightful place at the centre of the worldwide story of revolution,
empire, war and peace.

Spiced with tales of individual women who have shaped history,
celebrating the work and lives of the unsung female millions,
distinguished by a wealth of research, *The Women's History of
the World* redefines the concept of historical reality.

ISBN 0 586 08886 5

New Passages

Mapping Your Life Across Time

Gail Sheehy

The No. 1 U.S. Bestseller
Fully revised for the UK

'Stop and recalculate,' writes Gail Sheehy. 'Imagine the day you turn 45 as the infancy of another life.'

In the last twenty years an historic revolution has occurred in the adult lifecycle. Young people are waiting until their 30s to leave home and get married, more women are having children at 40 or over, 50-year-old men are being forced into early retirement, 60-year-olds feel like 50, and 70-year-olds feel like 60. People are taking longer to grow up, and much longer to grow old.

Healthy men or women who reach age 50 can now expect to live until their 80s or 90s. These people are now rejecting the whole notion of 'middle-aged decline' and heading for a completely new frontier – a Second Adulthood full of new passions, renewed enthusiasm, self-confidence and fulfilment.

But how are they coping with the new dilemmas and demands that Second Adulthood brings?

New Passages takes the stories of hundreds of people, backed up with extensive research and social analysis, to explore the new stages of adult life. Inspiring and informative, Gail Sheehy's insights will not only help you make sense of your own life by understanding others, but will permanently alter the way you think about yourself.

'An optimistic analysis of adult development in pessimistic times . . . grounded in the economic and psychological realities that make adult life so complex today'
New York Times Book Review

0 00 638676 8